T0133089

Annals of the American Society for Adolescent Psychiatry

ADOLESCENT PSYCHIATRY

DEVELOPMENTAL AND CLINICAL STUDIES

VOLUME 27

Editorial Board

Daniel F. Becker
Irving H. Berkovitz
Adrian Copeland
Leah J. Dickstein
Robert L. Hendren
Harvey A. Horowitz
Saul Levine
John G. Looney
John E. Meeks
Glen T. Pearson
Richard Rosner
Allen Z. Schwartzberg
Moisy Shopper
Max Sugar

Annals of the American Society for Adolescent Psychiatry

ADOLESCENT PSYCHIATRY

DEVELOPMENTAL AND CLINICAL STUDIES

VOLUME 27

LOIS T. FLAHERTY

Editor

THE ANALYTIC PRESS

2003   Hillsdale, NJ   London

© 2003 by The Analytic Press, Inc.

All rights reserved. No part of this book may be reproduced in any form, by photostat, microfilm, electronic retrieval system, or any other means, without prior written permission of the publisher.

Published by The Analytic Press, Inc.
Editorial Offices: 101 West Street, Hillsdale, NJ 07642
www.analyticpress.com
www.adolpsych.org

Typeset in Times New Roman by International Graphic Services, Newtown, PA.

ISBN 0-88163-393-3
ISSN 0226-24064-9

Printed in the United States of America
10 9 8 7 6 5 4 3 2 1

CONTENTS

Editor's Introduction

PART IV.   CLINICAL CONSIDERATIONS

PART V.   ASAP POSITION PAPER

EDITOR'S INTRODUCTION

LOIS T. FLAHERTY

Much of this volume of *Adolescent Psychiatry* focuses on trauma and violence. These are not new issues to psychiatrists, especially those who work with adolescents. Indeed, they are hardly new issues for the world. What is new is a growing awareness of the psychological, biological, and social impact of trauma on its victims, especially on the young. What awaits is the translation of this new knowledge into public policy, so that the effects of trauma can be mitigated and, ultimately, so that children and adolescents can be protected from harm.

The two Schonfeld Award papers in this volume deal with violence. Michael Kalogerakis has devoted much of his career to developing programs for violent youth in New York, where he served as Commissioner of Mental Health. He reviews the history of the pendulum swings in juvenile justice, revealing how far we have come from the original aims of the juvenile court. At the same time, the link between trauma and violence in adolescence is now firmly established, and there are programs that have good data for their effectiveness. My paper on terrorism attempts to show the appeal of ideologies that espouse violent revolution to young people.

Christopher Thomas et al. present a study from their groundbreaking work on youth violence in Galveston, Texas. The study links gang membership with serious violent crime, and by demonstrating the importance of the peer group, it points to ways that youth can be socialized away from gang membership.

The federal regulations on seclusion and restraint in inpatient settings that went into effect in 2001 were greeted with much apprehension. The study by Theodore Petti et al. shows that effective interventions can reduce the use of seclusion and restraint even with the most difficult state hospital adolescent populations. Most crucial to their findings is the importance of staff support.

Mani Pavuluri and colleagues present a comprehensive review of what we know about early-onset schizophrenia and bipolar disorders.

They discuss differential diagnosis and treatment strategies, with emphasis on newer pharmacological agents.

A series of papers by the Committee on Adolescence of the Group for the Advancement of Psychiatry deals with the nature, scope, and impact of trauma as well as implications of what we know for training and public policy. Freud's early discovery that histories of psychic trauma were prevalent among his patients—later put aside as he developed his theory of unconscious conflict—has been rediscovered as we have become aware of the appalling prevalence of child abuse and its lasting impact on its victims. Epidemiological studies have shown that traumatic stress is so prevalent in many societies and in subcultures of our own society that it can almost be considered a normative part of growing up. In areas as disparate as the inner cities of the United States and war-torn countries throughout the world, adolescents are traumatized by man-made violence. Natural disasters and disasters caused by human negligence take their toll everywhere.

Thanks to developments in neurobiology, we now have compelling evidence that this impact is in part mediated by measurable changes in brain function, as Patricia Lester et al. discuss in their paper on neurobiology and trauma. Cultural and gender issues are equally important in understanding the impact of trauma, as Warren Gadpaille demonstrates. These new awarenesses are being translated into clinical practice, as Monica Green's paper on intervention discusses. Finally, in this section, Max Sugar looks at the vulnerability of a particular group—late adolescents—to combat-related posttraumatic stress disorder, linking their vulnerability to developmental features of this period. His findings have particular significance for public policy, as late adolescents and young adults make up most of the frontline troops in combat.

Saul Levine dissects a multitude of self-deceptions and myths that he sees as having infected the mental health professions. Some of these involve beliefs (or purported beliefs) on the part of policymakers and funding agencies, others have been accepted uncritically by professionals themselves. All, in his view, have led to neglect of appropriate therapeutic care for adolescents.

James Gilfoil discusses the importance of families' attitudes toward psychotherapy in the outcome of therapy with teenagers. His paper includes a series of illustrations that constitute clinical pearls for the adolescent psychiatrist.

The final section consists of a resource paper on youth violence written by Charles Huffine, chair of the ASAP Topical Studies Council. This paper, which discusses the contributions of societal attitudes about youth to the perpetuation of violence and lack of appropriate interventions, was adopted as an official American Society for Adolescent Psychiatry (ASAP) position paper.

PART I

SCHONFELD AND KEYNOTE ADDRESSES

1   ADOLESCENT VIOLENCE IN AMERICA

A HISTORICAL PERSPECTIVE

MICHAEL G. KALOGERAKIS

There is no doubt that, for an adolescent psychiatrist in our nation, receiving the Schonfeld Award is the greatest honor that can be bestowed by one's colleagues, and I deeply appreciate having been chosen as the award recipient for this year. The significance of the honor is all the more impressive—and humbling—when one looks at the roster of previous award recipients: It is by any standard a veritable pantheon of professionals who have dedicated themselves to working with troubled adolescents during lengthy and distinguished careers.

Being so honored is all the more satisfying when the theme of the Annual Meeting is adolescent violence, a subject that has occupied me throughout my professional life. In thinking about what I might wish to address on this occasion, I opted for a historical approach rather than the usual clinical paper, because we have reached a point in the evolution of the problem at which a review of developments, even if brief, can provide a needed perspective from which to view the whole. I draw upon more than 15 years of experience as chief of service of an inpatient adolescent ward in a major municipal hospital, 4 years as a public health official in a state office of mental health, and more than 35 years as a private practitioner treating adolescents and adults, chiefly as a psychotherapist and psychoanalyst.

As historians sit down to chronicle the 20th century, the advances in science and technology and the maturation of political and social institutions will figure prominently among the many accomplishments that have defined the past 100 years. Sharing the spotlight with these incredible and unparalleled examples of human progress, however, is the long shadow cast by the violence that also characterized the century. The great wars, tribal enmity, pogroms, and political assassinations, though not new to human history, have permeated the century beyond all comprehension, detracting from the progress and affecting its final kaleidoscopic form. The passage of time may yet prove that the scientific achievements will have the more lasting impact, of course. But the violence to which our world has been subjected has cut so deeply into the psyche, taken such a toll on human life, and elevated hate and its expression to such unprecedented levels as to raise fundamental questions about our very nature and the ability of our species to survive.

Broad forces—economic, political and social—are generally credited with having spawned these major upheavals of our times. Yet, too often have we seen these forces exploited by the actions of a single individual, who, being in a position of power at a critical point in time, sought to impose a perverse, belligerent, and grandiose agenda on the people of that nation and, often, of neighboring countries. As social scientists and clinicians we have struggled to understand this inevitably self-defeating and thoroughly malignant warping of the human mind, whether we are looking at a political figure, a criminal, or, for our purposes today, a troubled youth.

We start with the recognition that every violent person was at one point an innocent child who, invariably, by the time he reached adolescence, was well on his way to a misanthropic relationship to the world. We are left to make sense of the pathological ontogeny that eventuates in the behavior we call violence. It has been said that violence has its roots in childhood, takes its form in adolescence, and finds its ultimate expression in adulthood. What have we learned about this trajectory?

Although violence has always been part of the human landscape, every American is by now painfully aware that we have been through a serious epidemic of adolescent violence in our country, deeply scarring families, schools, and communities. There is reason to believe that it is not quite over. However that may be, the decade from 1983 to 1993 was marked by the most serious outbreak of teenage violence in the nation's history. In turning our attention to this phenomenon, I shall for convenience divide our recent history into three periods: a pre-epidemic, an epidemic, and a post-epidemic era. I should like to review with you, then, the historical unfolding of the problem of adolescent violence, what factors may account for the course it has taken, what research has revealed, and society's current efforts to deal with it.

THE PRE-EPIDEMIC ERA

It has been more than 40 years since H. Rap Brown portrayed the violence in our country in words that have become legendary—"As American as cherry pie" (1967). He made it clear that he saw our nation as differing from other nations on this score. Indeed, the data give considerable support to his thesis, as Table 1, which compares statistics on homicide by adolescents in industrialized countries throughout the world, shows.

More recent data comparing adolescent violence in England and Wales, the Netherlands, Spain, and Italy with that in the United States showed prevalence rates that were 30% lower in the European nations. The samples involved 16- to 17-year-olds in 1992 or 1993 providing self-reports of serious violence (Junger-Tas, Terlouw, and Klein, 1994).

One important difference between the United States and other industrialized nations reported by the Centers for Disease Control and Preven-

TABLE 1

INTERNATIONAL COMPARISON OF HOMICIDE FOR MALES BETWEEN
15 & 24 YEARS HOMICIDES PER 100,000 POPULATION

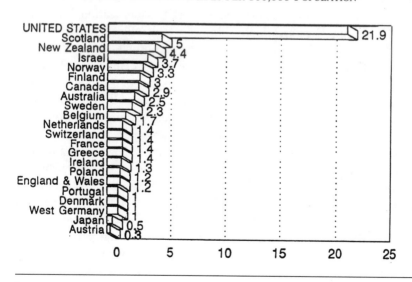

Data source: Fingerhut & Kleinman (1990).

tion (1997) is the ease of access to firearms. Between 1990 and 1995, the United States had the highest rate of firearm-related deaths among youths in the industrialized world, the rate for adolescents under 15 years of age being five times higher than that of 25 other countries combined.

The surgeon general concluded that although adolescent violence is international in scope, it is greater in the United States, is more likely to involve firearms, and is more lethal in its consequences (U.S. Department of Health and Human Services, 2001).

As early as the 1930s, there were sufficient problems with the generic population of antisocial or delinquent youths to spur the birth of a number of notable community-based efforts in cities facing the greatest incidence of juvenile crime. These were essentially social work initiatives growing out of sociological theory and political persuasions, which saw class inequality and social disorganization as primary causes of delinquency. Individual factors (whether physical or psychological) and family dynamics received little attention in these programs, with an occasional exception. They focused on urban areas that were the breeding grounds for the criminals of the future, including violent offenders. The Chicago Area Project (CAP) program, initiated in 1934, still stands as the first and most widely known delinquency-prevention program in American history. New York's Mobilization for Youth (MFY) and the Boston Midcity Project were similar communitywide efforts that tackled the same populations and problems.

A contemporary study of the history of gangs (Thrasher, 1927) was the first of many to bring to the fore an aspect of American society that had been with us for at least 200 years, virtually the full length of our existence as a nation. Gangs may have originated abroad, but they were to become a seemingly ineradicable part of the American scene. In the 1920s and 1930s, the typical gang was white and located chiefly in the major cities of the Northeast, but this was soon to change.

By 1967, criminologist Marvin Wolfgang was writing about our violent subculture (Wolfgang and Ferracutti, 1967), the United States having already earned the dubious distinction of being the most violent of the industrialized nations. The early 1960s saw the publication of another classical study of violent gangs by Yablonsky (1963) and a number of papers addressing the psychodynamics of youthful killers (Satten et al., 1960; Sargent, 1962; Smith, 1965).

Note that while previous decades had seen considerable work devoted to studies of aggression in children and adolescents, chiefly by learning

6

theorists, these did not address violence specifically (Bandura and Walters, 1959; Bateson, 1941; Dollard et al., 1939; Miller, 1941). Also, since most aggressive or behaviorally disturbed children do not become violent adolescents, they were of limited value in explaining violent delinquency.

Twenty years after the establishment of the first Juvenile Court in Chicago in 1899, 10 states were still permitting juveniles to be tried in adult courts under certain conditions. By 1940, an additional 10 states had passed statutes allowing transfer or waiver from the juvenile court. As was perhaps inevitable, distinctions were beginning to be drawn between different levels of seriousness of delinquent acts and of corresponding dispositions. Violent adolescents, though representing numerically a rather small group, were understandably a source of particular concern. Bender and Curran (1940) were probably the first to address the psychopathology of violence among hospitalized children and adolescents, initiating a continuing interest in this population at New York's Bellevue Hospital that was to span several decades (Bender, 1959; Kalogerakis, 1971a, b; Lewis and colleagues [e.g., Lewis, Pincus, Bard, et al., 1988]).

Asked by Family Court Judge Justine Wise Polier in the mid-1970s to name the most underserved groups of our hospitalized adolescents at Bellevue, I pointed to violent youths as the most problematic. This was not necessarily because they were all vicious, intractable youths, for some seemed little different from the rest of our population. But few treatment centers wanted them, especially if they were both violent and mentally disturbed (Polier, 1989).

We decided to establish a special unit at the hospital specifically designed for violent adolescents, but funding from the city was not forthcoming. Shortly thereafter (1976), a New York State–sponsored effort, spearheaded by the Office of Mental Health in cooperation with the Division for Youth, did see the light of day. Housed at the Bronx Children's Psychiatric Center, it was a small unit with a very high staff-to-patient ratio and was accordingly very expensive. At $60,000 per patient per year and with no expectation of immediate results, it was hardly slated to survive the scrutiny of budget officials and legislators for very long.

A less costly undertaking was opened in 1983 at another state mental health facility in New York (Queens Children's Psychiatric Center). It had a longer run and was one of very few such facilities anywhere (Faretra and Grad, 1989). At about this time, Governor Hugh Carey of New York established what may well have been the first statewide effort in the country to look at the problem—a Governor's Panel on Juvenile Violence on which I served as the lone psychiatrist among some 40 juvenile justice professionals. While such efforts were proceeding locally, little attention if any was being paid to the problem of juvenile delinquency, let alone adolescent violence, at the national level.

Faced with mounting public pressure to do something about the growing problems in the city's ghettos, the federal government finally took up the gauntlet and passed the landmark Juvenile Justice and Delinquency Prevention Act of 1974. With it came the hope that a full-scale assault on both delinquency and violence, properly funded, would finally be possible. Ironically, establishment of the Office of Juvenile Justice and Delinquency Prevention (OJJDP) did nothing to stave off the surge of adolescent violence that was to descend on the country scarcely a decade later.

In advance of the surge, a gradual escalation in juvenile crime had been proceeding apace, probably related to a number of factors. The baby boom of the 1960s, when the 13- to 17-year-old cohort increased to 10% of the population, was one of the factors that has been singled out as contributing to an increase in the total incidence of violence among adolescents, although the actual prevalence rates remained fairly stable through the 1970s and into the early 1980s (Zimring, 1998). Real increases have, in part, been ascribed to five developments:

1. Manufacturing jobs in the cities were declining as they were replaced by jobs in the suburbs in the technological and service industries that required more education, leading to a loss of job opportunities and increasing despair among the youth (Fagan, 1996).
2. Traditional family structure, at least among the poor, was changing, and a single-parent structure, with live-in fathers becoming increasingly rare, was becoming the norm, especially for African American youths.
3. Teenage pregnancy was on the rise.
4. Neighborhoods were deteriorating, and, concomitantly, gangs began increasing in numbers and in membership as well as changing their basic character.
5. Formerly stabilizing community institutions such as churches and community centers were disappearing.

More subtle changes were also occurring. Respect for authority—previously a given for most youths when it concerned teachers, doctors, nurses, and clergy—was steadily being eroded. This was a very palpable change on the adolescent ward at Bellevue, where our head nurse, always a beloved figure, was for the first time being subjected to hostile, threatening behavior. (What is not often recorded is that the same change was being observed, at least at New York University, among medical students and residents.) Was this an extension of the widespread rage over the Vietnam War? Assaults on the elderly were becoming commonplace. The answer to the age-old question, "Is nothing sacred?" was an emphatic "No!"—the only regular exception being mothers.

Other changes included a palpable increase in drug use, which evolved from glue-sniffing to marijuana to the hallucinogens and harder drugs, accompanied by a destructive impact on school attendance and overall adjustment. Public schools were becoming more crowded, their effectiveness progressively impaired. Handguns, which had slowly made their way into inner-city teenagers' life as a form of protection (including at school), had become readily available and more lethal. When the crack craze finally hit in the mid-1980s, with its accompanying illegal economy, one might well say that all hell broke loose.

Throughout this time, with the juvenile justice system at the federal level moving forward on a number of fronts, public health authorities were paying little attention to what was seen as largely a problem for social services, criminology, or law enforcement. The first official engagement of the public health system did not come until 1985 when Surgeon General C. Everett Koop established a Workshop on Violence and Public Health to look at the issue of violence in the country. This initiative, though an important first step, did not target youth in particular and was but a drop in the bucket, because what was needed was a major effort akin to those launched against tobacco use and drunken driving. But more of this in a moment.

As the psychopathology of adolescent violence began to be studied more intensively, often by mental health professionals working in juvenile justice, the question of what constituted appropriate treatment assumed increasing importance. This applied to both treatment programs and treatment modalities. The hue and cry had for some time been that nothing works with juvenile delinquents, and as I have already indicated, the violent youth was preeminently the persona non grata of all treatment facilities. Poor results led many in the juvenile justice system (legal aid lawyers and civil libertarians in particular) to reject the treatment or rehabilitation model and to turn to a correctional and even punitive model for disposition. Thoughtful mental health professionals, seeking a solution to the dilemma, were critical of the typical training school, which they saw as more custodial than therapeutic; on the other hand, they acknowledged that their own efforts were hardly more successful. The one-on-one, basically psychoanalytic model, even when modified from its use early in the century by Aichhorn (1935), had clearly been oversold and could not deal with the sheer numbers of youth in trouble. Pharmacological treatments were coming into use and cognitive-behavioral therapy was beginning to take a firm hold. Frustrated directors of training schools were coming to recognize that many of their charges were in fact psychiatrically disturbed (one director said to me that more than 40% of the youths in his training schools were depressed), believing strongly that they belonged in mental health facilities. In general, even good training schools lacked the resources to deal with disturbed chronically delinquent and violent juveniles. It was this situation that led to the establishment of the mobile mental health teams designed to assist the State Division for Youth in the diagnosis, treatment and (when necessary) alternative placement of these disturbed juveniles. This occurred in New York State in the late 1970s, while I was serving as Associate Commissioner for Children and Youth in the Office of Mental Health.

In the community at large, as truancy, "hanging out," drug use, and gang involvement began to replace traditional school attendance and learning as the primary developmental concern of adolescents, the life of many youths, especially in the ghettos of our nation, was beginning to heat up.

Such was the situation on the eve of the precipitous rise in arrests for violence by adolescents that brought both juvenile justice and mental health agencies to their knees.

THE EPIDEMIC ERA

Just how bad was it? Arrests of teenagers for violent crimes began to climb inexorably, attaining unprecedented levels. Figure 1 shows data culled from the Unified Crime Reports of the FBI (1998).

These data show that a very real rise in the incidence of arrests for violent crimes by adolescents occurred in the decade from 1983 to

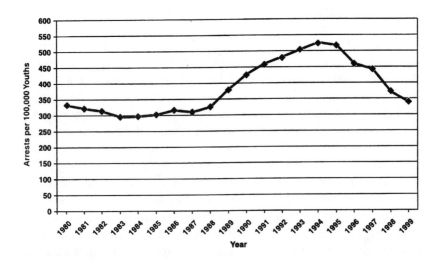

Figure 1 Arrest rate of youths age 10–17 for serious violent crime, 1980–1999.
Snyder 2001, Dept. of Health & Human Services.

1993. This was particularly true for the FBI Index crimes of homicide and aggravated assault, which rose 90% and 78% respectively, but also applied to robbery, which rose 63%. The greater part of these increases was registered among African American male adolescents in the inner cities who had a 61% rise in the rate for homicide, against 36% for Caucasians (1994). Though quite naturally the rates of violence were highest in the inner cities, where most of the high-risk adolescents resided, recent surveys covering much wider cohorts consistently show that about 30% to 40% of male youths have committed a serious violent offense by the age of 17. As astounding as this figure is, it is perhaps even more dismaying that 15% to 30% of girls report having committed a violent offense by age 17. Another change is that suburban and even rural whites began to show significant increases in their rate of involvement. The most visible and in many ways the most disturbing example of the epidemic of violence has been, for much of America, the spate of school shootings, which have generally victimized innocents, involved localities traditionally deemed safe and, as we know all too well, continue right down to the present.

As the rates for violence committed by youths began to rise, a need for answers as to why it was happening, what populations were involved, what factors were contributing, and what might be done to curb the problem finally brought some action from Washington. The first comprehensive effort by a federal government agency to study the problem systematically came in 1986, when OJJDP created the Program of Research on the Causes and Correlates of Delinquency, funding three coordinated, longitudinal research projects—at the State University of New York in Albany, at the University of Colorado in Denver, and at the University of Pittsburgh. For more than a decade, these centers collectively interviewed some 4500 youths 10 to 19 years old at regular intervals, in Rochester, Denver, and Pittsburgh, recording details of their lives. The wealth of data emerging from these studies confirmed many impressions from earlier studies but provided some surprises: The usually anticipated decline of violence in late adolescence was not observed; children as young as 10 were more involved in committing violence than had been thought; and the aforementioned prevalence of violence among girls was considerably higher than previously reported. In fact, in both Rochester and Denver, the prevalence of violence among 13- to 15-year-old girls was more than half the rate for boys in that age range. From 1991 to 1995, female juvenile arrests for FBI Index offenses increased 34%, while the rate for males increased only 9%.

The legislature decided to take action and, in 1992, passed amendments to the Juvenile Justice and Delinquency Prevention Act, directing the OJJDP to address the problem of juvenile violence specifically. It responded by setting up, in 1995, a Study Group on Serious and Violent Juvenile (SVJ) Offenders, bringing together a distinguished panel of researchers in juvenile justice and criminology. The Study Group met for two years, documented existing information about SVJ offenders, evaluated programs set up for them, and recommended further research. It issued its report in 1997, published in book form in 1998 (Loeber and Farrington, 1998).

The most striking correlation that came out of the burgeoning research into the whys and wherefores of the epidemic of juvenile violence was the fact that the use of firearms rose proportionately during the same period. The graph in Figure 2 makes this clear.

No other single factor showed a similar parallel. As an example, in Los Angeles, the proportion of gang-related homicides went from 71% in 1979 to 95% in 1994, mainly because of the increased use of handguns, especially semiautomatic handguns. Other factors were unquestionably involved, however. I shall single out only two of these for special comment, because they have figured prominently in the media coverage: gangs and drugs.

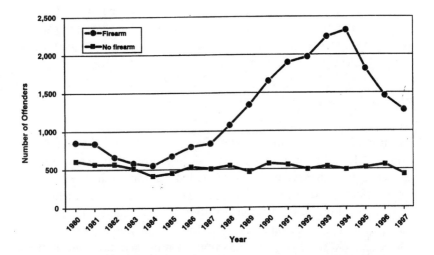

Figure 2 Firearm- and nonfirearm-related homicides by youths, 1980–1997. Snyder & Sickmund, 1999.

The Gang Factor

Just what was the impact of gangs? Though the media have unquestionably sensationalized drive-by shootings and drug wars, ascribing them to gangs (but not necessarily youth gangs), the fact remains that the increased violence that characterized the epidemic era was paralleled by a sharp increase in youth gang violence. In the Rochester study, gang members accounted for 68% of the serious violence; in Denver, self-reports indicated that adolescent gang members were responsible for 89% of all serious violent offenses. Evidence of gang migrations from core cities such as Los Angeles, of greatly increased membership, of heavy involvement in drug trafficking (46% of gang members, according to the 1996 National Youth Gang Survey), and of much increased use of firearms, was part of the reality of the decade, finally abating by the mid-1990s (National Youth Gang Center, 1999).

The Drug Factor

The demand for drugs was a critical factor in bringing on the epidemic, especially when crack hit the streets in the mid-1980s and became the

13

drug of choice in the inner cities. Gang rivalry for local markets often became lethal, with so much at stake. Yet most of the trafficking seems to have been carried out by adult gangs. Drug abuse itself had a less certain impact on the rates of violence.

Risk and Protective Factors

The principal goal of the NIJJDP Causes and Correlates study previously referred to was to identify risk and protective factors related to serious delinquency and violence, with the ultimate purpose of developing effective prevention strategies. These were sought in the five critical areas of child development: individual characteristics, family, peers, school, and community. The theoretical framework that was selected emphasized context and drew upon the seminal contributions of Bronfenbrenner (1979, 1986). Called a developmental-ecological perspective (Tolan, Guerra, and Kendall, 1995), it incorporated the essential features of the new discipline of developmental psychopathology (Loeber and Hay, 1994). Its focus was on the dynamic interplay between constantly changing risk factors, internal and external, as normal development unfolds. With this in mind, two distinct trajectories leading to a violent future have been identified: an early-onset form, beginning prior to age 13, that is associated with more serious and more chronic violent behavior; and a late-onset form starting in adolescence that appears to be more amenable to change. The risk factors for these two forms differ somewhat. Early-onset risk factors include involvement in delinquent activity, substance abuse, being male, physical aggression, poverty, and parental criminality. Late-onset factors include associating with delinquent peers, having weak ties to healthy peers, being a member of a gang, and involvement in other forms of delinquency.

As concerns protective factors, a number have been suggested but only two have been demonstrated to be consistently effective: an intolerant attitude toward deviance (in particular, violence) and commitment to school. Others will be referred to in the discussion of prevention.

Despite a research focus on the violent youth in searching for risk and protective factors, the factors that have emerged pertain generically to serious delinquency and are not specific for the violent individual. Further research is needed to shed light on points of differentiation. For the moment, some clues as to likely differences have emerged

14

from the Pittsburgh Youth Study component of the longitudinal research, which identified three distinct developmental pathways in boys' disruptive and delinquent behavior. They are 1) authority conflict, 2) covert acts, and 3) overt acts, the first two leading to milder forms of delinquency and the last involving increasingly aggressive acts such as annoying others, bullying, physical fighting, gang fighting, attacking someone, strong-arming, and forcing sex, leading potentially to serious violence (Kelley et al., 1997).

The Role of Public Health and the Professions

As the juvenile justice system conducted research that was increasingly intensive and sophisticated, the health and mental health agencies were nowhere to be seen. This was rather shocking given the fact that the roots of youthful violence lay in earliest childhood, long before any offense could occur that would involve law enforcement, and that since violent adolescents are frequently depressed, suicidal or mentally ill, they are often more appropriate for referral to the mental health system. In fact, the neglect by the public health system existed despite the fact that delinquent and violent youths had been routinely served by local and state mental health facilities for many years. (At Bellevue, for example, 40% of the annual admissions to the adolescent ward were remands from the Family Court, a good many of them with histories of violence.)

Psychiatric organizations, including the American Psychiatric Association (APA) and the then–American Academy of Child Psychiatry, were for many years equally guilty, because the subject of violence was seldom, if ever, addressed in conferences, studies, or published papers. The word violence rarely appeared in the psychiatric literature prior to the Kennedy assassination. The American Society for Adolescent Psychiatry (ASAP), with an interest in every variety of adolescent disorder, did better, as several of our members (Offer, Marohn, Rafferty, Kalogerakis, and others) turned their clinical and research skills to a serious exploration of delinquency and violence as forms of psychopathology. ASAP members were also prominent as founding members when the APA finally established a component to address juvenile justice issues, first as a task force in 1983, then as a permanent committee in 1987 (Buzogany, Kalogerakis, Marohn, Ratner).

When middle-class communities were struck, as in the school shootings at Columbine and elsewhere, a shocked public began to look for something other than a correctional response. In one fell swoop, individual and family psychopathology became a matter of urgent concern, and the mental health professional was sought out. Many of our own colleagues, as individuals, responded generously to these crises, both as clinicians and theoreticians. What was still missing was a concerted, coordinated, well-thought-out mental health strategy—federally mandated, funded, and administered, paralleling that of the juvenile justice system.

By 1993 to 1994, the wave of terrible violence that swept the country for one unforgettable decade seemed to abate. Once again, this paralleled an attenuation in the use of firearms. As we were soon to learn, however, there was little to cheer about, because unreported violence actually continued undiminished. But public concern had been galvanized, and previously somnolent government agencies were beginning to stir. All this notwithstanding, the hegemony of the justice system remained unchallenged.

THE POST-EPIDEMIC ERA

The arrest rates for violent juveniles actually did decline rather sharply after about 1993, suggesting that the epidemic of violence that had troubled the nation for a decade was coming to an end. Unfortunately, this was only partially true. When the figures for self-reported violence came in, it became clear that, for every arrest for violence, there were 10 instances of unreported violence. In addition, the incidence of homicide dropped to levels below those existing prior to the onset of the epidemic, but the incidence of aggravated assault remained as high as it had been in 1983. In a never-ending horror tale, we are regularly reminded that school shootings have hardly abated. If anything, they seem to have increased in frequency since the mid-1990s. Some researchers continue to predict a steady increase in the level of violence over the coming years (Snyder and Sickmund, 1999).

Prevention

With the deepening of our knowledge base, the focus has shifted to intervention strategies, with an emphasis on prevention. New initiatives are being tested, some highly touted and involving a variety of approaches. Many of these, on closer examination, have proved to be of little lasting value. Included are school-based programs on anger management and conflict resolution, boot camps and "tough love" programs in correctional settings, and waivers to the adult court. Out of this has come the realization that rigorous evaluation must be built into any intervention strategy if we are to learn what works.

With an emphasis on early intervention in the important areas of a child's life, a number of programs seem to have proved effective in addressing the identified risk factors. They are illustrated in Table 2.

Table 3 shows what has been found effective, partially effective, or not at all effective with these early interventions.

In actuality, 10 programs in current use have been identified as meeting the rigorous criteria set by the NIJJDP Causes and Correlates studies. These have been dubbed "Blueprints" (Mihalic et al., 2001) and are illustrated in Table 4.

What many of these programs share are a broad-based approach, a clear emphasis on the family, and work with youth that is rooted in a close, respectful, long-term relationship with a concerned adult. One particularly noteworthy intervention is Multisystemic Therapy (MST), a program developed at the Medical University of South Carolina, which has been evaluated in several clinical trials at different sites and has shown good results with conduct disorders, including violent behavior (Henggeler et al., 1997; Borduin, 1999). The program is home- and community-based and utilizes strategic family therapy, structural family therapy, behavioral parent training, and cognitive-behavioral therapy.

Three additional, highly successful programs differ significantly from each other, attacking different aspects of the many-headed beast that is adolescent violence. Each program is impressive in its own right. The first, the Boston Gun Project, is a gun suppression program targeting youth gangs. It was undertaken by the city of Boston after gun violence and killings in high-crime areas of the city had reached intolerable levels, leaving the residents constantly terrified. Multiagency in makeup, it featured, among other initiatives, a strong police involvement in which special police units met face-to-face with gang members and spelled out to them the legal consequences of continued gun use, emphasizing that these would be enforced. A very high reduction in gun violence, apparently around 80% over a five-year period, was the result (Kennedy et al., 1996; Clark, 1997).

TABLE 2

EFFECTIVE EARLY INTERVENTION PROGRAMS TO MEDIATE RISK FACTORS
KNOWN TO PREDICT SERIOUS AND VIOLENT JUVENILE OFFENDING

Involving parents:

- Parent management training
- Functional family therapy
- Family preservation

Involving children:

- Home visitation of pregnant teenagers
- Social competence training
- Peer mediation and conflict resolution
- Medication for neurological disorders and mental illness

Involving schools:

- Early intellectual enrichment (preschools)
- School organization interventions

Involving the community:

- Comprehensive community mobilization
- Situational crime prevention
- Intensive police patrolling, especially crime "hot spots"
- Legal and policy changes restricting availability and use of guns, drugs, and alcohol
- Mandatory laws for crimes involving firearms

Source: Loeber, R. and Farrington, D. P. eds., 1997. *Never Too Early, Never Too Late: Risk Factors and Successful Interventions for Serious and Violent Juvenile Offenders.* Final Report of the Study Group on Serious and Violent Juvenile Offenders. Washington, DC: U.S. Department of Justice, Office of Justice programs, Office of Juvenile Justice and Delinquency Prevention. Reprinted in Juvenile Justice Bulletin, May 1998.

The second program took place in Galveston, Texas, and also involved what would be considered tertiary prevention (or treatment), that is, intervention when the violence had already occurred. Named the Galveston Island Youth Program, it pulled together city government, law enforcement, juvenile justice, public recreation, public schools, the University of Texas Medical Branch, and concerned families in a collaborative and comprehensive effort involving five separate components (Thomas, Holzer, and Wall, 2002). The very impressive result

TABLE 3

EFFECTIVENESS OF INTERVENTIONS FOR SERIOUS AND
VIOLENT JUVENILE OFFENDERS

Treatment Type: Noninstitutionalized Offenders	Treatment Type: Institutionalized Offenders
Positive effects, consistent evidence	
Individual counseling	Interpersonal skills
Interpersonal skills	Teaching family home
Behavioral contracting	
Positive effects, less consistent evidence	
Multiple services	Cognitive-behavioral treatment
Restitution, probation/parole	Community residential programs
	Multiple services
Mixed but generally positive effects, inconsistent evidence	
Employment-related programs	Individual counseling
Academic programs	Guided group
Advocacy/casework	Group counseling
Family counseling	
Group counseling	
Weak or no effects, inconsistent evidence	
Reduced caseload, probation/parole	Employment-related programs
	Drug abstinence
	Wilderness/challenge
Weak or no effects, consistent evidence	
Wilderness/challenge	Milieu therapy
Early release, probation/parole	
Deterrence programs	
Vocational programs	

Note: Interventions were conducted primarily as single-component rather than multimodal programs. Results from multiple-services programs suggest that some of the interventions that showed less than consistent positive effects individually may have more significant effects when combined.

Source: Loeber, R. and Farrington, D. P. eds., 1997. *Never Too Early, Never Too Late: Risk Factors and Successful Interventions for Serious and Violent Juvenile Offenders.* Final Report of the Study Group on Serious and Violent Juvenile Offenders. Washington, DC: U.S. Department of Justice, Office of Justice programs, Office of Juvenile Justice and Delinquency Prevention.

TABLE   4

TEN MODEL PROGRAMS IN VIOLENCE PREVENTION: BLUEPRINTS

- Midwestern Prevention Program
- Big Brothers Big Sisters
- Functional Family Therapy
- Quantum Opportunities
- Life Skills Training
- Multisystemic Therapy
- Nurse Home Visitation
- Treatment Foster Care
- Bullying Prevention Program
- PATHS

These programs were chosen from a review of over 450 violence prevention programs, using rigorous criteria. Details can be accessed from the University of Colorado's Center for the Study and Prevention of Violence (http://www.colorado.edu/cspy/blueprints/model/Default.htm). See also Mihalic et al., 2001.

of this program was that between 1994 and 1999, when violent crime in the country dropped 19%, it dropped 78% in Galveston (American Medical Association, 2000).

The third program, generic in nature, is rare in that it represents a real primary prevention program. It is family centered and begins early, is aimed at strengthening families, and attacks one of the known precursors of serious delinquency and violence, child abuse, and neglect. Funded initially in 1979 by the National Institute of Mental Health (NIMH) and thus an exception to all the research being conducted under the aegis of the juvenile justice system, it is known as the Nurturing Parent Program. It uses a group- and home-based intervention approach and has recorded notable successes. Four patterns of abusive parenting were identified: 1) inappropriate parental expectations, 2) lack of empathy, 3) use of physical punishment, and 4) parental role reversal. Among the several assumptions made, the emphasis on empathy as the single most important element of nurturing parenting deserves special mention. Originally focused on 4- to 12-year-olds (average age, 6), it has since been expanded to include adolescents and a variety of ethnic and racial groups. Field tests have demonstrated very significant changes in self-awareness and parental expectations, in behavior management, and in the presence of empathy, and currently some 13 Nurturing

Parenting Programs are being implemented in the United States and abroad (Bavolek, Kline, and McLaughlin, 1979; Bavolek, 2000).

CONCLUSION

I have provided a brief review of developments related to the upsurge of youth violence in the United States that has been such a disturbing part of our recent history, and some examples of the associated societal response. A prodigious amount of research has produced an extensive literature that I could not even begin to cover. I have tried not to burden readers unnecessarily with endless statistics. More information can be readily accessed from the many publications of the OJJDP; from two very recent and important publications from health sources, the Surgeon General's Report on Youth Violence (U.S. Department of Health and Human Services, 2001) and the American Medical Association–sponsored report by a Commission for the Prevention of Youth Violence (American Medical Association, 2000); and from the Internet, for example, from the University of Colorado's Center for the Study and Prevention of Violence (http://www.colorado.edu/cspv).

The following are some personal impressions of a number of the issues just reviewed, based on my own observations as a clinician, public health official, and child advocate over the years. But first, here is a summary of some of the important facts relating to the prevention of violence, whether committed by children, adolescents or adults.

- Violence, as a form of human behavior, seldom has any re-deeming value. It is in fact invariably destructive, not only to the victim(s), but also to the perpetrator(s) and to many associated with both. There is consequently only one policy for individuals or society to have toward violence, and that is zero tolerance.
- In the overwhelming majority of cases, violence is preventable, and we have the requisite knowledge base to achieve prevention.
- The responsibility for violence prevention must be shared by all—first of all by government, but also by industry, social in-stitutions, communities, schools, professionals, families, and individuals.

- Collaboration toward the goal of violence prevention should, whenever possible, be voluntary, but failing that, it should be enforced by adequate legislation and the law.
- Regardless of the apparent etiology, a comprehensive strategy for intervention must be developmentally appropriate; must begin early in the life of the at-risk child; and must address the child, his or her family and peers, the school, and the community.
- Such efforts are unlikely to succeed without an equal commitment to address the broader issues of gun control; the role of media, movies, video, and popular music that glorify violence; and the Internet.
- Effecting prevention will require a huge investment of public funds over a long period of time, but this must somehow be budgeted, for there can be no higher priority for an enlightened society.
- Finally, continued research is needed to answer many remaining questions. Research must be adequately supported and address all aspects of the problem.

A review of this kind is, by its nature, somewhat frustrating in that it leaves little room to address important issues such as the nature of violence, why it is so much a part of the human experience, the human fascination with it, its relationship to life and death, and so on. The following are some clinical concerns that have preoccupied me as I have dealt with the subject over the past four decades. These are matters that I believe have received rather short shrift in the existing literature.

Having seen hundreds if not thousands of violent adolescents in my time, I have never ceased to ponder the question of what it actually takes to make a youth turn violent. In other words, in the pathways followed, what conditions differentiate the youth beset with violent impulses from the nonviolent delinquent or one who is disturbed in other ways? Considered from the standpoint of developmental psychopathology, three conditions seem to me to be necessary, though they are generally not sufficient:

1. In terms of normal development, the nurturing, caring qualities and empathy that characterize healthy child development have either failed to develop or have been severely compromised by later trauma.

2. Cognitively, a rationale has been internalized that justifies injuring another person or taking another life, for example, "He's not really human."
3. Emotionally, an impulse or desire to inflict harm on another has somehow evolved. Hate would be an example of this.

Whatever biological or environmental circumstances would lead to these conditions in the individual child would constitute the risk factors.

A second important area of concern has been the role of hostility in the causation of violence. It is not discernibly present in all violent adolescents but probably exists in the majority. Although considerable research has been conducted on the early roots of hostility in the first three years of life (Parens, 1991), we clearly need to have a better understanding of just how hostility develops in the growing child and of its subsequent pathways through adolescence.

Last, some comments on the place of psychodynamic psychotherapy in the treatment of the violent youth. Some meta-analyses of the literature have indicated that psychotherapy is of questionable value with this population (Lipsey, 1992). However, later studies of noninstitutionalized serious delinquents (Lipsey and Wilson, 1998) showed individual counseling to be one of the most effective interventions. It is apparent that the nature of the psychotherapy and the specific population it is used with are the relevant determinants of its value as a technique. I should add that any clinician who has worked with violent adolescents knows that for the conflict-ridden youth or one with an established personality disorder (which covers a large number of those involved in violent behavior) there is no other approach that offers hope for a definitive resolution to the problems. Is it always successful? Of course not. Is it cost efficient? Given the alternative—that is, inadequate interventions—yes. Is it worth it? That is a personal decision, but suppose it were your child?

Some important facets of the history of youth violence have not been dealt with here, although they are psychiatrically of great interest and significant enough socially to deserve a full airing. I include violence by satanic cults, neo-Nazis, skinheads, and other hate groups that commonly involve adolescents and have demographics and dynamics that differ from the groups focused on in this chapter. A future conference on these subjects would be welcome.

The AMA Commission report and the surgeon general's report do address some of these aspects. They are excellent resources, although the former is so comprehensive in its coverage that it may defeat its purposes by failing to identify priorities; the latter pointedly elects not to recommend policy initiatives and appropriate government action. It is unclear whether these shortcomings will be addressed in the near future.

As indicated here, our profession has been far from noble on the subject of adolescent violence. Official psychiatry, like national public health, has been asleep on the job as other professions have responded to the growing scourge of adolescent violence. There is no question that, on this matter, after an auspicious beginning in our involvement with delinquency at the start of the 20th century, we abdicated our responsibility until very late in the game. It is small comfort that the Public Health Service has now come through, for it took a full eight years after the alleged end of the epidemic of youth violence to issue a report on the subject—published only days before the outgoing administration (possibly the most socially conscious and compassionate we have ever had) folded up its tent! And what was the catalyst? A series of school shootings in white middle-class communities and long overdue outrage on the part of a suddenly terrified public.

I hope that this chapter leaves no doubt that the phenomenon of adolescent violence, by its very existence, constitutes a severe indictment of our society and of government. Let the responsibility fall where it belongs. However, serious criticism begins at home, and it would be an unfortunate error for adolescent psychiatrists to minimize our complicity. We are, after all, the self-appointed guardians of our youth's mental health. As we have seen, our leaders based in Washington, in a position to establish policy and set priorities, have been looking elsewhere for far too long. And we as individuals, with too few exceptions, have failed as scientists, failed as caretakers, and failed as advocates. Are we now prepared to rise to the challenge as the new administration in Washington asserts itself, seeing a lack of family values and godlessness as the culprits while in the same breath absolving the gun industry and the National Rifle Association of any responsibility for the continuing madness? To remain mute may be convenient, but it is unconscionable.

As for ASAP, those of us who have been entrusted with the legacy of what our founding fathers envisioned can feel proud that we have in many ways taken this organization beyond their wildest dreams. Yet, as concerns this most virulent of America's problems, arguably the greatest plague that has ever afflicted our young, our collective voice has been neither loud enough nor effective enough. This is all

24

the more sad when we consider that there is no group that knows adolescents better than we do.

Rather than wasting our energies on disillusionment and despair, let us record that real progress has been achieved, even if, to date, it is our colleagues in other fields who must, in the main, receive the credit for that. I hope that we will avoid meaningless genuflections and mea culpas, own up to our neglect, swallow our pride, and, however belatedly, assert our knowledge of adolescent development and psychopathology and our hard-earned clinical intuitions, to deliver on a potential unrealized and a commitment unfulfilled. It is a challenge we cannot afford to ignore.

REFERENCES

Aichhorn, A. (1935), *Wayward Youth.* New York: Viking Press.

American Medical Association (2000), *Youth and Violence: Report of the Commission for the Prevention of Youth Violence.* Chicago, IL: American Medical Association.

Bandura, A. & Walters, R. H. (1959), *Adolescent Aggression.* New York: Ronald Press.

Bateson, G. (1941), The frustration-aggression hypothesis and culture. *Psychological Review,* 8:350–355.

Bavolek, S. J. (2000), The nurturing parenting programs. *Office of Juvenile Justice and Delinquency Prevention Juvenile Justice Bulletin NCJ 172848.* Washington, DC: U.S. Government Printing Office.

——— Kline, D. F. & McLaughlin, J. A. (1979), Primary prevention of child abuse: Identification of high risk adolescents. *Child Abuse and Neglect,* 3(2):491–496.

Bender, L. (1959), Children and adolescents who have killed. *Amer. J. Psychiat.,* 116:510–513.

——— & Curran, F. (1940), Children and adolescents who kill. *Crim. Psychopathol.,* 1:297–322.

Borduin, C. M. (1999), Multisystemic treatment of criminality and violence in adolescents. *J. Amer. Acad. Child & Adol. Psychiat.,* 38:242–249.

Bronfenbrenner, U. (1979), *The Ecology of Human Development: Experiments by Nature and by Design.* Boston: Cambridge University Press.

——— (1986), Ecology of the family as a context for human development. *Devel. Psychol.,* 22:723–742.

Brown, H. R. (1967), Press conference 7/27/1967.

Center for the Study and Prevention of Violence (1999), *CSPV Blueprints Promising Fact Sheet: Preventive Intervention.* Boulder: Center for the Study and Prevention of Violence, Institute of Behavioral Science, University of Colorado at Boulder.

Centers for Disease Control and Prevention (1997), Rates for homicide, suicide, and firearm-related death among children: 26 industrialized countries. *Morbidity and Mortality Weekly Report,* 46:101–105.

Clark, J. R. (1997), LEN salutes its 1997 People of the Year, the Boston Gun Project Working Group. *Law Enforcement News,* 23(1):4–5.

Dollard, J. D. L., Doob, L. W., Miller, N. E., Mowrer, D. H. & Sears, R. R. (1939), *Frustration and Aggression.* New Haven, CT: Yale University Press.

Fagan, J. (1996), Legal and illegal work: Crime, work, and unemployment. In: *Dealing with Urban Crisis: Linking Research to Action,* ed. B. Weisbrod & J. Worthy. Evanston, IL: Northwestern University Press.

Faretra, G. & Grad, G. J. (1989), Special considerations in the inhospital treatment of dangerously violent juveniles. In: *Juvenile Psychiatry and the Law,* ed. R. Rosner & H. I. Schwartz. New York: Plenum.

Federal Bureau of Investigation. (1998), *Crime in the United States 1997.* Washington, DC: U.S. Government Printing Office.

Fingerhut, L. A. & Kleinman, J. C. (1990), International and interstate comparisons of homicide among young males. *J. Amer. Med. Assn.,* 263:3292–3295.

Henggeler, S. W., Melton, G. B., Brondino, M. J., Scherer, D. G. & Hanley, J. H. (1997), Multisystemic therapy with violent and chronic juvenile offenders and their families: the role of treatment fidelity in successful dissemination. *J. Consult. Clin. Psychol.,* 65:821–833.

Junger-Tas, J., Terlouw, G. J. & Klein, M. W. (1994), *Delinquent Behavior among Young People in the Western World: First Results of the International Self-Report Delinquency Study.* Amsterdam: Kugler.

Kalogerakis, M. G. (1971a), Homicide in adolescents: Fantasy and deed. In: *Dynamics of Violence,* ed. J. Fawcett. Chicago: American Medical Association, pp. 93–103.

——— (1971b), The assaultive psychiatric patient. *Psychiat. Quart.,* 45:372–381.

Kelley, B. T., Loeber, R., Keenan, K. & DeLamatre, M. (1997), Developmental pathways in boys' disruptive and delinquent behavior. *Juvenile Justice Bulletin, December 1997 (NCJ 165692).* Washington, DC: U.S. Department of Justice, Office of Justice Programs, Office of Juvenile Justice and Delinquency Prevention.

Kennedy, D. M., Piehl, A. M. & Braga, A. A. (1996), Youth violence in Boston: Gun markets, serious youth offenders, and a use-reduction strategy. *Law and Contemporary Problems,* 59:147–196. Special issue.

Lewis, D. O. & Balla, D. A. (1976), *Delinquency and Psychopathology.* New York: Grune & Stratton.

Lewis, D. O., Pincus, J. H., Bard, B., Richardson, E., Prichep, L. S., Feldman, M., & Yeager, C. (1988), Neuropsychiatric, psychoeducational, and family characteristics of 14 juveniles condemned to death in the United States. *Am. J. Psychiat.* 145:584–589.

Lipsey, M. W. (1992), The effect of treatment of juvenile delinquents: Results from meta-analysis. In: *Psychology and Law: International Perspectives,* ed. F. Losel, D. Bender, & T. Bliesener. New York: Walter de Gruyter, pp. 131–143.

———— & Wilson, D. B. (1998), Effective intervention for serious juvenile offenders: A synthesis of research. In: *Serious and Violent Juvenile Offenders: Risk Factors and Successful Interventions,* ed. R. Loeber & D. P. Farrington. Thousand Oaks, CA: Sage, pp. 313–345.

Loeber, R. & Farrington, D., eds. (1998), *Never Too Early Never Too Late: Risk Factors for Successful Interventions for Serious and Violent Juvenile Offenders.* Thousand Oaks, CA: Sage.

———— & Hay, D. F. (1994), Developmental approaches to aggression and conduct problems. In: *Development Through Life: A Handbook for Clinicians,* ed. M. Rutter & D. F. Hay. Oxford: Blackwell Scientific Publications, pp. 488–515.

Mihalic, S., Irwin, K., Elliott, D., Fagan, A. & Hansen, D. (2001), *Blueprints for Violence Prevention.* Bulletin. Washington, DC: U.S. Department of Justice, Office of Justice Programs, Office of Juvenile Justice and Delinquency Prevention.

Miller, N. E. (1941), The frustration-aggression hypothesis. *Psychol. Rev.,* 48:337–342.

National Youth Gang Center, (1999), *1996 Youth Gang Survey. Summary.* Washington, DC: U.S. Department of Justice.

Parens, H. (1991), A view of the development of hostility in early life. *J. Amer. Psychoanal. Assoc.,* 39 (Suppl.).

Polier, J. W. (1989), *Juvenile Justice in Double Jeopardy: The Distanced Community and Vengeful Retribution.* Hillsdale, NJ: Lawrence Erlbaum.

27

Sargent, D. A. (1962), Children who kill: A family conspiracy. *Soc. Work,* 7:35–42.

Satten, J., Menninger, K., Rosen, I. & Mayman, M. (1960), Murder without apparent motive. *Amer. J. Psychiat.,* 117:48–53.

Smith, S. (1965), The adolescent murderer: A psychodynamic interpretation. *Arch. Gen. Psychiat.,* 13:30–319.

Snyder, H. & Sickmund, M. (1999), *Juvenile Offenders and Victims: 1999 National Report.* Washington, DC: U.S. Department of Justice.

Thomas, C. R., Holzer, C. E. III & Wall, J. (2002), The island youth programs: Community interventions for reducing youth violence and delinquency. *Adolescent Psychiatry,* 26:125–143. Hillsdale, NJ: The Analytic Press.

Thrasher, F. M. (1927), *The Gang.* Chicago, IL: University of Chicago Press.

Tolan, P., Guerra, N. G. & Kendall, P. C. (1995), A developmental-ecological perspective on antisocial behavior in children and adolescents: Toward a unified risk and intervention framework. *J. Consult. Clin. Psychol.,* 63:579–584.

U.S. Department of Health and Human Services (2001), *Youth Violence: A Report of the Surgeon General.* Rockville, MD: U.S. Department of Health & Human Services.

Wolfgang, M. E. & Ferracutti, F. (1967), *The Subculture of Violence.* London: Tavistock.

Yablonsky, L. (1963), *The Violent Gang.* New York: Macmillan.

Zimring, F. E. (1998), *American Youth Violence.* New York: Oxford University Press.

2   YOUTH, IDEOLOGY, AND TERRORISM

LOIS T. FLAHERTY

Since September 11, 2001 many Americans, along with others around the world, have been preoccupied with the why of what happened. We wonder how Islamists could kill themselves and innocent people, believing they are doing this in the name of God. But terrorism is not new and exists everywhere. The radicalism of the late 1960s spawned its own terrorist movement, the Weather Underground. More recently the Unabomber—a lone individual with a history of mental illness—carried out successful terrorist operations and eluded capture over a period of many years. We saw another example in Oklahoma City in 1997. Terrorists have come from religious fundamentalist organizations, social protest groups, and radical political movements, both of the left and the right. Although many of the terrorists have been poor and uneducated, others have come from affluent, privileged circumstances. The fact that nearly all are late adolescents or young adults (or started their terrorist careers during this phase of their lives) raises the question as to whether there is something about youth that makes the lure of an ideology that promises a perfect society, together with the prospect of the violent overthrow of the existing world order, irresistible. If there is, can anything be done about it? This chapter is an attempt to explore this question and its implications.

TERRORISM

What Constitutes Terrorism?

The simplest definition of terrorism is the FBI's: "the unlawful use of force or violence against persons or property to intimidate or coerce

29

a government, the civilian population or any segment thereof, in further-ance of political or social objectives" (United States Department of Justice, 1999). However, the differentiation between terrorism and legit-imate political struggle is not easy. The saying, "One man's terrorist is another man's freedom fighter" illustrates the difficulty in knowing where to draw the line. Consider, for example, the following aspects of the American Revolution:

1. A series of underground cells were formed across Massachusetts with the goal of functioning secretly and independently of the political establishment.
2. A mob of men and boys began taunting a lone sentry at the Boston Customs House on March 5, 1770. When other British soldiers came to the sentry's support, the mob continued, daring the soldiers to shoot; a free-for-all ensued, and shots were fired into the crowd. Four died on the spot and a fifth died after four days. Six others were wounded.
3. Numerous other mob actions followed, involving destruction of homes of government officials and other buildings.
4. The colonies authorized the outfitting of privateers to prey on British ships, described as the enemies.

Terrorism is not a new phenomenon. The origin of the word terrorism comes from the period in France after its revolution, which became known as "the Terror." Terrorist groups have existed in the United States in many forms; examples include ecoterrorists, rightist militias, the Ku Klux Klan, Black Panthers, Weather Underground, and militant antiabortion groups. Worldwide examples include the Red Brigades, Islamic Jihad, Basque separatists, and the Irish Republican Army. We also speak of nonpolitical groups as terrorist, such as narcoterrorists, organized crime, and gangs. Although these groups resemble political terrorists in the methods they use and in many cases have similar dynamics, however they are usually thought of simply as criminals rather than terrorists.

Basically, terrorists are extremist groups with political agendas; their goal is to impose their views on others. The goal of theocracy is puritanism, that of Marxism is socialism, and that of groups such as the Aryan Nation is racial purity. All have a dream of what they consider to be an ideal society, and all believe that this ideal is achievable in reality, if only they can establish control. The goal of terrorism is to intimidate those whom they seek to influence. They do this by striking unexpectedly, creating a climate of fear and uncertainty—waiting for the other shoe to drop (Post, 2002). They choose targets that are symbolic, magnifying the perception of their destructive power. Thus, the influence of terrorist groups is often out of proportion to their numbers; a small group or even a single person can have a very large impact. The term asymmetrical warfare is an apt description.

Although not all radicals are terrorists, all terrorists are radicals. To understand terrorism, it is necessary to examine the nature of radical movements and why they often spawn terrorism.

Common Characteristics of Radical Movements

There is a sense of futility that anything other than extreme measures will work. A sizable contingent of American colonists urged negotiation with England, but those who favored declaring independence were opposed to any conciliation, maintaining that this would only be considered as proof of timidity and would encourage further repressive measures (McCullough, 2001). Thomas Paine (1776) exhorted the colonists to declare independence once and for all:

> Ye that tell us of harmony and reconciliation, can ye restore to us the time that is past? Can ye give to prostitution its former innocence? Neither can ye reconcile Britain and America. The last cord now is broken, the people of England are presenting addresses against us. There are injuries which nature cannot forgive; she would cease to be nature if she did. As well can the lover forgive the ravisher of his mistress, as the continent forgive the murders of Britain [pp. 41–42].

Destruction of the existing world order is seen as necessary. Fundamentalists maintain that modern society is degenerate and debased, the corruption of a golden age; the cure for this corruption is to return to the original state "before the fall." Marxists believe that society must progress toward an ideal state; they differ in whether this can occur in gradual fashion or must involve revolution. Racists maintain that racial purity must be restored through exclusion of

31

undesirable groups from the gene pool. All of these groups focus on destroying what exists, often with little sense of what will take its place. They speak of an apocalypse that will involve destruction of the existing world order, whether this be Armageddon, a race war, or a jihad.

Compromise and power sharing are rejected.   To compromise is seen as surrender, selling out, or allowing oneself to be corrupted. There is only good or evil, no in-between state. The struggle between good and evil is a zero-sum game—there can be only one winner. Thus, John Adams proclaimed, "The middle way is no way at all. If we finally fail in this great and glorious contest, it will be by bewildering ourselves in groping for the middle way" (quoted in McCullough, 2001, p. 101). Patrick Henry, in his famous give-me-liberty-or-give-me-death speech, pleaded, "Shall we try argument? Sir, we have been trying that for the last ten years." He concluded, "There is no longer any room for hope. . . . We must fight! . . . An appeal to arms and to the God of Hosts is all that is left us!" (Vaughan, 1997, p. 83)

A new world order is envisioned.   Thoreau, in advocating for civil disobedience, aligned himself with Christ, Copernicus, Luther, Washington, and Franklin (1849). Paine and many others saw the American colonies as linked historically to ancient Israel, and the new nation that would emerge from revolution as a "New Jerusalem," free of the corruption of Europe (indeed, the term New World reflects a similar connotation).

The end justifies the means.   A corollary of absolute conviction of the righteousness of one's cause is that extreme measures are justified in bringing about what is envisioned as a new world order, whether this be justice for the oppressed, a utopian society, a messianic age, or a theocracy. It is a short step to violence, if non-violent methods fail to work or work too slowly. Thoreau (1849), who never engaged in violent protest, saw opposition to unjust laws as necessary, "even if blood should flow" (p. 231). For the Taliban, the use of terror to enforce their interpretation of Islam is seen as necessary to free people from their addiction to sin (Maley, 1998).

There are impatience and a sense of urgency.   Radicals have no interest in waiting patiently for results. Thoreau (1849) argued that working from within to change the political system "takes too much time, and a man's life will be gone" (pp. 231–232). Just prior to the bombing of the New York City Police Department in 1970, Bernadette Dorn spoke for the Weather Underground, saying,

> Our job is to lead white kids into armed revolution. . . . Ever since SDS became revolutionary, we've been trying to show how it is possible to overcome the frustration and impotence that comes from trying to reform the system. . . . Tens of thousands have learned that protest and marches won't do it. Revolutionary violence is the only way [quoted in Powers, 1971, p. 212].

There is often a sense that the time is ripe. Paine (1776) urged the colonists to begin their violent revolt against England immediately, saying that the risk of failure would increase if they delayed and citing evidence that augured a quick victory. He wrote, "Now is the seed time of continental union, faith and honor. The least fracture now will be like a name engraved with the point of a pin on the tender rind of a young oak; the wound will enlarge with the tree, and posterity read it in full grown characters" (p. 22).

The prospect of violent change has its own appeal. Destroying entire buildings, disrupting social institutions, and striking terror into whole populations provides an unparalled sense of power, beside which the slow and incremental process of political change pales. Robespierre (1794) sounded the call to arms for the Reign of Terror, depicting the existence of the new French Republic as threatened by tyrants who encircled it from without and conspired from within to overthrow it and restore monarchy. He said, "We must smother the internal and external enemies of the Republic or perish with it" (p. 2).

In an astonishing juxtaposition of terms, Robespierre (1794) declared,

> If the spring of popular government in time of peace is virtue, the springs of popular government in revolution are at once *virtue and terror:* virtue, without which terror is fatal; terror, without which virtue is powerless. Terror is nothing other than justice, prompt, severe, inflexible; it is therefore an emanation of virtue;

YOUTH, IDEOLOGY, AND TERRORISM

it is not so much a special principle as it is a consequence of the general principle of democracy applied to our country's most urgent needs [p. 2, emphasis added].

Factors Contributing to a Rise in Terrorism

Tolerance and passive support.   There have been widespread concerns that terrorism is increasing worldwide. Arnold (1998) believes this is so and that it is due, at least in part, to tolerance and at least passive support for terrorism. He cites an erosion of the boundaries between violent and nonviolent behavior as an important factor. Our tolerance of borderline-violent protest—destruction of property, veiled threats, and harassment, for example—has led to social acceptance of more overtly violent behavior.

In addition, there is general moral support for the overthrow of unjust governments on the part of established social institutions; for example, Latin American clergy and churches in North America have supported Marxist rebellions in Latin America. This has been accompanied by ambivalence and confusion about holding terrorists accountable for their behavior because of sympathy for their causes and rationalization that their ends justify their means (Arnold, 1998). In the United States, our consciousness of our own history of armed struggle as underdogs who rebelled against an oppressive rule makes us sympathetic to others who depict themselves as victims or defenders of the oppressed (e.g., nature, the unborn).

Those who carry out terrorist acts are usually a relatively small number of people who are part of a much larger community that tolerates their activities or actually supports them. Political or religious leaders who support their goals serve to legitimize the zealots' radical actions. For example, the Ku Klux Klan operated in the South for the better part of a century, committing many terrorist acts. Arrests were rare and convictions almost nonexistent, because the elected political leaders, police, judges, and juries either were sympathetic or reluctant to speak out against them. Many members of the Weather Underground received lenient treatment from the courts in the 1960s and 1970s because of the widespread opposition to the Vietnam War. (This changed when they turned to bombing and armed robbery, activities which resulted in deaths.)

Finally, the institution of political asylum and the constitutional protections of free speech have allowed terrorist groups to operate in

34

Western democracies. The overall effect has been to create a certain permissiveness toward terrorism—at least prior to September 11, 2001.

IDEOLOGY

Definition

The term ideology is frequently used to describe an ideal or abstract speculation, especially one that is impractical, and it is usually used to describe a system of thought held by someone other than oneself. However, ideology may also be defined as a way of thinking about the world—the system of ideas an individual or group uses to make sense of everyday experience. Ideology forms the basis for understanding what one's place is in society and how one should live one's life (Silberstein, 1993). Stuart Hall (1985), a leading theorist of ideology, has defined ideologies as "the frameworks of thinking and calculation about the world—the 'ideas' people use to figure out how the social world works, what their place is in it, and what they ought to do" (p. 99). It tells us "who we are, how we are to relate to the world around us, what is real and true, what is good/bad, and what is possible/impossible" (Therborn, 1980, p. 78). Looked at in this way, it is clear that everyone has an ideology. Most people, however, do not spend every waking minute, or even significant amounts of time, thinking about their ideologies. One's personal ideology is in the background, generally not thought about very much, perhaps taken out and examined when challenged but nonetheless still operative, influencing important life decisions and views of oneself and others inside and outside one's primary social group. Ideology may be based on religious belief, an elaborate philosophical system, or it may be simple, even anti-intellectual. Mao Tse-Tung, for example, said in 1966 (at the height of the Cultural Revolution), "The more books you read, the stupider you become" (quoted in Chang, 1991, p. 426). This became the guideline for health and education.

How Ideology Maintains Control

Ideology is translated into practice and thus maintained by social institutions, schools and religious organizations, and the family (Hall, 1990).

These institutions in turn depend on language, or to be more precise, discourse. Foucault (1980), who coined the term discursive practices, described how discourse is the means by which social norms and organizations are organized and given legitimacy, creating a "regime of truth." (The truth of a statement, in Foucault's view, does not refer to anything intrinsic to the statement, but rather to a process by which propaganda in support of a particular view is produced and disseminated.) The relationship between truth and systems of power is circular; the power structure produces and sustains truth, and truth in turn supports power. Thus, beliefs are shaped by language and controlled and maintained by social institutions.

In the case of terrorist movements, language serves to justify and legitimize their violent actions. The reality or truth depicted by their discourse may be far removed from that of the larger society to which they belong. Captured Islamic terrorists, when asked how they could justify committing suicide when the Koran forbids it, denied that what they were doing was suicide, insisting rather that it was martyrdom, or self-sacrifice in the name of Allah (Post, 2002). For the Black Liberation Army, robbing banks was conceptualized as the expropriation of funds to finance a revolution (Castellucci, 1986). Language is used to cast the group in the role of victims, giving them permission—a duty, even—to retaliate and seek redress for injustice. Thus, the Islamists view the West as corrupt, evil, and threatening to Islam. The Black Liberation Army saw all blacks as oppressed and persecuted by the criminal justice system; those in jail were termed political prisoners. One can reasonably argue that each of these groups may have some valid points, but whether or not that is the case is beside the point—they are structuring reality for their followers in a way that resonates with the followers' experience and legitimizes terroristic actions.

The Ideology of Religious Fundamentalism

The early part of the 20th century saw the rise of political totalitarianism (socialism, communism, Naziism, and fascism), but the latter part of the century was characterized by the growth of religious fundamentalism. In recent years, the most extreme and destructive ideologies have been those of some religious fundamentalists. Although not all fundamentalist movements are linked to terrorism, some are; examples can be seen within each of the major religious traditions.

Fundamentalism Defined

Fundamentalists share a belief in an ideal religious-political reality that they are convinced has existed in the past or will emerge in the future. Fundamentalism is to a large extent a reaction against modernity; it exists in opposition to the perceived evils of the modern world.

Fundamentalism is not simply orthodoxy, although it is based in it; orthodoxy involves the evolution of a religion over time through a process of consensus, with adaptations to changes in society and modernization. Fundamentalism, in contrast, is "orthodoxy in confrontation with modernity.... What fundamentalisms share in common is the deep and worrisome sense that history has gone awry. What 'went wrong' with history is modernity in its various guises. The calling of the fundamentalist, therefore, is to make history right again" (Hunter, 1993, pp. 28–29). It is the imperative to make history right again that drives the fundamentalist to do whatever is possible to bring that longed-for world into existence.

All religious fundamentalist movements have sacred texts or oral traditions that are believed to be the revelation of the Word of God and require a leader to interpret them. (Note again the importance of language, both in terms of the sacred text and the interpretation of it.) These texts, and the interpretations of them by leaders of the movement, provide the ideological underpinnings of the movement.

One can see parallels between religious fundamentalism and extreme political views, and at times, the line between the political and religious spheres is fuzzy or nonexistent. Fundamentalism presupposes that the state has authority to enforce religious identity. Politics and religion are not separate; its aim is to remake the world. Lustick (1993) conceives of fundamentalism as a political style whose main goal is the transformation of society in accordance with "uncompromisable, cosmically ordained, and more or less directly received imperatives" (p. 105).

Examples

The Taliban. Ahmed Rashid (2001), a Pakistani reporter who has covered Afghanistan for over 20 years, has written an insightful book about the recent history of Afghanistan. *Taliban* (plural of *Talib*) means "students"; followers of the movement were recruited from madrassas, religious schools. Under the leadership of Mullah Omar, the Taliban's stated aims were to change the plight of people living under the corruption and excesses of the Mujaheddin by restoring peace, disarming the population, enforcing Sharia law, and defending the integrity and Islamic character of Afghanistan.

Rashid points out that the young students who joined the movement were ignorant of their own history, having only been taught about the ideal Islamic society created by the Prophet Mohammed 1400 years ago. Most were aged 14 to 24; neither they nor their teachers had any formal grounding in math, science, history or geography and many were barely literate: "They had no memories of their tribes, their elders, their neighbors, nor the complex ethnic mix of peoples that often made up their villages or their homeland" (Rashid, 2001, p. 32). War was the only occupation they were trained for—they knew nothing about farming or anything else. The ideology of the Taliban movement, "a simple belief in a messianic, puritan Islam" (p. 32) was the only thing that gave their lives meaning. Many had never lived with women, having grown up in refugee camps in which the sexes were segregated, and a sizable number were orphans who had never known any female relatives. The madrassas of course were only for boys, and they went from there into an all-male brotherhood created by the Taliban leaders. As a result, they readily accepted the necessity of the subjugation of women, who, they had been taught, posed dangers to men. They had no reason to question this teaching, having never known any women. (From a psychiatric standpoint, we might consider that their psychosexual development was somewhere between latency and preadolescence.) Within three months of the capture of Kandahar, 20,000 Afghans and hundreds of Pakistani madrassa students streamed across the border to join Mullah Omar. Their early victories reinforced their fundamentalist belief that God was with them. We have all become familiar with the atrocities they subsequently committed. Rashid points out that many of the Taliban's rules were based on Pashtun tribal mores rather than the Sharia, or Islamic law. The Taliban had no idea how to rule. Rashid also reports that an aide to Omar told him,

> The Sharia does not allow politics or political parties. That is why we give no salaries to officials or soldiers, just food, clothes, shoes, and weapons: We want to live a life like the Prophet lived 1400 years ago, and jihad is our right. We want to recreate the

time of the Prophet, and we are only carrying out what the Afghan people have wanted for the past 14 years [p. 43].

As Naipaul (1981) has also noted, Rashid points out that the obsession of radical Islam is not the creation of institutions, but the character and purity of its leader; it is "an all-inclusive ideology that rejects rather than integrates ... multiple social, religious and ethnic identities" (p. 80).

The overlap between religion and politics is exemplified by the Taliban, who Maley (1998) maintains were basically a totalitarian regime, considering it questionable whether they represented a religious movement or were really fundamentalists. Islamic resistance to the Soviet Union emerged soon after the 1978 coup in Afghanistan; the resistance inevitably had a religious dimension, because the Soviet system espoused atheism.

The values espoused by the Taliban were not the values of the village, as some maintained, but rather an interpretation of these values by those in refugee camps and madrassas in Pakistan who formed the nexus of this movement and recruited youth into it. The Taliban "are totalitarian in that they seek to monopolise the political sphere, and to assimilate all of social life to it. [They] recognize no private severe beyond the reach of political authority" (Maley, 1998, p. 21).

Gush Emunim. An example of radical fundamentalism within Judaism is Gush Emunim in Israel, popularly known as the Settlers Movement. Members of Gush Emunim hold a religious–Zionist perspective, that Jewish history is passing from exile to redemption and is now in the incipient stage of the end time or the "footsteps of the Messiah" (Sprinzak, 1993).

Gush Emunim's ultimate objective is the full redemption of the Jewish people and the entire world. They embody a religious transformation of secular Zionism into an instrument of messianic redemption. In their view, the role of the state is to secure the sovereignty of the Jewish people over the land of Israel.

By establishing settlements in the West Bank, Gaza, and the Golan Heights, Gush Emunim believe that they are helping to fulfill the will of God, who is behind the unfolding redemption of the land and people of Israel. They maintain that compromise with the Palestinians is impossible, that no territorial concessions are permissible, and that the

Arabs have no legitimate claims. Some members have even advocated extermination of the Arabs on grounds that the Palestinians are descendants of the Amalekites, and hatred of them is fully justified.

Gush Emunim has been described by scholars of such movements as a highly sophisticated political economic, and cultural network that dominates the life of nearly 100,000 settlers in Judea, Samaria, and Gaza; controls the yearly distribution of hundreds of millions of dollars; and significantly influences Israeli decisions. Gush Emunim contains an organizational core that is an umbrella organization of activists (20,000 in 1993); it is represented in parliament by right-wing parties (Lustick, 1993). The movement comprises an "invisible realm" as it operates through other organizations and influence on politicians (Sprinzak, 1993, p. 129). Through its efforts, settlements have received privileged status and economic benefits (including subsidies for settlements and financial incentives for settlers) from the government. Schools are a key component. They range from elementary schools to yeshivot, to adult education courses and Midrashot—short-term learning centers that offer courses on Judaism, Zionism, and the teachings of Rav Kook (the founder of Gush Emunim) for visiting groups. Schools are financed by the state as well as by generous donors.

Members of Gush Emunim consider themselves strictly observant Jews, although they have made some compromises, adapting orthodoxy to support their modus operandi. They tend toward disrespect of civil law, and have moved in the direction of challenging the legitimacy of the government; they would prefer Torah law (which is from God) and the halakhah. The settlements themselves involve extralegal activity (although they have at times been supported and actively encouraged by the government) (Sprinzak, 1993).

Gush Emumin have mainly engaged in vigilante activities—smashing car windows, breaking into houses, threatening Arabs—with few acts of severe violence. However, a radical component, the Jewish underground, was discovered in 1984 and has been involved in the premeditated killing of Arabs. A member of this extremist group assassinated Prime Minister Yitzak Rabin in 1995. Communities involve active zealots, sympathizers or passive zealots, and rabbinical patrons. The latter serve to legitimize the zealots' radical actions.

Ultraorthodox (Haredim). In contrast to Gush Emunim, the ultraorthodox Jews (although also fundamentalist) are very different

40

in that they oppose secular Zionism, some even referring to Zionists as atheists. They believe that it is sacrilegious for human beings to try to bring about a theocracy on earth by their own efforts. Rather, their goal in life is to be as observant as possible of Jewish laws, in the belief that this will hasten the coming of the Messiah. They idealize life as lived in the shtetls of medieval Eastern Europe and withdraw from modern life. Their schools do not teach secular subjects. Violent activities engaged in by this group have mainly involved throwing stones at cars traveling on the Sabbath; ultraorthodox Jews have never taken up weapons or used any means deliberately aimed at killing people (they also lack experience with or access to weapons, because they don't serve in the military). They have a sense of shared fate with other Jews despite their differences (Friedman, 1987).

Each of these groups is fundamentalist. There are striking similarities between the Taliban and extremists in Gush Emunim in terms of their views of political action toward the goal of bringing about God's reign on earth as opposed to those of the ultraorthodox Jews who retreat from the world (Maley, 1998). The Taliban, like Gush Emunim, want to change the world and impose theocratic rule. The differences between the ultraorthodox and settlers movements illustrate how much divergence can be based on the same religious tradition.

PSYCHOLOGY OF "TRUE BELIEVERS" AND MASS MOVEMENTS

Hoffer's The True Believer

Eric Hoffer, a self-educated son of German immigrants, published a classic study of mass movements in 1951. Writing in the years after World War II, trying to explain the rise of Naziism and Communism, he developed a theory that the emergence of such movements depended on the presence of large numbers of people who, feeling that their lives were "spoiled and wasted," were vulnerable to the influence of a charismatic leader who could exploit their emotional neediness. He saw fertile soil for all mass movements in an absence of self-esteem. Lacking inner resources to draw on for a source of self-worth and satisfaction, the vulnerable person readily turns outward toward movements that offer explanations. An ideology that offers a credible explanation as to why things are the way they are, and at the same time offers hope for change through collective action, is irresistible to disaffected people.

Hoffer saw essentially no difference between the great world religions and secular movements. He pointed out that all make a clear distinction between good and evil, offering the hope of replacing the current morass of moral decay and doom with the possibility of future redemption and fulfillment. Movements succeed if they can convince their followers that success is just around the corner and that they are living out glorious roles in bringing about the new reality.

The true believer is someone who has given up hope that things will ever improve and then miraculously finds a cause to join that relegates misery to the past, giving life a new meaning and purpose. Such a person is hooked for life, although he or she may change allegiances, moving to another group as social conditions change. Hoffer stressed the susceptibility to mass movements of those who feel that their lives are spoiled and wasted. Without using the terms, he described individual narcissistic vulnerability. One can see the parallels between what he described and the sudden illumination that comes with the elaboration of a paranoid delusional system in the progression of a psychotic disorder.

Hoffer (1951) also noted that adolescents and certain young adults are among those who are particularly prone to join mass movements, although, in contrast to the true believers, they usually move on when their circumstances change:

There are first the temporary misfits: People who have not found their place in life but still hope to find it. Adolescent youth, unemployed college graduates, veterans, new immigrants and the like are of this category. They are restless, dissatisfied and haunted by the fear that their best years will be wasted before they reach their goal. They are receptive to the preaching of a proselytizing movement and yet do not always make staunch converts. For they are not irrevocably estranged from the self; they do not see it as irremediably spoiled. It is easy for them to conceive an autonomous existence that is purposeful and hopeful. The slightest evidence of progress and success reconciles them with the world and their selves [p. 45].

Hoffer also noted that mass movements take root when societies are in the process of becoming more open, because freedoms and material possessions are more easily grasped. It is as if this opens people's eyes to what is lacking, what could be but is not, and deepens their longing and sense of deprivation. V. S. Naipaul (1981)—in a journey that began in Iran shortly after the revolution and took him through Pakistan, Malaysia, and Indonesia (all countries that fundamentalist Islamic movements have dominated)—noted that the rise of these movements to power occurred as the countries were emerging from colonialist domination and becoming increasingly westernized. One could make a case for this in Afghanistan as well, because the Soviets, notwithstanding their being hated as invaders, did introduce modernizations, including education for women.

GROUP PROCESS AND RADICAL MOVEMENTS

One can also understand radical political and religious groups in terms of group process. There is a natural tendency to form groups and to have enemies, reinforced by psychological forces that tend to promote cohesiveness among insiders and denigrate outsiders—what Pinder-hughes (1986) has termed "differential-aggressive bonding."

Meissner (2000) has expanded on the idea of differential-aggressive bonding to explain the formation of religious groups, describing what he terms "the cultic process" as "essentially a group process by which the group establishes and defines itself over and against other competing and oppositional groups" (p. 3). Projection and paranoid mechanisms are involved in this process. What is projected outward onto another group—the outgroup—are unacceptable aspects of the self as well as the destructive feelings and impulses toward these introjections. Projection plays a vital role in defining the group's identity and main-taining cohesiveness—who they are is defined in terms of who they are not. It allows for the displacement of destructive impulses away from a loved object onto a devalued object. These defense mechanisms are attempts to redeem damaged narcissism and regain a sense of self-esteem. They can provide a sense of inner worth and value in the service of preserving and sustaining a coherent and integrated sense of self. "The paranoid construction can, therefore, be envisioned as providing a context within which the organization of the self finds a sense of belonging, participation, sharing, meaningful involvement, and relevance" (Meissner, 2000, p. 16).

What keeps the group going is a belief system, "a paranoid construction that rationalizes, defends and justifies the projections" (Meissner, 2000, p. 29). Looked at another way, the belief system is the group's ideology, its stabilizing framework. Like the beliefs of delusional patients, extreme ideologies are not influenced by arguments against them or appeals to reason; their primary function is to serve an inner need rather than to reflect accurately an outer reality. Usually such groups manifest a paranoid style rather than clinical paranoia; they believe persecution to be directed at the group rather than at themselves as individuals. Thus, they may believe that their nation, culture, or way of life is threatened. The belief that the group rather than the individual is threatened can mitigate group members' need to retaliate violently and can channel their activities into nonviolent activism. But, if conditions are ripe, such a group can espouse violent activities directed at outsiders.

A group can develop "malignant prejudice" against another group (Meissner, 2000, p. 9). An egregious example is the set of beliefs about the Jews held by Christians until modern times, which led to centuries of persecution and formed the backdrop for the Holocaust. Erikson described as a predisposition the tendency for the other group to be dehumanized. If the process of dehumanization is complete, it becomes acceptable to kill members of the other group. Projection may occur onto other people, the social environment, social institutions, or governments (welfare mothers, big government, the media, and right-wing conservatives are recent examples in our own society). A key point is that the same process operates in pathological and nonpathological belief systems. Meissner has emphasized that such nonpathological paranoid processes are ubiquitous and operate in the lives of individuals as well as groups. He believes what makes them normal is being connected to a tradition, being consensually validated, and having an organized religious group as opposed to being idiosyncratic, unreal, and having elements of delusional wish fulfillment (although the definition of what is unreal and delusional depends on one's vantage point—mass movements such as Naziism might fit this description). There is a tendency for such groups to gravitate toward the mainstream over time.

Persecution, deprivation, or oppression in the sociopolitical realm . . . may interact with the individual's sense of victimization to intensify and radicalize his inner sense of humiliation, worth-lessness, and impotence, and provoke countermeasures intended to redress the psychic balance even as they lead to revolution or social disruption [Meissner, 2000, p. 13].

Meissner's insights into religious cults are helpful in understanding radical movements. Taken in the context of radical movements, reli-gious fundamentalism is simply one example of group processes involv-ing ideologies. Fundamentalist religious groups are the prototypes of the cultic process, but as we have seen, such groups can encompass secular ideologies.

LATE-ADOLESCENT AND YOUNG-ADULT DEVELOPMENT AND THE APPEAL OF IDEOLOGY

Counterculture movements in the 1960s focused attention on youth as a stage of life (Keniston, 1968). These movements were mainly formed by young people with privileged backgrounds who were college edu-cated and from the middle and upper classes. The movements coalesced around issues of social justice, especially for black Americans, and opposition to the Vietnam War. They rejected what they saw as the shallowness and materialistic values of American society. The vast majority of these young people were nonviolent, and indeed, the major form of social protest most engaged in was marijuana smoking. They were more apt to reject the dominant culture by dropping out of it than trying to change it. But a minority bent on changing society went from being reformists to revolutionaries. They began with peaceful protests but developed violent factions such as the Weather Underground, whose aim was to ignite a popular revolution that would lead to the overthrow of the government of the United States and spread throughout the world. These factions increasingly turned to terrorist tactics, first in protests that turned violent and later in isolated bombings, with tragic consequences. The public were mystified by the phenomenon of youth from affluent backgrounds joining terrorist groups. An understanding of development during this period of life can help to elucidate the attraction of radical movements for youth.

Postadolescence/Young Adulthood—A Time of Finding a Niche in Life

Developmental tasks.　Much as adolescence was understood as a result of social and cultural developments beginning in the 19th century, youth was conceptualized in the twentieth century as a further developmental stage that had emerged as a by-product of the ever-lengthening period between adolescence and the assumption of full adult responsibilities (Keniston, 1968). Without precise boundaries and not universal, youth comprises the early 20s, a time of further consolidation of identity and searching for commitment. During this period, many young people are still unsettled, trying to work out their relationship to the world. They are determined to make a difference, through changing themselves or the outside world.

By the time they reach the threshold of young adulthood, young people have usually completed the developmental tasks of late adolescence, including consolidation of identity and social roles and choice of life tasks (Erikson, 1958; Blos, 1962). Gender identity is usually firmly established by this point, and intimacy has been achieved. Ties with parents have been loosened.

The next phase involves figuring out how these tasks are to be accomplished—how one will live, love, and work to bring about what Vaillant (1977) has termed the "life dream." Blos (1962) termed this phase "postadolescence" and described it as a transitional period between late adolescence and adulthood. In contrast to earlier phases when instinctual conflicts dominate, ego-integrative processes are dominant during this period; resolution of earlier conflicts frees ego energy for this task.

Fitting in, being accepted, and feeling good about one-self—sustaining a sense of dignity and self-esteem—are the key developmental tasks of this era, which involves "the elaboration of a unique way of life" (Blos, 1962, p. 152). If all goes well, the end result will be "a patterned interaction with the environment and self" (p. 152). But if it does not, the result may be a sense of not fitting in, not accomplishing anything worthwhile, not making any difference, and being unimportant (what Hoffer termed a spoiled and wasted existence). Thus, future American patriot John Adams, at the age of 20, felt that life was passing him by. Dissatisfied with himself and his lack of accomplishment of anything significant or original, he wrote, "I have no books, no time, no friends. I must therefore be contented to live and die an ignorant, obscure fellow" (quoted in McCullough, 2001, p. 41).

Resolution of the dilemmas of this period. The dilemmas of the postadolescent period are resolved via experimentation with roles, milieu choices, and relationships. Young people choose what to identify with or what not to identify with (counteridentification). By doing so, they achieve a final stage in their detachment from the parents they once idealized. The selective acceptance of (as well as resistance to) identifications with past erotic object choices are the final steps in the detachment from infantile parental objects. Resistance occurs by externalization of what was once a part of object relations. Blos (1962) opined, "Conservatism and reformism may receive moral and emotional impetus from these sources" (p. 158).

This process is illustrated by the life of Henry David Thoreau. As a young man, he managed to graduate from Harvard College, although he found most of it boring and meaningless. Strongly rejecting what he saw as a culture obsessed with amassing wealth and ostentatious display, he refused an offer to work in his father's pencil factory, instead failing miserably at his first job, as a teacher. At the age of 28 he began a two-year stay in an isolated cabin he built himself, proclaiming in the book he wrote about the experience, "The mass of men live lives of quiet desperation" (Thoreau, 1854, p. 6). He went on to become a passionate advocate against slavery, going to jail for his refusal to pay taxes to what he considered an unjust state (he objected to the fact that taxes paid to Massachusetts went to support the federal government, which allowed slavery to continue).

Thoreau's 19th century example was echoed in the protest movements of the 1960s. For many Americans who were college students in the late 1960s, The United States seemed morally bankrupt—a society controlled by a military-industrial complex bent on destroying a small country on the other side of the world. Entering the workforce in such a society offered no hope for a meaningful life. They could scrape by on their own or with their parents' support well enough to have an extended moratorium before entering into obligations that would require them to become breadwinners. These students were drawn to movements that promised to work for peace and justice.

Counterculture movements had a particular appeal to young middle- and upper-middle-class white women. The late 1960s were a time of particular tumult for these women. Raised in the 1950s to be homemakers and mothers and not to make waves, they were suddenly told that they had been victims of male oppression and needed to revolt against it. With the backdrop of a country in turmoil over the Vietnam War, this was a time of uncertainty about identity and goals for many women. Traditional roles were denigrated, but options for new ones were still few. It is not hard to understand how these women could see their own experiences mirrored by what they imagined of those of black Americans and people in the Third World. Identifying with these groups and fighting for them allowed them to transmute their own discontent into a redemptive force. Diana Oughten was such a woman.

Born in 1942 to a wealthy family in a small midwestern town, she attended an elite college preparatory school and graduated from Bryn Mawr College, an equally elite women's college. She served in the Peace Corps in Guatemala and returned to the United States not sure of what she wanted to do. Desirous of helping the poor, she embarked on a career that led tortuously from community activism to the Weather Underground, dying at age 27 in the basement of a New York townhouse, where she had been attempting to assemble a bomb (Powers, 1971).

What stands out about the early part of Oughten's brief life is a pervasive sense of lack of direction and not fitting in. The latter dates back to her childhood, when she felt self-conscious about her family's wealth and was called "Moneybags" at school. She entered the Peace Corps for lack of a plan to pursue marriage or a career (an either/or choice being the general rule for women; see Flaherty, 1982), although she had opportunities for both. In Guatemala, she identified with the plight of the Indian people, feeling guilty about not suffering as they did, believing the work she was doing made no difference, and becoming increasingly drawn to revolution as the only way to effect change. The Students for a Democratic Society (SDS) offered her the chance to fulfill her desire to make a difference in the world and be part of a group who needed and accepted her. She hesitated when the Weathermen faction, having broken off from the SDS, embraced violent methods of achieving their goal of igniting a worldwide revolution led by youth. By the time this happened, however, she was a dedicated follower and too bound by ties of friendship and loyalty to extricate herself.

LOIS T. FLAHERTY

Developing a Cultural/Ethnic Identity

Consolidating an identity as a member of a cultural or ethnic group is another important feature of late adolescence. Cultural identity is closely linked to ideology; it involves the story of one's people and how they came to be where they now are in the world. Cultural identity is not fixed—not something transcending place, time, history, and culture— but is rooted in the narratives of the past (Hall, 1990).

The pluralism of our own society has provided a rich source of information about the multiplicity of identities of our youth. We are just beginning to understand the meaning of being an Asian youth, a black youth, a Hispanic youth, an immigrant youth, in our society, to give a few examples. We have become increasingly aware of the extent to which these identities influence self-appraisal, life choices, and behavior. The sense of identity that goes with these categories may be one of pride in one's success in spite of obstacles, or of self-denigration, low expectations, and/or victimization. The primary source of self-appraisal in the early years (of course, the family) becomes supplemented by that of cultural and social institutions (school, the workplace, the military, the gang in the wider sense of a group of supportive friends).

In the simplest of situations, a consonance exists between all of these points of reference. The views of one's family, school, and friends regarding life are basically similar, resulting in patterned interactions with the environment that reflect one's views of oneself and are mutually reinforcing. In times of rapid social change and a high degree of social mobility or when social institutions such as schools espouse different ideas from parents' about how to live and what is important, dissonance is likely to be the rule. Whatever the case, the individual is still faced with the task of sorting out for himself or herself a separate and unique identity. A daunting task at best, but much more difficult when the choices are seen as offering no rewards.

After rethinking earlier notions about parental and adult infallibility, the youth now must find something strong and dependable to believe in. This search for an ideal might be facilitated by a relationship with a mentor, membership in a group, a commitment to a cause, or some combination of these. The youth's choices are limited by the available possibilities, which are in turn determined by the culture. If the military is the only realistic option for young men, it is likely to be the one chosen. For many women, marriage and/or motherhood are virtually the only possibilities.

The search for an ideal is really a search for meaning. It is a creative process that involves the elaboration of a narrative about one's life—how one came to be the person one is now, who one is at this time, and where one is headed. The narrative, as others have described, is culturally determined (Esman, 1993; Rakoff, 1998; Galatzer-Levy, 2002). For youth who are feeling not so good about themselves and their lives, the script for the narrative may be that their miseries have been caused by some outside persons or groups. A sense of victimization can also be shared by an entire group, strengthened and reinforced within the community, and transmitted from one generation to the next. A charismatic leader can exploit the narrative and expand upon it, as Hitler did in post–World War I Germany, depicting the Germans as having been victimized by Jews.

In times of rapid social change, the old road maps to adulthood seem only to lead to a wasteland. Ideologies that pin the cause of anomie on an enemy (the system) and groups that offer the individual a sense of purpose and self-worth by rejecting the system are naturally appealing. Jerry Rubin (1969) asked, "Who the hell wants to 'make it' in America any more? . . . The American economy no longer needs young whites and blacks. We are waste material. We fulfill our destiny in life by rejecting a system which rejects us" (p. 27). Bruno Bettelheim (1971), writing about radical student protests of the late 1960s, attributed these radical movements to disappearance of the frontier—and the consequent lack of alternative means of finding oneself. His view (which Rubin's statement supports) was that youth felt that they were becoming obsolete because of technology: "Their existential anxiety is that they have no future in a society that does not need them to go on existing" (p. 18). He noted ominous similarities between these student protesters and the youth of Nazi Germany, who bought into Hitler's rhetoric about helping the suffering of the German people. Needless to say, another generation of young people embraced technology and flocked to careers created by the explosion of this new field. The source of the anomie was not technology itself but the rapid societal changes it engendered and the dissonance between society and its youth.

LOIS T. FLAHERTY

Youth and Radical Movements

Thus, we have seen some of the forces that drive disaffected youth in any society into mass movements. These movements appeal to youth whose lives lack a sense of direction and meaning by virtue of their own particular psychology. But there are whole societies that are unable to supply youth growing up in them with the ingredients of healthy narcissism: a sense that who they are and what they do matters. Cut off from their historical past and cultural traditions, living in the shadow of the industrialized world, they have nothing. Extremist groups are particularly likely to appeal to youth in such societies. By belonging to these groups, youth put on the trappings of power and superiority by adopting an ideology that tells them they are special, important, and have a glorious role to play. The cultic aspects of extremist groups serve to delineate group members from outsiders, who are seen as corrupt, unclean, and inferior. By doing so, they further define identity and provide social support (Meissner, 1985). Thus, belonging to the group and believing in its ideology protect against the shame and humiliation that the youth would otherwise feel.

The appeal of such groups to poor, uneducated youth for whom there are few, if any, alternatives is obvious. However, the seeming enigma of relatively well-educated terrorists can also be partly explained on the basis of a similar developmental trajectory. We know all too well that young people can grow up in what appear to be optimal circumstances and still be afflicted by an ennui for which extremist movements provide an antidote.

Fundamentalist ideologies offer ready-made answers to make sense of the world and one's role in it. As pure, theoretical frameworks, they do not necessarily have to work in practice. They are beautiful in their perfection as only ideas can be. One need not bother to figure out how people will actually live on a day-to-day basis in a theocracy. An Islamic state, led by an imam, with strict enforcement of the rules of the Koran as expostulated by the Sharia, will result in a perfect society. If people lead virtuous lives, everything else will take care of itself. Late adolescents, with their newly developed powers of abstract thinking that enable them to imagine a perfect world, are suckers for ideologies. The price they pay, a willing suspension of disbelief, seems small to them in comparison with the emotional and social rewards they gain.

Given the susceptibility of youth to ideology, it is natural that those who would recruit them to their cause focus on education as the means of gaining adherents (indoctrination is a more accurate term). The Taliban movement included schools for children and youth in Afghanistan and Pakistan. These schools, sponsored by one of the political parties, were aimed at orphans and children from poor families. Their teachings were based on the Deobandi school (founded in Deoband, India, 1867), a branch of Islam emphasizing the importance of ritual. In the Deobandi teaching, evil is equated to a departure from ritual; therefore, enforcing adherence to proper ritual is paramount. The Taliban movement itself included others besides students in these schools—former communists, more secular Pashtuns—and was transformed by aid from Saudi Arabia and Pakistan into an organized political force (Maley, 1998). Although the appeal of Islamic fundamentalism as an ideology lies in its presentation of a pure faith together with a rejection of the corruption of modern industrial and technological society, the power of Islamism comes from its totalitarian institutions, which in turn could only come about with massive funding. Thus, a "regime of truth" was created and sustained.

The Course of Individuals Involved in Radical Movements

Involvement in radical movements, whether cults or political groups, is temporary for many of the young people who join them and is not necessarily a sign of psychopathology (Levine, 1992). As I have shown, some who join, like Diana Oughten, subsequently become caught in a web of tangled interpersonal relationships from which they are unable to extricate themselves; they continue with the group out of fear of leaving and group loyalty, even though they begin to have misgivings about the group. The process of extricating oneself is likely to be slow and painful, complicated by the fact that the young person has dropped out of the mainstream of life for a period of time and may not have job opportunities (analogous to the situation of gang members). How much more difficult it is for young people to leave the group in areas where radical fundamentalism has taken hold.

Given the tremendous grasp that such groups have on their members—the pull of ideology plus that of a social network—one wonders how members do leave and if there are clues in their leaving that would be helpful in combating extremist movements. We might look at dissidents, who conclude through a slow and painful process that the movement's premises are false, despite the immense support for it by totalitarian social structures, the lack of freedom to join or to leave, and the indoctrination they receive from childhood on.

Consider, for example, the Chinese author Jung Chang. Born in 1952, raised by parents who were totally committed to the communist regime in China, she was a dedicated Red Guard as a teenager, during the Cultural Revolution. She willingly bore the hardships associated with being reeducated in the primitive remote western part of the country. As a young adult, she began to question the regime. She began to wonder what was so bad about the West after reading some of the books that were allowed into the country in conjunction with President Nixon's visit in 1972, such as *The Best and the Brightest, The Rise and Fall of the Third Reich,* and *The Winds of War.* (Reading of these books was encouraged so that the Chinese would not appear to be ignorant before foreign visitors.) She was most impressed by the fact that dissent was tolerated. The idea of the universality of human rights illuminated her consciousness, confirming Paine's prophecy: "The cause of America is in a great measure the cause of all mankind" (p. xi).

Chang (1991) wrote,

With the help of dictionaries which some professors lent me, I became acquainted with Longfellow, Walt Whitman, and American History. I memorized the whole of the Declaration of Independence, and my heart swelled at the words "We hold these truths to be self-evident, that all men are created equal," and those about men's "unalienable Rights," among them "Liberty and the pursuit of Happiness." These concepts were unheard of in China, and opened up a marvelous new world for me. My notebooks, which I kept with me at all times, were full of passages like these, passionately and tearfully copied out [p. 473].

It is noteworthy that Chang was not influenced by formal propaganda from the West, but rather by her own reading of literary works. Similarly, the fall of the Soviet Union occurred after it became increasing permeable to information from the outside. This suggests that the flow of information across borders can have powerful effects, even in societies that attempt to control what their people see and hear and read. Even as Islamic fundamentalists strive to control (or maintain control) over their countries and people, there are powerful crosscurrents pushing toward liberalization, as in the case of Iran. Totalitarian regimes can only partially block out ideas from the world beyond their borders. Such ideas are contained in all media, of course, but they are nowhere more concentrated and articulate than in books, especially those in the liberal humanistic tradition.

SUMMARY

Terrorism is a widespread phenomenon that, although existing throughout history, has taken on more malignant possibilities because of globalization and modern technology. Although economic support for terrorism is the fuel that keeps its flames burning, its basic substrate lies in group dynamics and social and cultural narratives that exert a powerful influence on vulnerable individuals and indeed whole populations. Ideology, an essential component of terrorism, has a uniquely powerful appeal to older adolescents and young adults. Youth is a time when ideology plays a central role. Its appeal is greatest to those for whom other life goals are unattainable or lack meaning. Those who are searching for a place in the world are easily drawn to ideologies that promise to change their social reality and give them a meaningful role in it.

Dynamics of trauma and revenge are also important and facilitate an intergenerational transmission of violence. A sense of having been unrightfully deprived of what is legitimately one's own—one's birthright—serves as an explanation for present misery. Focusing on the alleged external source of misery justifies taking action against the enemy who has caused it. Narratives of persecution and oppression cry out for redress. The next chapter of these narratives is always revenge. All that remains is to translate the idea into action. Youth are all too willing to play the roles scripted for them, even if these roles include suicide bombings.

Terrorism takes place in the context of a belief that nothing else will work or has worked and/or that one cannot take the time to wait for results by working through the system. In addition, because compromise is not an acceptable option, there is no point in trying to bring about incremental or partial change. Violent revolutionary means of accomplishing goals are particularly likely to appeal to people who have little tolerance for delay and who have not learned that patience can pay off—these features characterize many youth throughout the world.

WHAT CAN BE DONE?

Obviously, containment of terrorism is a paramount and immediate issue, both within our own borders and outside. In the West, our tolerance of borderline-violent protest has led to an erosion of the boundaries and social acceptance of more overtly violent behavior. Just as a decreased tolerance for petty crimes is widely believed to be a factor in falling crime rates nationally in the United States, we need to think in similar terms about the activities of domestic extremist movements and determine where to drawn the line between criminal behavior and tolerance of dissent. Those who work with adolescents who have been violent know that clear limits and consequences for behaviors such as verbal threats are important deterrents to escalating violence.

The Weather Underground fell apart when law enforcement efforts to combat it increased, and many leaders were arrested and given lengthy jail terms. At the same time, many adherents began to question its commitment to violence, particularly after some of its members were killed making bombs. In the United States and Canada, a major rethinking has occurred regarding the extent to which our commitment to openness and concerns about individual rights have allowed terrorists to enter our countries and operate freely within them. We cannot have total safety without abolishing democracy, but we can increase our level of safety.

Opinions vary widely as to how much infringement on civil liberty should be tolerated, but it is clear that we will have to reach a new equilibrium between the ideals of maintaining safety and protecting individual freedoms. In a more long-term approach, we need to understand the dynamics of terrorism. This includes an appreciation of the importance of a victim identity in perpetuating and legitimizing violence against those who are perceived to be the enemies. Such an identity is rooted in cultural traditions transmitted from one generation to the next and sustained by group dynamics that inevitably cast outsiders as different and inferior. Claims of having been victimized (being deprived of one's land is among the most common) are not amenable to reason and logic, because they are linked to an even more pervasive and essential sense of lack of worth. Such a lack of self-esteem is perhaps greatest among young people in areas where a sense of community has been lost (or, in some cases, may never have existed). It is hard to imagine a more fertile breeding ground for extremist ideologies than refugee camps. Terrorists' attainment of their goal of destroying an enemy will not eliminate the problem of their own lack of community.

Considering the psychological, social, and cultural influences on those drawn to ideologies that espouse terrorism helps to explain why efforts to get at its root causes by promoting economic development and increasing literacy and secular education are essential. These efforts, if successful, will help young people find meaning in their lives through being productive members of communities that offer them opportunities to love and to work. Perhaps most important is building true communities that are based on mutuality between leaders and people rather than on terror, with a sense of internal cohesion that does not depend on the existence of a "great Satan."

REFERENCES

Arnold, T. E. (1998), *The Violence Formula: Why People Lend Sympathy and Support to Terrorism.* Lexington, MA: D.C. Health.

Bettleheim, B. (1971), Obsolete youth: Toward a psychograph of adolescent rebellion. *Adolescent Psychiatry,* 1:14–39. New York: Basic Books.

Blos, P. (1962), *On Adolescence.* Glencoe, IL: Free Press.

Castellucci, J. (1986), *The Big Dance: The Untold Story of Kathy Boudin and the Terrorist Family that Committed the Brink Robbery Murders.* New York: Dodd, Mead.

Chang, J. (1991), *Wild Swans: Three Daughters of China.* Simon & Schuster.

Erikson, E. (1958), *Young Man Luther: A Study in Psychoanalysis and History.* New York: Norton.

Esman, A. (1993), G. Stanley Hall and the invention of adolescence. In: *Adolescent Psychiatry,* 19:6–20. Chicago: University of Chicago Press.

Flaherty, L. T. (1982), To love and/or to work: The ideological dilemma of young women. *Adolescent Psychiatry,* 10:41–51. Chicago: University of Chicago Press.

Foucault, M. (1980), *Power/Knowledge: Selected Interviews and Other Writings, 1972–1977*, ed. & trans. C. Gordan. New York: Pantheon Books.

Friedman, M. (1987), Life tradition and book tradition in the development of ultraorthodox Judaism. In: *Judaism Viewed from Within and Without*, ed. H. E. Goldberg. Albany: State University of New York Press.

Galatzer-Levy, R. (2002), Created in others' eyes. *Adolescent Psychiatry*, 26:43–72. Hillsdale, NJ: The Analytic Press.

Hall, S. (1990), Signification, representation, ideology: Althusser and the post-structuralist debates. *Critical Studies in Mass Communication*, 2:99–112.

Hoffer, E. (1951), *The True Believer: Thoughts on the Nature of Mass Movements*. New York: Harper & Row.

Hunter, J. D. (1993), Fundamentalism: An introduction to a general theory. In: *Jewish Fundamentalism in Comparative Perspective*, ed. L. J. Silberstein. New York: New York University Press, pp. 27–41.

Keniston, K. (1968), *Young Radicals: Notes on Committed Youth*. New York: Harcourt Brace & World.

Levine, S. (1992), Cults revisited: corporate and quasi-therapeutic co-optation. *Adolescent Psychiatry*, 7:63–73. Chicago: University of Chicago Press.

Lustick, I. S. (1993), Jewish fundamentalism and the Israeli-Palestinian impasse. In: *Jewish Fundamentalism in Comparative Perspective*, ed. L. J. Silberstein, pp. 104–116. New York: New York University Press.

Maley, W. (1998), *Fundamentalism Reborn? Afghanistan and the Taliban*. New York: New York University Press.

McCullough, D. (2001), *John Adams*. New York: Simon and Schuster.

Meissner, W. W. (1985), Adolescent paranoia: Transference and countertransference issues. *Adolescent Psychiatry* 12:478–508. Chicago, University of Chicago Press.

——— (2000), *The Cultic Origins of Christianity*. Collegeville, MN: The Liturgical Press.

Naipaul, V. S. (1981), *Amongst the Believers: An Islamic Journey*. New York: Knopf.

Paine, T. (1776), *Common Sense*. Amherst, NY: Prometheus Books, 1995.

Pinderhughes, C. A. (1986), Differential bonding from infancy to international conflict. *Psychoanal. Inq.*, 6:155–173.

Post, J. M. (2002), Killing in the name of God: Osama Bin Laden and radical Islam. *Group for the Advancement of Psychiatry Circular Letter #580:* 9–11.

Powers, T. (1971), *Diana: The Making of a Terrorist.* Boston: Houghton Mifflen.

Rakoff, V. (1998), Neitzsche and the Romantic construction of adolescence. *Adolescent Psychiatry,* 22:39–56. Hillsdale, NJ: The Analytic Press.

Rashid, A. (2001), *Taliban: Militant Islam, Oil and Fundamentalism in Central Asia.* New Haven, CT: Yale Nota Bene.

Robespierre, M. (1794), Speech on the moral and political principles of domestic policy. In: *The French Revolution,* by P. Dawson, Englewood Cliffs, NJ: Prentice-Hall 1967. pp. 132–136.

Rubin, J. (1969), An emergency letter to my brothers and sisters in the movement. *New York Review of Books,* New York City, February 13, p. 27.

Silberstein, L. J. (1993), Religion, ideology, modernity. In: *Jewish Fundamentalism in Comparative Perspective,* ed. L. J. Silberstein. New York: New York University Press, pp. 3–26.

Sprinzak, E. (1993), The politics, institutions, and culture of Gush Emunim. In: *Jewish Fundamentalism in Comparative Perspective,* ed. L. J. Silberstein. New York: New York University Press.

Therborn, G. (1980), *The Ideology of Power and the Power of Ideology.* London: Verso.

Thoreau, H. D. (1849), *Civil Disobedience.* New York: W. W. Norton, 1966.

——— (1854), *Walden, An Annotated Edition,* ed. W. Harding. New York: Houghton Mifflin, 1995.

United States Department of Justice, Federal Bureau of Investigation (1999), *Terrorism in the United States 1999.* Electronic text. Available at http://www.fbi.gov/publications/terror/terror99.pdf. Accessed January 9, 2003.

Vaillant, G. E. (1977), *Adaptation to Life.* Boston: Little, Brown.

Vaughan, D. J. (1997), *Give Me Liberty: The Uncompromising Statesmanship of Patrick Henry.* Nashville, TN: Cumberland House.

PART II

ORIGINAL ARTICLES
AND REVIEWS

3 SERIOUS DELINQUENCY AND GANG MEMBERSHIP

CHRISTOPHER R. THOMAS, CHARLES E. HOLZER, III, AND JULIE A. WALL

Youth violence and serious delinquency increased dramatically in the 1980s. Over the same period, youth gangs increased in number and membership (Table 1). Previously found only in large inner cities, youth gangs appeared in smaller cities and suburban communities. Some researchers (Sickmund, Snyder, and Poe-Yamagata, 1996) consider the rise in youth gangs a contributing factor to the increase in youth violence. Gang members are more likely than other delinquents to have and use guns (Maxson, Gordon, and Klein, 1985; Hutson et al., 1995).

TABLE 1

INCREASE IN GANGS AND GANG MEMBERS IN THE UNITED STATES

Study	Year	Gangs	Members
Miller (1975)	1975	2,700	81,500
Miller (1982)	1982	2,285	97,940
Spergel and Curry (1988)	1988	1,439	120,636
Curry et al. (1996)	1993	4,881	249,324
OJJDP (1997)	1995	25,000	665,000
OJJDP (1999)	1997	30,533	815,896
OJJDP (2000)	1998	28,700	780,200

Adapted from: Office of Juvenile Justice and Delinquency Prevention.

This research was funded by the Moody Foundation of Galveston and the John D. and Catherine T. MacArthur Foundation. The authors gratefully acknowledge the assistance of Roberta Lee, R.N., Dr.P.H., and Freddy Paniagua, Ph.D.

Others (Blumstein, 1995) point to the increase in illegal drug trade, particularly crack cocaine, as a cause for the increases in gangs, guns and juvenile homicide. In their study of Chicago gangs, however, Block and Block (1993) found that the relationship between gangs, drugs, and homicide was weak and did not explain the increase in youth homicide. Although juvenile homicides dropped in the late 1990s, the presence of gangs in American communities has not. The most recent survey by the National Youth Gang Center of U.S. law enforcement agencies reported 28,700 youth gangs with 780,200 members for 1998 (Office of Juvenile Justice and Delinquency Prevention, OJJDP, 2000). The survey found that youth gangs are present in all states, with 4463 cities and counties experiencing gang activity. Although these numbers decreased slightly from their peak in 1996, they still document a substantial increase and spread in gang presence over the past two decades.

Youth gangs are not a new phenomenon in society. London in the 1600s had groups calling themselves names like the Dead Boys, committing acts of vandalism and engaging in fights with each other and the watch (Pearson, 1983). Gangs may have appeared in the United States in the 1780s (Sheldon, 1898). As a factor in the development of antisocial behavior, gangs have been a focus of sociological research since the 1920s (Thrasher, 1927; Shaw and McKay, 1943). Jenkins and Hewitt (1944) described membership in delinquent peer groups as an important aspect in the psychiatric classification of behavioral problems in youth. Their work, along with other studies (e.g., Argyle, 1961), served as the basis for the "group delinquent reaction" diagnostic category in the American Psychiatric Association's (APA) 1968 *Diagnostic and Statistical Manual for Mental Disorders,* second edition *(DSM-II)*. Gangs were viewed not only as a causative factor in delinquent behavior, but also as predictive of a potentially better outcome than the "unsocialized, aggressive delinquent reaction" (Meeks, 1975). Robins (1966) did not find gang involvement to be of any predictive value for adult antisocial behavior, however. In her longitudinal study of boys referred to a child guidance clinic, antisocial boys who participated in gangs were not significantly more likely to be sociopathic adults than other antisocial boys, nor were gang members, when compared with boys who did not belong to a gang. The concept of deviant peer groups as important to the classification of antisocial behavior in youth persisted with the subcategory of "group type conduct disorder" in the *DSM-III-R* (APA, 1987) but was dropped from the *DSM-IV* (APA, 1994).

Part of the difficulty with understanding youth gangs is the difference in opinion as to what constitutes a gang as opposed to a deviant peer group (Klein, 1995; Curry and Decker, 1998). Most researchers recognize a youth gang as a distinct group recognized by its members and the community and involved in criminal acts. Other groups are involved in crime (such as hate groups, motorcycle gangs, and prison gangs), but these are generally considered distinct from youth gangs. Joining a gang, like antisocial behaviors in general, tends to be more common in males than females, but there appears to be an increase in both female gang members and female gangs (Winfree et al., 1992; Curry, Ball, and Decker, 1996). Most gang members are between the ages of 12 and 24 years old, with an average age of 18 (Curry and Decker, 1998). Recent trends in age distribution within gangs indicate that membership may be aging (OJJDP, 2000).

Contrary to popular belief, most gang members do not belong for life but only for a year or so (Esbensen and Huizinga, 1993). The size of a gang can vary greatly but generally ranges from 10 to 25 members, and larger gangs tend to be composed of smaller cliques. A gang, in contrast to a delinquent peer group, is typically characterized by a name, a recognized leader or leadership, and home territory or turf (Klein, 1995). Gangs also establish their identity through the use of dress, speech, signs, and graffiti (Knox, 1991). Gangs tend to be ethnically homogeneous and composed of minorities, reflecting the neighborhoods where they are more likely to be found and to recruit their members (Spergel, 1993).

Substantial information exists about delinquent behavior by youth gangs in established communities, but information is limited concerning the new youth gangs and gang members in emerging gang communities. It is unclear whether the recent spread and rise in number of youth gangs reflected a marked change in youth gangs or an expansion of previous patterns. In addition, there is little information regarding gang members' personality characteristics or psychopathology.

METHOD

Galveston, Texas, is representative of many communities that experienced the appearance of youth gangs and an increase in youth crime in the late 1980s. It is a city of 59,000 residents located on a barrier island off the Texas coast about 50 miles southeast of Houston. The juvenile population between the ages of 10 and 17 was 6050 according to the 1990 census and ethnically diverse with approximately one-third each of African American, Hispanic, and white youth. According to census data, 40% of Galveston children live in single-parent homes, and 36% live in poverty. Juvenile crime rose by 60% in Galveston County between 1988 and 1992. In 1988, no homicides were attributed to Galveston City youth, but in 1992, there were 57 drive-by shootings, 15 juvenile arrests for murder and attempted murder, and 109 arrests for aggravated assault. There were no established youth gangs in the early 1980s, but by 1992, there were about 350 gang members and 10 to 12 recognized gangs with an average size of 20 members, according to the Galveston Police Department. The Galveston gangs quickly exhibited the organization and activities of established gangs in larger urban centers, including the use of names, signs, dress, and graffiti to identify themselves. Although the Galveston gangs copied many of the attributes of the older gangs, they were not a product of gang members from those cities relocating in this community.

Design

Information regarding peers, antisocial behaviors, other youth problems, and family interactions and communication obtained from serious delinquents and their designated parents or guardians was compared with respect to gang membership. Data analyzed for this study were collected as part of the baseline interviews for a prospective randomized trial of multisystemic therapy based on methods developed and supervised by Henggeler and colleagues (1986). Because baseline information was collected prior to assignment, treatment is not relevant to this analysis.

Sample

The subjects were 66 serious delinquents and their parents or guardians living in a small city (population 59,000) with an emerging youth gang problem. Potential subjects were referred by juvenile probation after sentencing. Eligible youth had at least one conviction for a violent offense or a conviction for any offense with a history of at least two additional offenses. (Serious delinquency is usually defined as violent or frequent juvenile offenses.) Youth whose sentences included placement out of the home were excluded. One eligible youth was excluded because a sibling and parent were already participating in the prospective treatment study.

Recruitment

After the first meeting with a referred youth's probation officer, a member of the research staff met with the youth and the parent or guardian to explain the study and obtain written consent if they agreed to participate. About 75% of eligible youth and a parent or guardian agreed to participate over the two and one-half years of recruitment. The 25% who refused to participate were similar in offense history to those who agreed. The study was approved by the University Institutional Review Board and County Juvenile Justice Board and protected by a Federal Certificate of Confidentiality.

Interviews

Families who agreed to participate were interviewed in their homes. A team of two trained lay interviewers conducted separate and simultaneous interviews with each youth and the designated parent or guardian. Interviews lasted 45 minutes to one hour with youth and one and one-half to two hours with adults. All instruments were translated for use with subjects whose primary language was Spanish.

Instruments

Basic demographic information, reports on the youth, and descriptions of family interactions were collected from both the youth and parent or guardian. Youth instruments included the Child-Life, or C-Life, an instrument we have developed to collect basic demographics, Youth Self-Report (YSR, Achenbach, 1991b), Family Adaptability and Cohesion Scales, third edition (FACES-III, Olson and Tiesel, 1991), Self-Reported Delinquency Scale (SRDS, Elliot, Huizinga, and Ageton, 1985), Parent–Adolescent Communication instrument (PAC, Barnes and Olson, 1982). Parent or guardian instruments included basic demographics (A-Life), Child Behavior Checklist (CBCL, Achenbach, 1991a), supplement questions to the CBCL on antisocial behaviors (Loeber et al., 1991), FACES-III, and PAC.

A Gang Survey (GANGS) was developed for this study by the authors. The gang assessment survey includes 33 questions on gang awareness, reasons for joining and leaving, involvement, and activities. Gang membership status for delinquents was based on the self-report of gang membership in this section. This method is the most common and recommended in gang studies (Fagan, 1990). The survey also incorporates 18 questions regarding positive and negative peer attributes and interactions with parents from Part B of the Family, Friends, and Self Assessment created by Simpson and McBride (1992) of Texas Christian University.

Analysis

Prior to analysis, data were placed in Statistical Analysis System (SAS) data files, scales were scored, and the scores from youth and parents were merged. Participants were categorized by gang membership status as current, past, and never members of a gang. These groups were then compared on youth reports of antisocial behaviors, other youth problems, peer associations, and family interactions by ANOVA (Duncan Multiple Range Test). Similar comparisons were then made for parent reports.

RESULTS

Gang Membership

Of the 66 delinquents, 9 reported current gang membership and 15 reported past gang membership. Of the delinquents, only five were female, and all of them denied any current or past membership in gangs. Two females reported being involved in a gang fight, one had friends who were gang members, and one had family members who belonged to a gang. The female delinquents were not included in further comparison analysis. Table 2 presents the demographics for the 61 male subjects by gang membership. The median age was 15, with no significant differences based on gang membership status. Fifty youth (82%) reported current enrollment in school, with the ninth grade being the average highest grade attended. Again, there were no differences in highest grade attended when compared by gang membership. Fourteen youth (25%) reported having a job. Current and past gang members

TABLE 2

DEMOGRAPHICS

Gang Membership	Never $n = 37$	Past $n = 15$	Current $n = 9$	Total $n = 61$
Age				
12 yrs.	1	—	—	1
13 yrs.	5	1	—	6
14 yrs.	8	5	2	15
15 yrs.	11	4	2	17
16 yrs.	9	5	5	19
17 yrs.	3	—	—	3
Race and ethnicity				
White	5	—	—	5
African American	25	11	4	40
Hispanic	6	2	5	13
Other	1	2	—	3
Highest grade attended				
6	—	1	—	1
7	6	2	—	8
8	10	6	2	18
9	16	4	6	26
10	2	2	1	5
11	3	—	—	3
Living with natural parents				
Both parents	6	1	1	8
Father only	2	—	1	3
Mother only	26	13	6	45
Neither	3	1	1	5

reported joining a gang at a median age of 12 years and an average duration of gang membership of 2.47 years.

Comparison of Problem Behaviors Reported by Youth

The 61 male subjects reported diverse, frequent, and severe antisocial behaviors. Current gang membership was associated with significantly more aggressive and antisocial behavior. Current gang members also reported significantly more deviant peers, fewer good peers, and poorer communication with their parents than past gang members.

Current gang members had significantly higher scores than past and never gang members on the YSR delinquency, aggression, externalizing, and total problem scales summarized in Table 3. There were no significant differences on the same scales between delinquents who were past or never members of a gang. The scores for all three groups on the four scales were comparable to the mean scores reported for a referred population (Achenbach, 1991b). Interestingly, there were no significant differences associated with gang membership for the YSR internalizing scales, and those scores were comparable to the mean scores reported for a nonreferred population (Achenbach, 1991b).

Current gang members reported significantly more offenses than past and never gang members on the SRDS scales for public disorder, minor and serious property theft, minor and serious assault, and total number of offenses, as summarized in Table 4. There were no significant differences on the SRDS scales between delinquents who were past gang members and delinquents who were never members of a gang. Current gang members reported significantly more status and drug-sale offenses than delinquents who were never members of a gang. Past gang members did not differ from current or never gang members in their reports for status and drug-sale offenses.

Comparison of Peer Associations Reported by Youth

Youth reports about their peers are summarized in Table 5. Current gang member delinquents reported significantly more bad peers than delinquents who were past or never members of a gang. There were

TABLE 3
Youth Self-Report

Gang Membership	Never (N) ($n = 37$)		Past (P) ($n = 15$)		Current (C) ($n = 9$)		Comparisons Reaching Significance ($p < 0.05$)
	Mean	STD	Mean	STD	Mean	STD	
Withdrawn	3.4	2.1	3.5	2.5	5.0	3.3	
Somatic	3.0	2.7	2.4	2.2	3.4	3.2	
Anxious/ depressed	4.3	4.8	3.9	4.5	6.0	4.1	
Social problems	2.8	2.1	2.6	2.1	3.6	2.2	
Thought problems	2.5	2.6	2.6	2.0	4.6	4.0	
Attention problems	4.7	3.5	4.2	2.3	6.0	2.9	
Internalizing	10.5	7.6	9.7	7.3	13.9	8.7	
Delinquency	4.9	3.1	4.3	2.4	8.9	4.4	C > P; C > N
Aggression	8.6	6.4	7.7	5.1	15.0	8.3	C > P; C > N
Externalizing	13.5	8.8	12.1	6.4	23.9	12.0	C > P; C > N
Total problems	38.9	24.1	38.3	15.4	60.4	28.9	C > P; C > N

no differences in the number of bad peers reported by delinquents who were past or never members of a gang. This pattern corresponds with that found for youth reports of antisocial behaviors. As expected, current and past gang member delinquents also reported having more friends who were gang members than the delinquents who were never members of a gang. Past gang members reported significantly more good peers than current gang members. Delinquents who were never members of a gang did not differ from current or past gang members in their reports

TABLE 4

SELF-REPORTED DELINQUENCY SCALE

Gang Membership	Never (N) ($n = 37$)		Past (P) ($n = 15$)		Current (C) ($n = 9$)		Comparisons Reaching Significance ($p < 0.05$)
	Mean	STD	Mean	STD	Mean	STD	
Status	0.6	0.7	0.9	0.6	1.3	1.0	C > N
Public disorder	0.4	0.6	0.8	0.9	1.4	1.3	C > P; C > N
Minor property theft	0.8	1.3	0.7	0.8	2.3	1.7	C > P; C > N
Serious property theft	0.6	1.3	0.5	0.7	2.8	2.5	C > P; C > N
Minor assault	0.4	0.6	0.3	0.6	1.0	0.9	C > P; C > N
Serious assault	0.3	0.5	0.7	0.8	1.4	1.2	C > P; C > N
Drug sales	0.2	0.5	0.3	0.6	0.8	0.8	C > N
Total SRDS offenses	3.9	4.5	4.5	3.7	11.8	8.3	C > P; C > N

of good peers. Surprisingly, the three groups did not differ in their reports of peer–parent interactions.

Comparison of Family Interactions Reported by Youth

Youth reports on the PAC scale for primary and secondary parental figures are summarized in Table 6. Past gang members reported significantly more open communication and better total communication with the primary parent on the PAC than current gang members. No differences associated with gang membership were found for reports of

TABLE 5

GANG SCALE

Gang Membership	Never (N) (n = 37)		Past (P) (n = 15)		Current (C) (n = 9)		Comparisons Reaching Significance (p < 0.05)
	Mean	STD	Mean	STD	Mean	STD	
Good peers	2.7	0.6	3.0	0.6	2.4	0.7	P > C
Bad peers	2.4	0.8	2.5	0.8	3.4	1.0	C > P; C > N
Peer-parent interaction	3.7	0.8	3.9	0.6	4.0	0.7	

problem communication with the primary parent on the PAC. In comparison to national norms for the PAC, current gang members were at the 33rd percentile, never members of a gang at the 55th percentile, and past gang members were at the 79th percentile (Barnes and Olson, 1982). Overall, the pattern for youth reports about communication with the secondary parent were the same as with the primary parent except for problem communication. Current gang members reported more problems in communication with the secondary parent than past gang members. There were no significant differences based on gang membership for the FACES-III adaptability, cohesion, or family-type scales summarized in Table 7. The youth described their families as disengaged to separated in cohesion, structured to flexible in adaptability, and midrange in family type, using Olson's linear scoring system (Olson and Tiesel, 1991).

Comparison of Youth Problem Behaviors Reported by Parents

No significant differences were associated with gang membership in parent or guardian reports, in contrast with the reports by youth. Parents and guardians reported internalizing problem scores consistent with nonreferred youth and externalizing problem scores consistent with referred youth on the CBCL, as summarized in Table 8 (Achenbach,

TABLE 6

PARENT ADOLESCENT COMMUNICATION SCALE

Gang Membership	Never (N)		Past (P)		Current (C)		Comparisons Reaching Significance ($p < 0.05$)
	Mean	STD	Mean	STD	Mean	STD	
Youth Report Primary Parent							
	$n = 36$		$n = 15$		$n = 9$		
Total	67.3	12.9	75.6	10.5	61.3	14.6	P > C
Open	38.8	10.0	42.3	6.3	33.0	10.0	P > C
Problem	30.8	7.4	26.7	6.2	31.7	9.3	
Secondary Parent							
	$n = 33$		$n = 12$		$n = 7$		
Total	67.4	13.2	77.8	10.1	56.6	18.8	P > C
Open	38.4	10.3	43.5	5.6	31.4	9.6	P > C
Problem	29.3	9.4	24.8	7.1	34.9	10.3	C > P
Parent Report							
	$n = 35$		$n = 14$		$n = 9$		
Total	70.8	11.4	73.6	10.3	66.2	12.0	
Open	38.7	6.4	42.6	5.1	37.1	7.3	P > C
Problem	27.9	7.4	28.9	7.0	30.9	8.7	

1991a). The CBCL supplemental antisocial behaviors and offense-type scales that correlate to the SRDS are presented in Table 9. Although parents and guardians described diverse offenses, there were no significant differences based on gang membership, as seen with the SRDS.

Comparison of Family Interactions Reported by Parents

Responses on the PAC open-communication scale comprised the only significant difference between parent reports with respect to gang membership (Table 5). Parents of past gang members reported significantly

TABLE 7

FAMILY ADAPTABILITY & COHESION SCALE-III

Gang Membership	Never (N)		Past (P)		Current (C)	
	Mean	STD	Mean	STD	Mean	STD
Youth Report	$n = 37$		$n = 14^a$		$n = 9$	
Cohesion	3.2	1.9	3.2	1.8	2.6	1.5
Adaptability	5.0	1.6	5.1	1.8	4.6	1.3
Type score	4.1	1.4	4.2	1.3	3.6	1.1
Parent Report	$n = 37$		$n = 15$		$n = 9$	
Cohesion	3.4	1.8	3.5	1.2	2.9	0.9
Adaptability	4.7	1.8	5.1	1.7	5.3	1.8
Type score	4.1	1.4	4.3	1.1	4.1	0.9

[a]15 for Adaptability.

TABLE 8

CHILD BEHAVIOR CHECKLIST

Gang Membership	Never $n = 37$		Past $n = 15$		Current $n = 9$	
	Mean	STD	Mean	STD	Mean	STD
Withdrawn	4.1	3.1	4.3	2.7	5.2	3.6
Somatic	2.6	2.9	3.5	3.1	3.9	2.9
Anxious/depressed	5.2	4.8	7.1	6.4	7.3	5.5
Social problems	2.8	2.5	3.3	2.2	3.0	2.2
Thought problems	1.8	2.3	2.0	1.6	1.9	2.1
Attention problems	6.4	4.5	7.3	4.1	6.3	4.2
Internalizing	11.4	8.3	14.5	10.3	15.6	10.6
Delinquency	6.9	4.5	8.1	4.2	8.8	5.4
Aggression	13.3	8.6	12.7	7.4	5.4	7.3
Externalizing	20.3	12.3	20.8	11.0	24.2	12.2
Total problems	44.8	27.8	48.9	25.6	53.6	28.2

TABLE 9

PARENT-REPORTED DELINQUENCY

Gang Membership	Never n = 37		Past n = 15		Current n = 9	
	Mean	STD	Mean	STD	Mean	STD
Status	1.0	0.9	1.5	1.0	1.6	0.7
Public disorder	1.1	0.8	1.5	0.8	1.7	0.7
Minor property theft	2.1	2.7	1.9	1.9	3.6	3.7
Serious property theft	0.4	0.6	0.6	0.9	0.9	1.2
Minor assault	1.6	1.3	1.7	1.7	1.9	2.0
Serious assault	0.3	0.6	0.5	0.5	0.6	0.7
Drug sales	0.1	0.2	0.1	0.4	0.1	0.3
CBCL supplement items	42.2	25.2	48.5	25.4	53.1	32.1

more open communication with their sons than parents of current gang members. Parents of delinquents who were never members of a gang did not differ on this scale from parents of either current or past gang members. Parents gave the same range of descriptions as their sons for cohesion, adaptability, and overall family type on the FACES-III, summarized in Table 6.

DISCUSSION

Delinquents who were current gang members had significantly higher levels of self-reported aggression and delinquency than delinquents who had never been gang members or were no longer gang members. The finding that gang members commit more offenses and are more aggressive than other delinquents is consistent with studies in larger urban centers with a longer history of gang presence (Klein and Myerhoff, 1967; Esbensen and Huizinga, 1993; Spergel, 1993; Huff, 1996). The finding that past gang members reported the same levels of antisocial behaviors as those delinquents who never were members of a gang suggests that active gang participation exacerbates delinquency and aggression. Although this study is cross-sectional in design, longitudinal research has found the same pattern (Thornberry et al., 1993). Current gang members did not differ from other delinquents on characteristics that might provide alternative explanations, including demographics such as age, school, or length of gang involvement, and internalizing youth problems such as depression or anxiety. Clearly, efforts to prevent gang involvement would have a dramatic impact on the frequency and severity of youth offenses, given the disproportionate rate reported by gang members, especially violent crime. Programs that focus on ending gang involvement would also help, because past gang members do not differ in offense patterns of delinquents that were never gang members.

Some previous research has indicated that gang youth have more problems with social relationships, lower self-esteem, and more symptoms of depression than youth that are not gang members (Yablonsky, 1962; Wang, 1994; Thornberry, 1998). It does not appear that internalizing problems or symptoms are associated with gang membership in the serious delinquents in this study. There was no significant difference for specific or overall internalizing problem scales between the comparison groups, although there was a trend toward slightly higher scores for current gang members. None of the groups differed in the level of internalizing problems from general community reports on the same scales. This finding is consistent with other recent studies comparing the individual features of gang members with youth that are not gang members in both emerging and established gang communities (Hill et al., 1999; Maxson, Whitlock, and Klein, 1998). The difference in reports may reflect the survey methods and questions of the various studies.

The influence of delinquent peers on adolescent antisocial behavior is not unique to gangs (Elliot et al., 1985). Deviant peers alone cannot explain the differences found between the groups in this study, as all of the delinquents described some number of bad peers and friends who were gang members. Others have suggested that the influence of gangs is quite different from that of delinquent peers (Klein, 1995). In a detailed analysis of data from the Seattle Social Development Project, Battin and colleagues (1998) found that gang membership independently predicted both self-reported and officially recorded delinquency beyond the influence of delinquent peers. All delinquents in this study described some number of bad peers and friends who were gang members. The higher level of delinquent and aggressive behavior by current gang members may simply reflect the greater number of antisocial peer contacts provided by gang involvement. Higher frequency and severity of antisocial behaviors by gang members may also exert a stronger influence on new members. It could be argued that this association is a result of self-selection by delinquents with severe antisocial behaviors, but past gang members reported the same level of antisocial behaviors as delinquents who never were members of a gang. Rutter and Giller's (1983) review of delinquency studies concluded that changes in social groups influenced changes in behaviors, even if the change in peer group was involuntary.

It is interesting that past gang members reported significantly more good peers than current gang members. This implies that leaving the gang involves not only reducing bad-peer associations, but also increasing good-peer associations. The related finding, that delinquents who never were members of a gang had similar numbers of good peers as current or past gang-member delinquents, supports this explanation. Having positive peers may facilitate leaving a gang. Developing ways to provide positive peers for target youth may benefit interventions directed at ending gang involvement.

Another important aspect of peer relationships is the influence of parents (Poole and Regoli, 1979). Current gang members did not report their peer–parent interactions as different from other delinquents despite having significantly more bad peers. Either the current gang members did not perceive parental disapproval, or their parents did not perceive a problem with their sons' associates. The poorer communication reported by current gang members and their parents supports both possible explanations. The possibility that parents of current gang members did not perceive a problem with their sons' peers is supported by the finding that they did not report a higher rate of their sons' antisocial behavior in comparison to the other parents. These observations are consistent with other studies that have reported poor parental monitoring and involvement as risk factors for gang membership (Bowker and Klein, 1983; Campbell, 1990; Moore, 1991).

Parent reports did agree with youth reports for internalizing youth problems, family interactions, and problems in open communication. Parents also described a high level of aggressive and antisocial behavior in the delinquents, but without differences for gang membership. The discrepancy between parent and youth reports of antisocial behaviors for current gang members might be understandable in light of other findings. As with peer–parent interactions, the parents of current gang members might be less well informed of the extent of their sons' antisocial activities. The finding of poor communication reported by both current gang members and their parents in contrast with past gang members and their parents supports this explanation.

Another aspect to leaving a gang may be that better communication was reported by past gang members and their parents than by current gang members and their parents. The youth and their parents indicated no other differences in family structure with respect to gang membership. Efforts to improve family communication and involvement may benefit interventions involving the family to reduce gang participation.

Future Research and Clinical Implications

The study indicates that reducing gang involvement may decrease the frequency and severity of offenses in delinquents. It follows that the reasons for delinquents' quitting gangs are as important as the ones for joining. Differences between past and current gang members in associations with peers and communication with parents may be reasons for leaving a gang.

This study was only with serious delinquents. Further prospective study including nondelinquent youth is needed to clarify these factors influencing gang membership. Interventions directed at increasing associations with positive peers and improving parental communication may be a promising approach to reducing gang involvement and related delinquency in youth.

REFERENCES

Achenbach, T. M. (1991a), *Manual for the Child Behavior Checklist/ 4–18 and 1991 Profile*. Burlington: University of Vermont Department of Psychiatry.
——— (1991b), *Manual for the Youth Self Report and 1991 Profile*. Burlington: University of Vermont Department of Psychiatry.
American Psychiatric Association (1968), *Diagnostic and Statistical Manual of Mental Disorders*, 2nd ed. (*DSM-II*). Washington, DC: American Psychiatric Association.
——— (1987), *Diagnostic and Statistical Manual of Mental Disorders*, 3rd ed., revised (*DSM-III-R*). Washington, DC: American Psychiatric Association.

———— (1994), *Diagnostic and Statistical Manual of Mental Disorders*, 4th ed. (*DSM-IV*). Washington, DC: American Psychiatric Association.

Argyle, M. (1961), *A new approach to the classification of delinquents with implications for treatment.* California Board of Corrections, Monograph No. 2.

Barnes, H. & Olson, D. H. (1982), *Parent-Adolescent Communication.* St. Paul: Family Social Science, University of Minnesota.

Battin, S., Hill, K., Abbott, R., Catalano, R. & Hawkins, J. (1998), The contribution of gang membership to delinquency beyond delinquent friends. *Criminology,* 36:93–115.

Blumstein, A. (1995), Violence by young people: Why the deadly nexus? *Natl. Inst. Justice J.,* 229:2–9.

Block, R. & Block, C. (1993), *Street gang crime in Chicago.* Research in brief. Washington, DC: National Institute of Justice.

Bowker, L. & Klein, M. (1983), The etiology of female juvenile delinquency and gang membership: A test of psychological and social structural explanations. *Adolescence,* 18:739–751.

Campbell, A. (1990), Female participation in gangs. In: *Gangs in America,* ed. C. Huff. Newbury Park, CA: Sage, pp. 163–182.

Curry, G. D. (1995), *National Youth Gang Surveys: A Review of Methods and Findings.* Washington, DC: Office of Juvenile Justice and Delinquency Prevention.

———— Ball, R. A. & Decker, S. H. (1996), *Estimating the National Scope of Gang Crime from Law Enforcement Data.* Research in brief. Washington, DC: National Institute of Justice.

———— ———— & ———— (1996b), *Developing National Estimates of Gang-Related Crime.* Washington, DC: National Institute of Justice.

———— & Decker, S. (1998), *Confronting Gangs: Crime and Community.* Los Angeles, CA: Roxbury.

Elliot, D., Huizinga, D. & Ageton, S. (1985), *Explaining Delinquency and Drug Use.* Beverly Hills: Sage.

Esbensen, F. & Huizinga, D. (1993), Gangs, drugs and delinquency in a survey of urban youth. *Criminology,* 36:799–828.

Fagan, J. (1990), Social processes of delinquency and drug use among urban gangs. In: *Gangs in America,* ed. C. R. Huff. Newbury Park: Sage, pp. 183–222.

Henggeler, S., Rodick, J., Borduin, C., Hanson, C., Watson, S. & Urey, J. (1986), Multisystemic treatment of juvenile offenders: Effects on adolescent behavior and family interactions. *Develop. Psychol.*, 22:132–141.

Hill, K., Howell, J., Hawkins, J. & Battin-Pearson, S. (1999), Childhood risk factors for adolescent gang membership: Results from the Seattle Social Development Project. *J. Res. Crime & Delinquency,* 36:300–322.

Huff, C. (1996), The criminal behavior of gang members and nongang at-risk youth. In: *Gangs in America*, ed. C. R. Huff. Thousand Oaks, CA: Sage.

Hutson, H., Anglin, D., Kyriacou, D., Hart, J. & Spears, K. (1995), The epidemic of gang-related homicides in Los Angeles County from 1979 through 1994. *J. Amer. Medical Assn.,* 274:1031–1036.

Jenkins, R. & Hewitt, L. (1944), Types of personality structure encountered in child guidance clinics. *Amer. J. Orthopsychiat.,* 14:84–94.

Klein, M. (1995), *The American Street Gang.* New York: Oxford University Press.

———— & Myerhoff, B. (1967), *Juvenile Gangs in Context: Theory, Research, and Action.* Englewood Cliffs, NJ: Prentice Hall.

Knox, G. (1991), *An Introduction to Gangs.* Berrien Springs, MI: Van de Vere.

Loeber, R., Stouthamer-Loeber, M., Van Kammen, W. & Farrington, D. (1991), Initiation, escalation and desistance in juvenile offending and their correlates. *J. Criminal Law & Criminology,* 82:36–82.

Maxson, C., Gordon, M. & Klein, M. (1985), Differences between gang and nongang homicides. *Criminology,* 23:209–222.

———— Whitlock, M. & Klein, M. (1998), Vulnerability to street gang membership: Implications for practice. *Soc. Serv. Rev.,* 72:70–91.

Meeks, J. (1975), Group delinquent reaction. In: *Comprehensive Textbook of Psychiatry-II,* 2nd ed., ed. A. Freedman, H. Kaplan, & B. S. Sadock. Baltimore: Williams & Wilkins, pp. 2136–2142.

Miller, W. B. (1975), *Violence by Youth Gangs and Youth Gangs as a Crime Problem in Major American Cities.* Washington, DC: Office of Juvenile Justice and Delinquency Prevention.

———— (1982), *Crime by Youth Gangs and Youth Groups in the United States.* Washington, DC: Office of Juvenile Justice and Delinquency Prevention.

Moore, J. W. (1991), *Going Down to the Barrio: Homeboys and Homegirls in Change.* Philadelphia: Temple University Press.

Olson, D. H. & Tiesel, J. (1991), *FACES-III: Linear Scoring & Interpretation.* St. Paul: Family Social Science, University of Minnesota.

Office of Juvenile Justice and Delinquency Prevention (1997), *1995 National Youth Gang Survey* (NCJ Publication No. 164728). Washington, DC: OJJDP.

———— (1999), *1997 National Youth Gang Survey* (NCJ Publication No. 178891). Washington, DC: OJJDP.

———— (2000), *1998 National Youth Gang Survey* (NCJ Publication No. 183109). Washington, DC: OJJDP.

Pearson, G. (1983), *Hooligan: A History of Reportable Fears.* New York: Schocken Books.

Poole, R. & Regoli, R. (1979), Parental support, delinquent friends, and delinquency: A test of interaction effects. *J. Criminal Law & Criminology,* 70:188–193.

Robins, L. (1966), *Deviant Children Grown Up.* Baltimore: Williams & Wilkins.

Rutter, M. & Giller, H. (1983), *Juvenile Delinquency, Trends and Perspectives.* New York: Guilford Press.

Shaw, C. & McKay, H. (1943), *Juvenile Delinquency and Urban Areas.* Chicago: University of Chicago Press.

Sheldon, H. (1898), The institutional activities of American children. *Amer. J. Psychol.,* 9:424–448.

Sickmund, M., Snyder, H. & Poe-Yamagata, E. (1996), Juvenile Offenders and Victims: 1996 Update on Violence. *OJJDP Statistical Briefing Book.* Washington, DC: Office of Juvenile Justice and Delinquency Prevention.

Simpson, D. D. & McBride, A. A. (1992), Family, Friends, and Self (FFS) assessment scales for Mexican American youth. *Hispanic J. of Behavioral Sciences,* 14(3):327–340.

Spergel, I. (1993), *Gang Suppression and Intervention.* Washington, DC: Office of Juvenile Justice and Delinquency Prevention.

Spergel, I. A. & Curry, G. D. (1988), Gang homicide, delinquency, and community. *J. Criminal Law & Criminology,* 20:381–405.

Thornberry, T. (1998), Membership in youth gangs and involvement in serious and violent offending. In: *Serious and Violent Offenders: Risk Factors and Successful Interventions,* ed. R. Loeber & D. Farrington. Thousand Oaks, CA: Sage, pp. 147–166.

———— Krohn, M., Lizotte, A. & Chard-Wierschem, D. (1993), The role of juvenile gangs in facilitating delinquent behavior. *J. Res. Crime & Delinquency,* 30:55–87.

Thrasher, F. (1927), *The Gang.* Chicago: University of Chicago Press.

Wang, A. (1994), Pride and prejudice in high school gang members. *Adolescence,* 29:279–291.

Winfree, T., Fuller, K., Vigil, T. & Mays, G. (1992), The definition and measurement of gang status: policy implications for juvenile justice. *Juv. & Fam. Ct. J.,* 43:29–37.

Yablonsky, L. (1962), *The Violent Gang.* New York: Macmillan.

4 A CHRONICLE OF SECLUSION AND RESTRAINT IN AN INTERMEDIATE-TERM CARE FACILITY

THEODORE A. PETTI, JOHN SOMERS, AND LINDA SIMS

The use of restrictive practices, particularly seclusion and mechanical restraint (S&MR), in psychiatric hospitals and residential treatment centers for children and adolescents has generated considerable controversy and consternation for policymakers, providers, consumers, and other interested parties. Health and mental health professionals have argued for employment of these restrictive interventions as therapeutically necessary. Advocacy and consumer groups have lobbied strenuously for their attenuation (American Psychiatric Association, 2001). The Joint Commission on the Accreditation of Hospital Organizations (JCAHO) has been urging reductions of restrictive practices in hospitals and residential treatment centers for many years through their standards. The Health Care Financing Administration (HCFA), in a sudden and surprising move, changed the entire landscape with regulations promulgated in August 1999. These regulations have had a major impact on S&MR utilization policies and practices. Confusion and widespread changes in procedures resulted from these changes in hospital and residential treatment of adolescents with severe psychiatric disorders.

The use of seclusion as a form of control has its roots deep in American history. The practice of seclusion for disruptive behavior can be dated to the first schoolhouse in the United States, located in what is now the historical district of St. Augustine, Florida. There,

Appreciation is expressed to the patients and staff of Larue Carter Hospital, particularly Diana Haugh, M.S., R.N., Paul Wagner, A.C.S.W., Robert TenEyck, Ph.D., Roger Nelson, B.S. and to our consultant and colleague Wanda K. Mohr, Ph.D., R.N.

down an alley, can be found the building, with a closet specifically designated for managing unruly youth. The modern use of S&MR as medical or nursing interventions evolved following a pattern described by Gair (1980). He describes their initial use as measures to ensure the safety of youth in residential care. These measures evolved to become standard psychiatric treatment. Gair notes the poorly articulated rationale for this standard of practice. He considers seclusion to be a therapeutic necessity that becomes an endpoint of limit-setting following the failure of alternative interventions to control dangerous or disruptive behavior toward self or others. Restraint serves as a means to interrupt determined efforts at self-mutilation. S&MR have become routine practices in most institutional and residential programs for juveniles (Zusman, 1997). There are no rigorous methodological studies comparing S&MR to other interventions for youth undergoing psychiatric treatment or residential placement; only case reports, program descriptions, and overviews are available (Cotton, 1989; Garrison et al., 1990; Troutman et al., 1998; Singh et al., 1999; Petti et al., 2001; American Academy of Child and Adolescent Psychiatry, AACAP, 2002).

The paradigm shift reflected in rising S&MR utilization since the 1970s and accompanying concerns of advocacy groups suggested a need for S&MR reassessment. Since 1995, JCAHO has issued many Type 1 recommendations for noncompliance following accreditation reviews indicating that immediate improvement needs to be addressed to JCAHO standard on S&MR (Zusman, 1997). Guidelines for the use of S&MR continue to be promulgated in the tug-of-war between practitioners allied with professional organizations and consumers allied with advocacy groups. To date, HCFA and JCAHO regulations and standards seem more stringent than those desired by many professionals and providers, and less stringent than those desired by patient advocacy groups. The AACAP has developed the "Practice Parameter for the Prevention and Management of Aggressive Behavior in Child and Adolescent Psychiatric Institutions, with Special Reference to Seclusion and Restraint" (2002) to address this issue. We present a university-affiliated, intermediate-term state hospital's successful efforts, initiated in 1995 and continuing to this time, to decrease S&MR utilization. We expect that the approaches employed and lessons learned in the process are similar to those experienced by many programs in managing the increasing numbers of more severely ill, destructive, violent, and dangerous youth in settings that must adjust to the changing fiscal and political climate in the human services system. We intend to chronicle these efforts and provide insights to those interested in understanding and learning from these experiences and advancing the field to be more effective and efficient in the care of such youth.

THE HOSPITAL AND ITS HISTORY

The evolution of the hospital, regarding the population of patients it serves and the dramatic shifts in role within the system of care in which it operates, is similar to that experienced by many other state hospitals throughout the nation. In the 1960s to 1980s, the Youth Service (YS) of Larue Carter Hospital (LCH) served youngsters of average intelligence who were often acutely disturbed or belonged to special clinical populations and came from relatively intact family systems. In the 1980s, the burgeoning public mental health centers and private hospital beds to serve these youngsters resulted in increasing referrals of more treatment-resistant, developmentally disabled patients. In the 1990s, the hospital began admitting droves of more severely ill youngsters who had demonstrated ineffective response to multiple acute, brief hospitalizations, residential and out-of-home placements, and/or prescription of multiple psychotropic agents and intensive outpatient treatment. Many of these youth had been physically and/or sexually abused. The adolescents included those who had been sexual predators, those who were severely violent and aggressive towards others, and those with dangerous self-injurious behavior, including females who would ingest foreign objects (e.g., paper clips, staples, tooth brushes, plastic utensils, batteries). Many had histories of injuring hospital or residential staff and/or regular S&MR utilization to control their behavior.

The following case represents a significant, small percentage of patients referred to our service. Chantelle was a large-for-her-age 15-year-old African American female when she was court-committed to Youth Service. During her 16-month residence in a for-profit hospital, her violence and aggression resulted in the hospitalizations of several staff members and peers. Her presenting symptoms included explosive, violent, and self-injurious behaviors. She had been hospitalized at the age of 13 for aggressive behavior, and two times thereafter. Her history was significant for suicidal ideation, homicidal threats, acute anxiety attacks, dissociative episodes, flashbacks, memory lapses, and trauma induced by sexual and physical abuse. Behavior problems of temper outbursts and stubbornness dated to the age of two. At the time of admission to LCH, she was on thiothixene 15 mg three times per day and albuterol as needed for asthma. Shortly after admission, she attacked and severely injured a nurse and assaulted a peer, who was not so badly injured. No psychotic symptoms were present, nor did she show remorse at the time of either attack. Her admission Axis I diagnoses were conduct disorder, mixed type, severe, and a number of rule-outs for depressive and anxiety disorders. She received an Axis II diagnosis of borderline personality disorder.

Chantelle came from a chaotic home situation. Her family of origin was very violent, abusive, and dysfunctional. Both parents had served prison time for violent acts. Removed from her mother's care as a baby because of the mother's physical abuse of Chantelle and her siblings, she lived with relatives for several years before returning to reside with mother in preadolescence. Following this, she reported being sexually abused by her mother, her mother's lesbian lover, and, at the age of 13, by her uncles. The family denied this and reported that they were afraid of Chantelle because she had threatened to kill them and had lied about them. During Chantelle's hospitalization on Youth Service, her mother was very inconsistent in her visits and phone contacts, which created a significant stressor for Chantelle and often served as a trigger for aggressive behavior.

Upon admission, Chantelle was evaluated on a number of measures. Her projective assessment showed significant deficits in connecting cause and effect, attaching to others, engaging in empathy or under-standing the perspective of others, and coping with intense emotions. Her thinking was contaminated by strong interfering emotions that prevented her from processing reality accurately, although she showed no psychotic symptoms. She viewed her external environment as being restrictive and dangerous; she appeared to be evasive and defensive and gave up quickly on challenging tasks. Her resources to cope with emotions were impoverished and her thinking rather concrete in nature. On communication assessment, she showed significant verbal language deficits in both receptive and expressive domains. Such deficits compro-mised her ability to process emotions and express them in a socially acceptable manner. It was also noted that she had difficulty retrieving information efficiently and in a timely manner, which made her school experience problematic and challenging. Chantelle was enrolled in intensive language therapy to address these deficits as well as a number of other communication issues.

Psychometric assessment revealed a significant improvement in functioning from the time of admission to discharge. Upon admission, she showed a full scale IQ of 78 with verbal IQ of 72 and performance IQ of 90. At the time of discharge, Chantelle revealed a full scale IQ of 91 with a verbal IQ of 86 and performance IQ of 100.

Chantelle's course of treatment was unique due to her dangerous and violent behavior. After injuring the nurse and a peer, threatening others, and exhibiting self-injurious behaviors, she was placed on a strict behavioral protocol that included placement in wrist-to-waist restraints to keep her and others safe. This measure was taken after much deliberation with her physicians and treatment team members. The protocol allowed Chantelle to earn an hour out of restraints for each day she did not engage in abusive loudness or physical or verbal threats toward others, and complied with the unit rules. If she engaged in such adverse behaviors, she returned to ground zero, lost all accumulated time out of restraints, and began the process over again. Concomitant with the restraint protocol, Chantelle engaged in therapy that focused on anger control management, relaxation techniques, and supportive reinforcement of appropriate behavior. Over the course of about three months, with a number of ups and downs, she earned her way out of restraints and was able to tolerate a more normalized system of rewards and consequences.

The initial days of being restraint-free proved stressful for Chantelle due to her need to take personal responsibility and to exercise self-control through internal mechanisms rather than external ones. In order to assist her, restraints were made available to her and she could voluntarily ask for them. However, she never asked for or needed them. At the termination of the restraint protocol, significant changes occurred. She seldom struck out at others, she demonstrated less frequent violent or threatening posturing, and her anger shifted toward inanimate objects such as trash cans, pictures, or walls, or toward herself. She engaged in superficial mutilation of her arms, which usually consisted of using a pencil eraser "to erase myself." All of these episodes eventually subsided. In addition, her speech was noted to be softer and more melodic, and she became less intrusive. Her personal hygiene improved, and she kept her bedroom tidier. In the three months before discharge, she had two episodes of challenging behavior and one incident of superficial self-mutilation that resulted in two room confinements, which she handled without incident. These three episodes coincided with court review dates and missed appointments by her mother. At the end of hospitalization, Chantelle's behavior had improved to the point that she was accepted by three different residential placement facilities. She and her treatment team chose a therapeutic group home placement distant from her family, which Chantelle decided would be less stressful to her well-being. She was discharged on the following medications: albuterol inhaler, two puffs three times per day, diphenhydramine 50 mg at bedtime, lorazepam two mg every four hours as needed for severe agitation, clindamycin 1% to face daily, multivitamins, and lactase enzyme tablets. For a few years following discharge, she would visit YS regularly and proudly review the progress she had made.

The use of a rigid behavioral protocol using ambulatory wrist-to-waist restraints in combination with psychoeducational interventions was instrumental in helping Chantelle transfer external control measures to internal ones. In addition, her work in language therapy enabled better self-expression, which increased her ability to manage conflict and to engage more insightfully with psychotherapy. This case is meant to illustrate when restraint is the "least restrictive alternative for managing aggression" (Troutman et al., 1998, p. 557).

The intellectual level of youth admitted to the YS program has steadily dropped into the borderline range. This change has had a major impact on the S&MR rate. Many of these patients, like Chantelle, have developmental receptive and expressive language disorders. The proportion of families able to work regularly with staff for their children's transition back to home and community has decreased markedly. The average length of stay had climbed to a year and more.

Our YS is located within a heavily bureaucratized state hospital. It consists of 42 beds, 31 of which are devoted to middle and high school populations. The patients are housed in three clinical units by school classification. In relation to the other Indiana state hospital programs serving youth, YS provides the only services for adolescent girls, is one of two hospitals providing inpatient services to elementary-age children, and is one of three programs serving adolescent boys.

During the period in which major effort was devoted to decreasing the S&MR rates and duration of use, many changes occurred. These included adjusting to the closing of another state hospital that led to the subsequent expansion of beds from 34 to 42 and a significant upheaval in staff composition. The eight additional beds were used to create a unit to house boys and girls of middle-school age. This unit had significantly higher rates of S&MR than did the other two units. Two years into this report, LCH moved away from the university campus and into a former Veterans Administration Hospital.

The new facility, a designated historical site, was notable for its "soft" interior as contrasted with the institutional hardness of the former state hospital, and for environmental blind spots that reduced the ability to monitor patients. In addition, the hospital itself experienced erosion in numbers of professional and direct care staff after the relocation. We unofficially estimate the turnover as about 60% due to replacement of LCH YS staff by those with greater seniority from the closed non-university-affiliated hospital. This merging of staff culminated in a significant blending of two different cultures. The occasional confusion and lack of consistency resulting from the merging process contributed to the perceived increasing need for restrictive interventions.

The use of S&MR became increasingly more problematic with these changes. Risk management data showed that YS accounted for over 70% of hospital S&MR episodes even though it represented only 30% of total hospital beds. Additionally, the data indicated that the high use of S&MR correlated significantly with staff and patient injuries. These factors raised concern in all involved, including consultants and evaluators during formal accreditation procedures.

INTERVENTIONS AND STRATEGIES EMPLOYED OVER SEVEN YEARS

Youth Service leadership committed itself in 1995 to decrease escalating S&MR rates. Multiple efforts were made to achieve this goal by focusing attention on the extant culture supporting excessive S&MR utilization. Presented sequentially, many of the approaches are similar to those attempted by other hospitals and residential treatment centers. In retrospect, they mirror and adhere to the principles presented in AACAP's (2002) practice parameter addressing this issue. Early interventions from 1995 are discussed in the following sections.

A Mandate from on High

The hospital superintendent requested that the entire hospital decrease S&MR rates. She voiced concern about the escalating rates on Youth Service.

Feedback on Performance

An improvement of organizational performance (IOP) office systematically collected S&MR data from July 1996. Feedback to staff of S&MR rates were routinely provided quarterly, then monthly, and finally on a weekly basis in 1999.

Accentuating the Positive

A strength-based treatment approach was initiated to deal with the changing nature of the population served. In-service training was conducted hospitalwide, and consultants with relevant expertise were invited to assist in using strength-based strategies and techniques.

Outside Assistance

A group was developed to provide an outside perspective, promote family and community involvement, and guide policies and procedures. This began as an effort to develop a parent advisory group in an attempt to elicit their views for YS direction. But we were rarely able to engage parents in this endeavor. The group began to evolve into an advisory group of advocates, consumers, and members of YS clinical leadership. It ceased to exist during early parts of the move but was later reconstituted after the move.

More Assistance

Consultation was obtained from a senior Indiana Division of Mental Health administrator/nurse with extensive experience in long-term psychiatric care of juveniles. Concrete suggestions regarding YS structure and procedures were provided, and attempts were made to implement the recommendations.

Decreases in S&MR frequency were noted during 1995 and early 1996. The YS leadership felt that significant progress was being made until announcement of the hospital relocation in mid-1996. Improvement had been seen even as changes of staff occurred, with the blending of a traditional state hospital (which had closed under a cloud of allegations) and a university-affiliated hospital with a major research and training mission. However, S&MR rates soon escalated, beginning in July 1996. Figures 1 (mechanical restraint) and 2 (seclusion) illustrate restrictive incidents from July 1996 through December 2001. Data collection prior to that time was insufficient for evaluation purposes. Interventions A, B, and C are noted in the figures. Figures 3 (restraint) and 4 (seclusion) provide the data in hours of restrictive intervention.

Following announcement of the impending move away from the academic campus, patients and staff became anxious and apprehensive. The tensions of moving and subsequent perception by both patients and staff of an unsafe environment in the new facility led to even more dramatic increases in S&MR rates, as demonstrated in Figures 1 through 4. The hospital relocated in November 1996. In the new facility, YS occupied the space formerly used as a nursing home for veterans. The youth learned quickly that they could punch holes in walls, climb into the space above dropped ceilings, and hide from staff in environmental blind spots. This arrangement significantly increased acuity and made behavior management extremely difficult.

Following the relocation, concerted efforts to reduce S&MR rates were initiated as follows (see Interventions B in Figures 1 and 2):

- *Aversive paperwork through an overcorrection-like policy.* Staff members were mandated to go beyond the customary documenta-

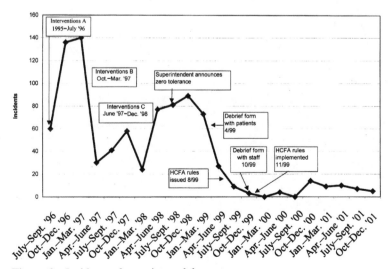

Figure 1   Incidents of restraint—adolescent.

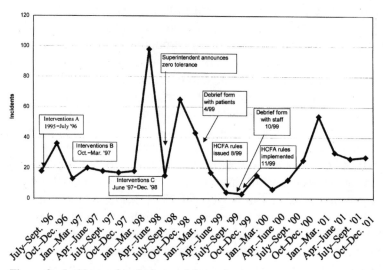

Figure 2   Incidents of seclusion—adolescent.

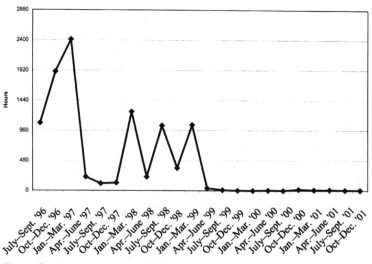

Figure 3   Restraint hours—adolescent.

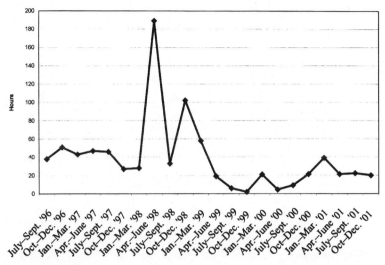

Figure 4 Seclusion hours—adolescent.

tion process with each S&MR incident. They were required to complete an additional form after each incident, indicating how S&MR would be avoided in the future.

- *Prevention training.* Staff received annual hospitalwide Conflict Prevention Institute (CPI©) training on early behavior awareness and nonphysical interventions. Booster CPI© sessions were provided to YS staff to review principles and, significantly, approved physical intervention techniques. The training emphasized anticipation of potentially explosive situations and use of techniques to lessen anxiety and agitation, thus preventing incidents likely to call for seclusion or restraint. A take-down procedure (known and used by many state hospital staff when confronting assaultive patients) was prohibited. This prohibition resulted in staff anger and feelings of frustration. The change in approach to violent patients required substantial effort by clinical leadership to demonstrate the utility and efficacy of the new approach.
- *Indiana Division of Mental Health mandate.* The state issued directives to decrease documented excessive S&MR rates.
- *Staff empowerment.* A model was implemented to give frontline staff more clinical responsibility and enhanced understanding of principles and practices of quality care through consultation

with senior clinicians. This initiative was unsuccessful and short-lived, due to the failure of both staff and senior clinicians to accept it.

The interventions described above had little lasting impact in lowering S&MR rates or attitudes towards their use during the early post-move years. The following interventions did change the culture and entrenched attitudes, and S&MR rates decreased slightly (see Interventions C, Figures 1 and 2).

Addressing Self-Injurious Behavior (SIB) Directly

Female adolescents who had been engaging in self-cutting and ingestion of various objects such as batteries, plastic knives and forks, and pieces of jewelry were being admitted in increasing numbers. Such SIB is particularly difficult to manage in a residential setting that houses adolescent females with borderline personality disorder psychopathology. Copycat behavior or imitation results in the behaviors becoming endemic. The adolescent unit implemented a program for borderline personality disorder symptoms to reduce SIB, a frequent precipitant to use of mechanical restraint. As a framework of intervention, we adopted a model described by Barstow (1995). The goals of the intervention are to assist the patient to identify feelings that precede the SIB and to develop higher self-esteem by identifying positive qualities conveyed about her by staff and peers. Staff assisted in this process by 1) encouraging the patient to identify thoughts preceding the SIB; 2) asking the patient to stop any SIB and move to a neutral location; 3) assisting the patient in identifying feelings that trigger negative cognitions and replacing them with positive ones; 4) helping the patient to cope by encouraging her to communicate thoughts and feelings rather than engaging in harmful behavior; 5) inviting her to participate in unit activities, volunteer work, or peer interactions to reduce social isolation; and 6) encouraging the patient to engage in self-care activities (e.g., grooming and hygiene) and to record daily thoughts and feelings in a journal.

Increasing Predictability

A YS-wide behavioral-level system was instituted in 1998 to increase staff consistency, to reward constructive and compliant patient behaviors, and to decrease destructive modeling by the sickest or angriest patients.

Decreasing Punitive Features of the Program

A consultant with expertise in behavioral management of group living helped us in 1996 define bottom-line behaviors, stop strategies, and group and community rewards. Prior to this, the program depended upon privileges of restricted buildings or ground passes as rewards (motivators) and room confinement or "chair time" as consequences for negative behaviors. Greater emphasis was placed on implementing this more positive approach.

Providing Additional, Alternative Programming

Recreational therapy staff increased gym time and outside activities. In a general hospital, pediatrics generally needs to exert considerable effort to get the environment, support services, and other resources appropriately allocated to meet the needs of their pediatric patients. A similar situation exists when a youth service is housed within a general psychiatric hospital. Ongoing initiatives are necessary to get scheduled, usable time in the gym, opportunities for progression of independent functioning in the hospital setting, and related support.

Obtaining More Outside Assistance

A reactivated advisory committee, comprised of members from consumer and advocacy groups, Indiana Division of Mental Health, University Schools of Education and Nursing, parents, and YS senior staff, provided guidance for modifying YS policies and procedures. The committee was highly critical of our programming and of the level system, which the members viewed as punitive and negative. They were especially dismayed by Level Red (the bottom level), which was used to restrict students with dangerous behavior from participation in programming. Our staff had commented that these difficult-to-treat patients were unable to achieve the points or behaviors required to access the positive constructive rewards or reinforcers available. The group also felt that there were too few differences in the upper levels of the system to be meaningful to the youngsters. Fine-tuning was done, and the level system appeared to work especially well for adolescent boys as privileges were tied directly to level attained.

Although significant changes were made, high S&MR rates persisted. Lack of change was attributed to an influx of particularly difficult patients, including clusters of females with serious SIB, along with especially large-for-their-age, violent, assaultive boys who generally felt abandoned by their families. These youngsters had learned to depend on restrictive, coercive measures as their means of self-control. They were highly resistant to accepting responsibility for their actions. Patient and staff injuries and external pressures catalyzed reassessment of our strategies and demanded development of new approaches to reduce S&MR rates to more acceptable levels. Additional measures were then introduced, as noted in the following sections.

Changing the Locus of Control over the Decision to Use S&MR

Any ongoing restrictive intervention (i.e., 24-hour mechanical restraint program for dangerous behavior) had to be cleared through the YS medical director. This mandate was meant to eliminate the practice of mechanically restraining assaultive boys and SIB girls with repetitive ingestion of foreign objects to the bed for extended periods.

S&MR Elimination as Mandate

A zero-tolerance policy for S&MR was announced by the superintendent in 1998, and in-service training was accelerated.

Medication as an Aid

The use of as-needed (PRN) medication was encouraged to help decrease the agitation and anger experienced by the youngsters before they lost complete control and to shape their ability to regain control. Considerable discussion took place to legitimize the use of PRN medication, particularly for situations in which the adolescent requested medication. Many RNs and other staff believed that such a patient request was akin to a manipulation of sorts and should not be honored. Others felt that if the teens had sufficient control and were aware enough to ask for a PRN, that they should then be able to exert the effort to calm themselves and seek alternative ways to manage their problems. Nurses were directed to give PRN medication when requested or when the patient's behavior was escalating to loss of control. They were also to note on the 24-hour sheet and elsewhere whether the PRN had been effective. Physicians became more willing to prescribe PRNs, and nurses ultimately began to administer PRNs with increasing frequency. As the youngsters were able to request PRN medication before they exploded, the incidence of S&MR seemed to decline.

Several dynamics may be operating in such a situation. These include a possible placebo effect (Vitiello, Ricciuti, and Behar, 1987; Vitiello et al., 1991; Petti et al., 2003) and the impact of the patients' feeling that they may be making a contribution to their care. The simple act of honoring their requests may enable or assist them to be more active in helping themselves. Being able to monitor oneself is the first step in change for most psychotherapies. This ability to recognize an internal state that can result in loss of control is a major step in the treatment process. In a later study specifically addressing perceptions of the PRN medications they received, most hospitalized youth felt that the PRN medication was helpful (Petti et al., 2003). Unfortunately, many felt that there was no viable option besides the medication to assist them from losing control and hurting someone or damaging things. We are currently studying these perceptions over a period of 12 weeks to begin to understand the meaning of PRN medications and how they may change over time.

More Meetings and Paperwork

Systematic reviews of the care plan were mandated for any patient requiring three seclusions or restraints in a period of one week. The expectation was that understanding of the behavior would be shared with staff and that alternatives to help the youth in the situation would be developed.

Despite such concerted efforts, the S&MR rate doubled between July 1998 and March 1999. The senior leaders then initiated a set of interventions that seemed to demonstrate positive results. The first and perhaps most important was instituted in April 1999.

Debriefing Questionnaire

A structured debriefing questionnaire was developed, piloted and administered to patients as soon after their S&MR incidents as possible. The instrument is found in Appendix 1. The patients were generally very cooperative in responding to the questions. A decrease in incidents followed.

Summary Data

Summary data of the youth perceptions of S&MR from April through September 1999 were presented to unit staff for feedback and discussion in October 1999. Ongoing presentation to staff of the data followed. However, it was decided to broaden the debriefing effort to include staff, the other side of the S&MR equation.

Interviews with Staff

An analogous instrument was developed to interview staff participating in the S&MR incidents (see Appendix 2). These interviews began shortly after the summary results of the patient survey interviews were presented to staff in October 1999. A dramatic reduction of S&MR rates followed (see October to December 1999 in each figure).

Responses to the survey by the youth and staff involved in S&MR episodes are of interest. The results and a lengthy discussion can be found in an earlier work (Petti et al., 2001). Safety was the major item on the minds of both the youth and staff. Over 50% of patients (33 definite and 11 somewhat less definite of the 81 responses) reported that the restrictive intervention resulted from assaultive behavior or verbal aggression. Staff reported safety as the basic reason for the use of seclusion or restraint in 53 of the 81 responses. Noncompliance with staff request was the reason for S&MR use given by 15 patients, and anger by 5 others. Sixteen youth could not or would not provide a perceived reason for the restriction.

In constructing the questionnaire, we were most interested in the question asking about alternatives that could have prevented the seclusion or restraint. The largest number of responses to this item was of the generic variety, representing 21 of the 81 respondents. Examples included "Could have done what staff said" (from a 14-year-old white male), and "Ignored everything" from a 17-year-old white female. Nine youth were more specific in the alternatives they suggested; for instance, "Apologize to Sara and handle myself and think before [I] act" from a 15-year-old white female. Compliance with staff requests was suggested by 23 of 81 respondents, with 12 being specific to the situation and 11 more generic (e.g., to obey and do what staff asked). Directives to staff were reported by four patients (e.g., "Talk to me"). The qualitative difference between generic and specific responses in these cases related to the evidence that the youth had given thought to actually linking the behavior and consequences to the alternative as compared to simply giving a rote response from discussions they had had with staff or from their therapy sessions.

It is encouraging that most of the patients' responses indicated that the solution to the situation should be with the teen himself or herself. The failure of the remaining 28 youth to give useful responses is a matter of concern, especially the 4 defiant responses ("Nothing; no one can help me when I'm angry"), the 10 coded denial or deflection ("I don't know" or "Leave me alone"), and the 4 non sequiturs ("I got a shot, I was held down"). Perhaps of even greater concern are the staff responses to the same question. Over half of the staff (9 members) blamed the patient, the system (9), or the medication level (7), whereas 10 staff members reported being at a loss as to what could have been done differently. Only 12 staff members accepted responsibility for finding an alternative solution, and an equal number had no recorded responses. Sadly, one staff member, with regard to the episode of a 12-year-old African American male, responded, "Nothing, really." A small percentage of such responses clearly indicated that much remained to be accomplished in this area.

When asked about what interventions were employed prior to the use of S&MR for the incident under discussion, discrepancies were noted between staff and patient perceptions. Because many patients responded with several answers for this question, more than 81 patient responses were coded. Confinement, broadly defined to include directing the patients to their room or quiet room by staff, was perceived to have been used by 37 youth as contrasted to 58 staff. Medication employed as a PRN was the intervention reported by 31 patients and 54 staff. Verbal interchange was reported by far more staff than patients. Therapeutic verbal interactions (e.g., one-to-one talks) were reported by 50 staff but only 18 youth; on the other hand, directives to behave from the staff were given as an answer by 21 staff and 9 youth. Other verbal interactions, such as verbal contracts and attempts to offer alternative activities, were reported by 21 staff. Coping skills are taught as a means to manage frustration or anger; five youth reported that deep breathing, counting to 10, and going off the unit to run were offered and attempted prior to the use of S&MR.

Given the horror stories surrounding the S&MR issues, including the number of deaths reported elsewhere with the use of seclusion or restraint in institutional settings (Ross, 1999), we queried youth and staff about the perceptions of safety during the seclusion or restraint process. Psychological adverse effects of S&MR have not been adequately researched. Feeling unsafe is a potential adverse effect of S&MR. Therefore, we wanted to determine if patients felt safe during the S&MR intervention. Even though 65% of patients reported that they had felt safe during the S&MR process, 25% said that they had not. Likewise, only 53% of staff reported feeling safe during the implementation of seclusion or restraint, with 36% reporting not feeling safe. No injury during the restrictive episode was reported by almost 75% of both patients and staff. Injury to staff or patient was reported by 12% of patients and 14% of staff. These findings have implications that require further exploration.

This study reveals the need to understand the underlying perceptions of both patients and staff concerning the use of seclusion or restraint. The employment of a formal debriefing process geared to the issues of relevance to our youth was highly useful in understanding the restrictive event and working with both youth and staff in developing more appropriate interventions. The form is no longer in use because the state has mandated that a uniform form be administered in the debriefing process. Though this statewide form is modeled after our interview, it contains extraneous questions that render it much less useful for our purposes.

Time-out frequently preceded loss of control, and we found this was of especial interest. Our inference is that time-out is often perceived as a form of punishment and isolation from support; this leads to increased anger and frustration. This reasoning is consonant with findings in younger children (Natta et al., 1990; Measham, 1995). As a result, we reexamined our policies and procedures regarding the use of time-out and assisted staff in understanding that time-out is an aversive consequence and may serve as a form of rejection for our youth. We were unable to determine the variables (e.g., tone of voice, demeanor, wording, or the directive itself) that could affect the manner in which the request or demand for taking a time out was made, or whether such factors influenced the perception of the time-out intervention that ultimately led to seclusion or restraint. We were also unable to determine the extent, if any, that a hands-on escort may have had on the subsequent need for a more restrictive intervention. These are questions that need to be considered in future studies in this area, because time-out has also been wholeheartedly embraced by milieu staff and families as a reasonable and effective intervention for agitated behavior. Children, however, prefer medication to time-out as a response to their inability to control themselves (Kazdin, 1984).

All of our efforts were occurring in a rapidly changing human services system. As we were making changes in the structure and process of our service delivery, JCAHO and HCFA were increasing the demand to eliminate restrictive practices in hospitals and residential centers.

Using Outside Pressure

The mandate to lower S&MR rates via the HCFA regulations (which were announced on August 1, 1999, and went into effect in November 1999) was duly noted. The hospital, along with all other entities receiving federal funding, significantly increased the effort invested in this task. An HCFA requirement limited the initiation of S&MR to a physician order, upon recommendation by a registered nurse, and mandated that a physician had to observe the patient within one hour after the youngster was placed into S&MR. The YS medical director also required physicians to routinely question any nursing request for S&MR orders with the following suggested list:

Have the staff:

1. Talked to the child in a quiet, neutral manner?
2. Asked the child what we can do to help him or her?
3. Suggested the usefulness of taking time to "chill out" and "get it back together"?
4. Offered a PRN?
5. Used a PRN?

Revamping the Level System

Considerable staff time and effort were devoted to modifying the level system for the middle school boys. With the patients offering their suggestions and feedback regarding various aspects of the changes, the program was simplified for this group and included an award chart. The program allowed the boys to earn points for appropriate behaviors on the half hour during waking hours. This change considerably reduced negative interactions with staff, reduced time out of school, and resulted in improved morale for the patients and staff.

Overall, the S&MR rates varied over the seven years, with notable peaks and valleys in response to changes in the hospital, changes in patient population, and admission of youngsters with challenging behavior. The trend in both rates and duration of S&MR is decidedly down. Periods of days and weeks without need for S&MR are common. Information collected prior to July 1996 has missing data points and cannot be considered. The average numbers of S&MR episodes by quarters from July 1996 through December 2001 are detailed in Figures 1 through 4. These data demonstrate the relationships between restrictive episodes, hours spent in each, and related injury rates for patients and staff. The data demonstrate substantial decreases in S&MR, even before the HCFA regulations were promulgated. Moreover, lower rates have been sustained since June 1999 and appear correlated with the initiation of formal, structured debriefing of patients and staff involved in S&MR episodes. Related injuries to patients and staff varied in association with changes in S&MR rates and demonstrated a slightly decreasing trend correlated with a decrease in both S&MR episodes and total hours. Change in mechanical restraint use is particularly dramatic. As noted above, the seclusion rate returned to low levels, except during periods when especially high-risk youth were admitted and then failed to become engaged in the program.

Our experience confirms an earlier report demonstrating that S&MR rates can be decreased even in a highly bureaucratized system (Singh et al., 1999). Goren, Abraham, and Doyle (1996) and Singh et al. (1999) decreased, then eliminated S&MR in their public, acute-care child and adolescent psychiatric hospital, which was threatened with a federal investigation regarding its excessive use of S&MR. This reduction was accomplished through planned programmatic change (i.e., implementing a number of interventions, including a discussion

102

team that empowered direct line staff). Our study employing a different approach demonstrates similar results in a much larger intermediate-term care state hospital that includes a youth service. Our population is likely more chronic and treatment resistant, given the intensity and extent of interventions, including the number of prior hospital admissions.

However, even with total commitment of professional staff and senior administrators, there is a tendency to revert back to old habits. This reversion to restrictive and coercive interventions may occur even as decreased injuries to patient and staff accompany decreases in S& MR rates. The failure to demonstrate a significant increase in staff injuries as anticipated by the staff as a result of the zero-tolerance policy is a critical finding. Such data indicate that the measures to reduce restrictive interventions may ultimately decrease injuries to both patients and staff. Such an effort requires attention to the home and community as well as the patient or resident and institution staff.

Eliminating restrictive practices except when absolutely needed remains the challenge. We have placed greater emphasis on working with families and communities before the actual hospital admission, to address the resistance of some families and community agencies to having the most violent and impulsive youngsters return to the home community from the hospital. The preadmission procedures mandated as a component of the admission process have helped to identify salient treatment issues, to determine which interventions have worked or might work to reduce agitation, and to outline disposition options and to assign responsibility should further residential care or alternative placement be required in order to avoid having the youth wait for funding to occur once the decision is made that the patient is ready for discharge from the hospital. This approach ensures quicker, appropriate disposition when maximum hospital benefit is achieved and decreases the too-often-observed plateau of gains followed by behavioral regression and need for S&MR when a youngster remains in the institutional setting beyond that time.

We have noted the frequently occurring phenomenon of plateauing, during which a youngster who has achieved the objectives of the hospitalization must remain hospitalized for some reason. This is usually related to our inability to secure funding for a less restrictive intervention or to the family's concern about their inability to manage the youth. The therapeutic and behavioral gains generally have been maintained for a finite period, but then the youth becomes discouraged and begins to use more primitive defenses to deal with the frustration and anxiety related to the lack of movement in returning home or back into the community. When the associated anxiety becomes too great, the youth regresses to earlier psychopathic behavior including aggression, violence, and destructive behavior. At that point in the hospitalization, under such circumstances, the need for seclusion or restraint is likely to recur. Having clear options for posthospital disposition is also important to alleviate the associated anxiety of patients who have done well but fear failing in the community. (This phenomenon is frequently experienced in nonhospitalized children with psychiatric disorders enrolled in special education when it is time for them to be mainstreamed back to their local schools.)

Hospital staff require frequent updates and boosters to maintain gains in improving the environment or milieu. Such updates include CPI© training; YS Advisory Committee feedback, structured interviews of those experiencing S&MR with feedback; level system review and inservices focused on specialized issues and populations (e.g., middle school boys and self-injuring adolescent girls). Creative strategies to assist those charged with direct care of these patients must be developed and tested to address the changing population of psychiatric patients admitted to hospitals and treatment centers. Altering established cognitive and behavioral patterns of patients and staff by modifying the culture in which they operate is difficult. The debriefing questionnaires have been used sporadically since completion of the original interventions because the modified form as noted above made it less useful and because S&MR rates maintained their decline. However, the modified form is used whenever rates begin to increase.

The findings relating S&MR episodes to the use of time-out in a quiet room resulted in attempts to find alternative solutions to disruptive behaviors before they elevate to the level of a restrictive intervention. Direction to take time in an unlocked room may be perceived as punitive by the youth and lead to escalation of dyscontrol by young adolescent psychiatric inpatients. Such perceived punitive or isolating staff behaviors towards them can be predicted to result in negative behavior by the youngsters (Natta et al., 1990). Employing an assessment of conditional probabilities of sequences of staff and child interaction, Natta and associates (1990) demonstrated with child psychiatric inpatients that positive staff behaviors tend not to be associated with subsequent changes in negative or positive patient behaviors. However, punitive and isolating behaviors (e.g., forced time-outs by staff holding the door) lead to decreases in child positive behaviors and increases in negative behaviors. Such negative behaviors in our study seemed to frequently precipitate seclusion. The relationship of holding the door and related coercive staff behaviors to increased restrictive interventions is tenuous but supported by the literature, even when safety is the issue (Singh et al., 1999). To associate it with regression in staff attitude towards condoning S&MR is speculative at best, because there are so many confounding variables. The more judicious use of time-out or isolation from the program will also need to be examined further.

Related S&MR issues are myriad and emotionally charged. Internal attempts to change the institutional culture exemplified by S&MR practice may be ineffective or brief unless accompanied by external threats or sanctions. Illustrations abound (Singh et. al., 1999). Our experience adds support to the value of external sanctions in encouraging residential programs to make necessary changes under a given set of circumstances. S&MR reduction was occurring in our case but might have been short-lived without the clout of HCFA regulations. There is no doubt that situations exist in which seclusion or mechanical restraint may be required (Singh et al., 1999; Troutman et al., 1998). The patient, Chantelle, described above and the case reported by Troutman and colleagues (1998) demonstrate the therapeutic value of mechanical restraints when applied judiciously.

Both Chantelle and the patient described by Troutman et al. (1998) were violent, aggressive, and explosive. Both cases demonstrate the utility of walking restraints to assure both safety and therapeutic caring. The danger associated with S&MR (Kennedy and Mohr, 2001) adds to the complexity of making the decision about when and when not to consider their use. The associated adverse effects of physical and/ or mechanical restraint have been recently reviewed (Mohr, Petti, and Mohr, 2003). Considerations such as psychological trauma with S& MR, or cardiac arrest, asphyxia, aspiration, and rhabdomyolysis (muscle breakdown) that can lead to death in adolescents as well as adults should be cause for concern and for reassessment of the use of mechanical restraint (Mohr et al., 2003). It is especially imperative that medical staff educate front-line caregivers concerning the adverse effects associated with the use of mechanical restraints or holding procedures. There is little in the literature concerning the effects of seclusion on adolescents. However, posttraumatic symptoms and lack of trust in mental health professionals have been reported by children and adolescents who have been physically restrained as a therapeutic measure in psychiatric facilities (Mohr, Mahon, and Noone, 1998). Traumatic symptoms were present in those same youngsters on 5-year follow-up (Mohr and Pumariega, 2002). In addition, deaths resulting from mechanical restraint or from holding techniques employed with younger children should be of serious concern; these require dissemination of information as we were able to do through grand rounds presentations.

The perceived need to find an effective response to increases in aggressive, assaultive, and self-injurious patients may explain critical attitude changes in nurses and nursing staff, over the past 25 years, related to limit-setting and restrictive authority. S&MR have become standard interventions in many facilities and have resulted in a change in culture from therapeutic milieu to one of coercion and quasi punishment. Because a rapid response to aggression or threat of such has been viewed as critical, the authority to initiate S&MR had moved from the physician and nurse and was increasingly delegated to front-line staff as a preventive measure against the imminent breakdown of a patient's self-control. Historically, the failure to act quickly when patients begin losing self-control was considered to undermine patient and staff morale. Employing restrictive interventions was seen as reassuring to all involved. Physicians, if asked to authorize these decisions, were faced with a dilemma when justification for a seclusion or restraint order was ambiguous or questionable. Physicians usually erred in favor of supporting staff. Advocacy groups believe the authority to initiate S&MR has been abused and is detrimental to patient welfare. Reestablishing physician authority, with the advice of nurses, to order S&MR played a deciding role in our ability to maintain the gains in reducing S&MR rates. The debriefing exercise provided a better understanding of the issues necessary to make needed changes in policies and procedures (Petti et al., 2001). A strength-based program of interventions proved successful, in conjunction with planned decreases in the S&MR rate to zero in one case report (Singh et al., 1999).

Many factors continue to operate that can threaten the success of maintaining and further reducing the attenuation of S&MR rates in our service. One of these factors is that staff feel that they have lost their most effective means of control when faced with psychotic or angry youngsters who feel the need to hurt or be punished (Millstein and Cotton, 1990). Ongoing staff training must be implemented to counteract such perceptions. This training needs to focus on detecting early signs of frustration or agitation that precipitate destructive or assaultive behavior, and on interventions to redirect the patient. This training must also assist staff in understanding the dynamics of a changing population admitted to psychiatric hospitals and the clinical skills that must be employed to divert violent behavior. Marohn (1992), for example, notes the need to consider violent adolescents' desire and need for affectionate contact, their lack of insight into their own psychological world, and their difficulties in differentiating thoughts from feelings and action in evaluation and treatment of the assaultive adolescent.

Leadership and staff involvement are also keys to reducing and eliminating unnecessary restrictive practice (Singh et al., 1999). Training and continuing education about the counterproductive nature of such coercive interventions as S&MR and their adverse effects must be offered. The reduction of injuries accompanying decreased S&MR use, noted in this chapter and the case study offered by Singh and associates (1999), must be emphasized. Likewise, the task of acute and intermediate-term hospitals, residential treatment centers, and schools in teaching youngsters to control themselves rather than to be controlled by others must be given the highest priority.

The following situation illustrates the manner in which early efforts can serve as the base for interventions when slippage occurs.

The adolescent boys' unit was experiencing a number of assaultive incidents resulting in restrictive consequences, including seclusion and restraint. The problematic behaviors included fighting, arguing, destruction of property, lack of respect for self and others, no investment in using therapy or groups for therapeutic benefit, and a decreased personal responsibility to make good choices. As a response to this increase in challenging behavior, members of the treatment team met to analyze environmental variables and to fashion a response to decrease dangerousness.

The tenor and thinking in the meeting reflected the work that had been accomplished in approaching challenging behavior in a more reflective and functional-analytic manner. The meeting began by identifying the four boys who were creating the majority of the violence and serving as provocateurs. Each boy's behavior was delineated into concrete descriptors, which could serve as target behaviors. In addition, environmental variables were identified that could be contributing to the milieu's deterioration. The team's discussion represented a more problem-solving and supportive approach, which echoed the in-services on positive behavior interventions and feedback from the debriefing questionnaires.

The team also brought to light that the provocateurs were receiving a greater portion of the attention than the patients who were complying with the program. This recognition of disproportionate differential reinforcement led the team to think about how to reward patients who were adhering to the program and how to assist those patients who were causing chaos. This shift in focus represented a dramatic change in behavior-change philosophy and strategies. The team recognized that intense support rather than intense punishment was the answer to meeting behavior challenges. This is not to say that restrictive measures are not necessary to contain dangerous and violent behavior, but such interventions require concomitant positive behavior-intervention strategies.

The team made a decision to increase supportive therapeutic interventions by instituting the following changes:

- *Helping program.* The boys were asked to help staff plan a program that would increase safety on the unit.
- *Peer monitoring program.* A staff member became a peer buddy for each boy who posed the greatest challenge. The staff agreed to see the patient each day and spend brief quality time together. One of the authors chose a boy who had a very violent history before admission to the hospital. The author met with the patient each day for brief talks, checked in to see how he was doing, and played checkers on a periodic basis. Since that time, this boy has increased his level and has had no occurrences of aggressive behavior. He was able to earn a home visit rather quickly after the mentoring began.
- *Intensive group programs.* The charge nurse on the boys' adolescent unit coordinated intensive programs for the most challenging patients. These programs were held off the unit, in the school area, to implement a divide-and-conquer strategy and to give the higher-functioning boys an opportunity to earn staff time and attention. The program consisted of groups for anger management, a focus group titled "stop the violence," social skills, manners, and physical activity. During the first week of implementation, no aggressive episodes occurred during the day. The program was then extended into evening programming.
- *Positive staff attitude.* Staff were asked to adopt an attitude that conveyed to the boys, "The new intensive program will work,

and everyone needs to support it." This request represented a united and positive front, conveying an attitude that was expected to become contagious for the boys.

- *Community meeting.* A community meeting with the boys and girls was held to discuss their perspective of the situation and how they could help to reduce dangerousness and violence.
- *Assignment of staff.* A special staff was identified for each shift to coordinate and direct requests from the boys. This assignment reduced staff splitting by the boys and increased consistency. The staff members were instructed to check with the primary staff person before granting any privileges or requests.
- *Privilege room.* A room that had been reserved for higher-functioning boys now became an activity room where staff could interact with those boys who were demonstrating self-control. This change increased the ability to engage the patients on a more frequent and sustained basis.
- *School programming.* A plan was put into place that would place a nursing staff member as an assistant in every classroom. The plan was partially in place at this time and was viewed as helpful in decreasing disruptive behavior and increasing academic engagement.
- *Consolidation of staff.* A plan was discussed to close two of four patient units during the day to increase the number of staff available to program patients who were sick or could not attend school or activities due to precautions.

Although these strategies are certainly not novel, they represented a change in thinking for this team and a more positive approach to programming for disruptive adolescent patients. The array of interventions reduced the coercive practices that often increase resistance and retaliation by patients. It was encouraging to see staff think about behavior differently and to focus on supportive interventions rather than on punitive ones. The psychiatrist must be prepared to facilitate and support such a process in order for an appropriate intervention to be implemented.

As the authority of physicians and nurses is being reasserted into the process of initiating restrictive interventions in hospitals, day treatment, and residential treatment centers, the psychiatrist and other team leaders must continue to address the moral, ethical, and clinical factors influencing S&MR. We must continue to develop innovative strategies to study S&MR parameters, reasons for the use of restrictive practices, and outcomes of S&MR implementation that will inform and guide current and future practice. However, restrictive interventions need to be available when truly needed in situations where safety of patients and staff are at risk. This position has been supported by a leading advocate for the mentally ill (Ross, 1999). Guidelines for the use of restrictive interventions and development of a culture that questions the efficacy of such practice will be critical in assuring that S&MR are used only for emergency purposes. Internal and external pressure for change within facilities and professions may be required to effect such change.

REFERENCES

American Academy of Child and Adolescent Psychiatry (2002), Practice parameter for the prevention and management of aggressive behavior in child and adolescent psychiatric institutions, with special reference to seclusion and restraint. *J. Amer. Acad. Child & Adol. Psychiat.*, 41(2S):4S–25S.

American Psychiatric Association. (2001), HCFA issues rules on restraints with amendments to ease staffing requirements. *Psychiat. Serv.*, 52:986.

Barstow, D. G. (1995), Self-injury and self-mutilation. *J. Psychiat. Nurs.*, 33(2):19–22.

Cotton, N. (1989), The developmental-clinical rationale for the use of seclusion in the psychiatric treatment of children. *Amer. J. Orthopsychiat.*, 59:442–449.

Gair, D. G. (1980), Limit-setting and seclusion in the psychiatric hospital. *Psychiat. Opinion*, February: 15–19.

Garrison, W. T., Ecker, M. A., Friedman, M. D., Davidoff, M. D., Haeberle, K. & Wagner, M. (1990), Aggression and counteraggression during child psychiatric hospitalization. *J. Amer. Acad. Child & Adol. Psychiat.*, 29:242–250.

Goren, S., Abraham, I. & Doyle, N. (1996), Reducing violence in a child psychiatric hospital through planned organizational change. *J. Child & Adol. Psychiat. Nurs.*, 9:27–36.

Kazdin, A. (1984), Acceptability of aversive procedures and medication as treatment alternatives for deviant child behavior. *J. Abnorm. Child Psychol.*, 12:289–302.

Kennedy, S. S. & Mohr, W. K. (2001), A prolegomenon on restraint of children: Implicating constitutional rights. *Amer. J. Orthopsychiat.*, 71:26–37.

Marohn, R. C. (1992), Management of the assaultive adolescent. *Hosp. Community Psychiat.*, 43:622–624.

Measham, T. J. (1995), The acute management of aggressive behavior in hospitalized children and adolescents. *Can. J. Psychiat.*, 40:330–336.

Millstein, K. H. & Cotton, N. S. (1990), Predictors of the use of seclusion on an inpatient child psychiatric unit. *J. Amer. Acad. Child & Adol. Psychiat.*, 29:256–264.

Mohr, W. K., Mahon, M. M. & Noone, M. J. (1998), A restraint on restraints: The need to reconsider restrictive interventions. *Arch. Psychiat. Nurs.*, 12:95–106.

—— Petti, T. A. & Mohr, B. D. (in press), Adverse effects associated with the use of physical restraint. *Can. J. Psychiat.*

—— & Pumariega, A. J. (2002), Post restraint sequelae five years out: Concerns and policy implications. In: *The 14th Annual Research Conference Proceedings, A System of Care for Children's Mental Health: Expanding the Research Base,* ed. C. Newman, C. J. Liberton, K. Kutash & R. M. Friedman. Tampa: University of South Florida, pp. 437–439.

Natta, M. B., Holmbeck, G. N., Kupst, M. J., Pines, R. J. & Schulman, J. L. (1990), Sequences of staff–child interactions on a psychiatric inpatient unit. *J. Abnorm. Child Psychol.*, 18:1–14.

Petti, T. A., Mohr, W. K., Somers, J. & Sims, L. (2001), Perceptions of seclusion and restraint by patients and staff in an intermediate-term care facility. *J. Child & Adol. Psychiat. Nurs.*, 14:115–117.

—— Stigler, K., Gardner-Haycox, J., & Dumlao, S. (2003), Perceptions of p.r.n. psychotropic medications by hospitalized child and adolescent recipients. *J. Am. Acad. Child & Adol. Psychiat.*, 42:434–441.

Ross, E. C. (1999), Death by restraint. *Behav. Healthcare Tomorrow*, 9:21–23.

Singh, N. N., Singh, S. D., Davis, C. M., Latham, L. L. & Ayers, J. G. (1999), Reconsidering the use of seclusion and restraints in inpatient child and adult psychiatry. *J. Child & Fam. Stud.*, 8:243–253.

Troutman, B., Myers, K., Borchardt, C., Kowalski, R. & Bubrick, J. (1998), Case study: When restraints are the least restrictive alternative for managing aggression. *J. Amer. Acad. Child & Adol. Psychiat.*, 37:554–558.

Vitiello, B., Hill, J. L., Elia, J., Cunningham, E., McLeer, S. V. & Behar, D. (1991), P.r.n. medications in child psychiatric inpatients: A pilot placebo-controlled study. *J. Clin. Psychiat.,* 52:499–501.

———, Ricciuti, A. J. & Behar, D. (1987), P.r.n. medications in child state hospital inpatients. *J. Clin. Psychiat.,* 48:351–354.

Zusman, J. (1997), *Restraint and Seclusion: Improving Practice and Conquering the JCAHO Standards.* Marblehead, MA: Opus Communications.

Appendix 1. Debriefing Questionnaire
PATIENT'S VIEW

A clinical staff member (not directly involved with the incident) should interview the patient and complete this form within 24 hours of the conclusion of each incident of seclusion or restraint.

Interviewer: _____ **Date of Interview:** _____

Patient Name: _____ **Date/Time of Incident:** _____
Restraint/Seclusion

Staff Involved:

---

1. Explain the reason restraint or seclusion was used.
   Patient's view:

2. What could have been done to prevent the use of restraint/ seclusion?
   Patient's view:

3. What alternatives were provided prior to the use of restraint/ seclusion?
   Patient's view:

4. Did you receive: (Circle)
   A. PRN Medication   Before   During   After   NA
   B. Explanation of reason for use of restraint/ seclusion   YES   NO
   C. Explanation of release criteria   YES   NO

5. Did you (patient) feel safe while you were restrained/
   secluded?   YES   NO
   (If no, provide explanation)

6. Were you (patient) injured during the use of restraint/seclusion?
   (Patient)   YES   NO

7. Was your dignity and privacy respected during the use of
   restraint/seclusion? (If no, provide explanation)
   Patient's view: YES   NO

DATE REVIEWED BY TREATMENT TEAM: _____

Actions taken: (Circle)

   1. Modification of treatment plan
   2. Change in Medication
   3. Other alternatives identified
   4. None required at this time
   5. Other _____

Appendix 2. Debriefing Questionnaire
STAFF'S VIEW

A clinical staff member (not directly involved with the incident) should interview the staff involved and complete this form within 24 hours of the conclusion of each incident of seclusion or restraint.

Interviewer: _____ **Date of Interview:** _____

Patient Name: _____ **Date/Time of Incident:** _____
Restraint/Seclusion

Staff Involved/Interviewed:

_____

(circle staff interviewed)

1. Explain the reason restraint or seclusion was used.
   Staff's view:

2. What could have been done to prevent the use of restraint/ seclusion?
   Staff's view:

3. What alternatives were provided prior to the use of restraint/ seclusion?
   Staff's view:

4. Did the patient receive: (Circle)
   A. PRN Medication   Before   During   After   NA
   B. Explanation of reason for use of restraint/
      seclusion   YES   NO
   C. Explanation of release criteria   YES   NO

5. While restraining/secluding the patient, did you (staff) feels safe?   YES   NO
   (If no, provide explanation)

6. Was staff injuring during the use of restraint/seclusion?
   Staff's view: YES   NO

7. Was the patient's dignity and privacy respected during the use of restraint/seclusion? (If no, provide explanation)
   Staff's view: YES   NO

Submit completed forms to the Service Line Manager.

1999

5 EARLY RECOGNITION AND DIFFERENTIATION OF PEDIATRIC SCHIZOPHRENIA AND BIPOLAR DISORDER

MANI N. PAVULURI, PHILIP G. JANICAK,
MICHAEL W. NAYLOR, AND JOHN A. SWEENEY

Pediatric schizophrenia (Volkmar, 1996; Kumra, 2000) and pediatric bipolar disorder (Lewinsohn, Klein, and Seeley, 1995) are uncommon disorders with incidence rates of approximately 1%. Both are chronic illnesses associated with severe psychosocial morbidity (Werry, McClellan, and Chard, 1991; Andreasen, 1999; McClellan et al., 1999) and high utilization of mental health services (Murray and Lopez, 1996). It is often difficult to differentiate pediatric schizophrenia (PS) and pediatric bipolar disorder (PBD), especially in cases where symptoms of psychosis predominate. The distinction is important, however, given that PS and PBD respond to different psychopharmacological interventions, and PBD has a better long-term outcome (Werry et al., 1991; McClellan et al., 1999). Several studies comparing PS and PBD phenotypes indicate a strong bias against diagnosing bipolar disorder in youth (Joyce, 1984; Werry et al., 1991; Carlson, Fennig, and Bromet, 1994; Carlson, Bromet, and Sievers, 2000). This is illustrated by a major follow-up study in which earlier results (Kydd and Werry, 1982) were proclaimed invalid when about half of the schizophrenic cases were subsequently rediagnosed as bipolar disorder (Werry et al., 1991). In this study, 61 hospitalized children with initial diagnoses of schizophrenia, schizophreniform psychosis, bipolar disorder, schizoaffective disorder, or psychotic depression were evaluated. All those with follow-up diagnoses of schizophrenia had been correctly identified, but this was not the case in bipolar disorder, for which the initial diagnosis was frequently schizophrenia. This also explains the results of the initial study, which suggested a good outcome for schizophrenia in children under 16 years of age, associated with higher premorbid level of functioning, rapid onset of illness, and the presence of affective symptoms (Kydd and Werry, 1982). Furthermore, with the advent of recent data, there is another challenge to differentiate PBD from attention-deficit hyperactivity disorder (Wozniak et al., 1995; Biederman et al., 1996; Geller et al., 1998; Geller et al., in press). This will be briefly addressed in the "Recognition of Pediatric Bipolar Disorder" section. Apart from criteria that help to recognize and differentiate these disorders at a very young age, there is now evidence that even prodromal symptoms of psychosis can be identified (McGlashan, 1998; McGorry, 2000). It is uncertain, however, how accurately PS and PBD can be differentiated at this prodromal stage. This chapter reviews the critical issues in recognizing PS, PBD, and their prodromal symptoms, and how best to differentiate them.

Included are results from key studies that characterize the following:

1. Pediatric schizophrenia
2. Prodromal symptoms of pediatric schizophrenia
3. Pediatric bipolar disorder
   a) Prepubertal and early-adolescent-onset bipolar disorder
   b) Adolescent onset
4. Prodromal symptoms of pediatric bipolar disorder

RECOGNITION OF PEDIATRIC SCHIZOPHRENIA

Pediatric schizophrenia, also referred to as childhood-onset schizophrenia (Alaghband-Rad et al., 1995) or very-early-onset schizophrenia (Werry et al., 1991), is characterized by psychotic symptoms at or before 12 years of age. Phenomenological, neuroimaging, other biological, and outcome data found PS to be continuous with the later-onset disorder (Frazier et al., 1996; Jacobsen and Rapoport, 1998). Furthermore, PS resembles poor-outcome adult cases with a more severe premorbid course (Watkins, Asarnow, and Tanguay, 1988; Asarnow et al., 1994).

Symptoms and course are the two defining features of this disorder in both children and adults. *DSM-IV-TR* criteria (American Psychiatric Association, APA, 2000) include delusions, hallucinations, and thought disorder. The remaining symptoms (such as disorganized behavior, negative symptoms, and impaired functioning) are nonspecific in very young children. Poor motivation, silly or disorganized behavior, and declining or lower school grades cannot be specifically attributed to schizophrenia in a developing child. For such a diagnosis, the six-month duration of illness criterion sets a high bar for diagnosis in children, unless symptoms are severe and persistent (Werry et al., 1991). Therefore, the emphasis remains on the precise recognition of core symptoms to make a definitive diagnosis.

Age-Specific Presentation of Core Features

Delusions. Delusions are present in 54% to 63% (Kolvin, 1971; Green et al., 1984; Russell, Bott, and Sammons, 1989) of youth with PS. The delusions tend to be simple and less elaborate in young children than in adults. Persecutory, somatic, bizarre, and grandiose delusions are predominant, with child-oriented themes involving monsters, pets, toys, and family members (Russell et al., 1989). Clinical examples include: "Mom is mixing the cleaning agent in my milk and poisoning me," "Electricity is going through my body," "There is a devil in my dog," and "They are talking about me." Often, the child may shout at the suspected people.

Hallucinations. Auditory hallucinations, seen in 79% to 82% of patients with PS, are the most common psychotic symptoms (Kolvin, 1971; Green et al., 1984; Russell et al., 1989). Visual hallucinations are the second most common type of perceptual abnormality in 30% to 46% and are almost exclusively seen in patients who also experience auditory hallucinations (Russell et al., 1989). Children are less able to describe them, and they also tend to be less complex and nonaffective in nature. Examples include seeing "bad guys in white suits"; feeling as though "a shadow is following"; seeing eyes move across the room along with one eye and a leg; hearing unfriendly voices; changing volume of auditory hallucinations, normal conversations, and moving cars; hearing footsteps behind, which become louder and then gradually softer; seeing geometric figures and white circles.

Thought disorder. There is some variability in the prevalence of thought disorder, with estimates varying between 40% and 100%, depending on the definition used (Kolvin, 1971; Green et al., 1984; Russell et al., 1989; Caplan, 1994). Thought disorder has been variously defined as incoherence, marked loosening of associations, talking past the point, derailment, and illogical thinking. The concept of thought disorder in childhood links the loosening of associations with distractibility and illogicality with poor abstract thinking (Caplan, 1994). Impaired maturation of underlying cognitive and linguistic skills can be reflected outwardly as developmental delays and persistent formal thought disorder, which differs from the episodic worsening of thought disorder seen in adult schizophrenia. Deficits in information processing and abstract thinking (Asarnow et al., 1994), in combination with other psychotic symptoms, may manifest as disorganized thinking. Poverty of thought content and incoherence may be less frequent (Russell et al., 1989). An example of formal thought disorder is as follows: "I am not a city person; I would like to live in a country because the city is noisy. Country has big roads, animals; I hate snakes, though. When the snake comes in one way, I go in the opposite direction. When the truck ran over the snake, the snake was about to bite. Teresa is weird. Teresa and I went into the bush and she got really scared. I always check if there is a snake and walk the other way; you are not supposed to scare the snake, then it won't hurt you. What did you *ask*?"

Associated Features of PS

Specific developmental disabilities.   Approximately half of those with PS have some form of developmental delay, with speech and language the most commonly delayed milestones (Kolvin, 1971; Green et al., 1984; Alaghband-Rad et al., 1995).

Delay in language development.   Common problems include articulation delays and stuttering. Expressive and mixed expressive and receptive language delay are seen in up to 40%, with a significant delay in spoken language. In a study of 61 consecutively admitted youth with PS, Hollis (1995) compared subjects with childhood-onset (age 7 to 13) and adolescent-onset (age 14 to 17) PS to clarify the pattern of age- and gender-based variations in developmental impairment. He found that impaired language and speech development were significantly higher in childhood-onset schizophrenia than in adolescent-onset schizophrenia. There was no significant difference in the occurrence and pattern of psychotic symptoms or other developmental problems such as motor or social impairment. There was no evidence to support gender-based differences in developmental impairment (Alaghband-Rad et al., 1995; Hollis, 1995).

Borderline to low-average IQ (range of 60–135). School-performance-based intelligence estimates show generally low-normal IQ (Alaghband-Rad et al., 1995). Often, prepsychotic IQ testing is not available to examine any cognitive decline secondary to the disorder, but in patients for whom results from multiple testing was available, no deterioration in the cognitive functioning was noted.

Insidious onset. More than half of the children with PS have an insidious onset. In one study that attempted to retrace the prodromal period after first hospitalization for psychosis, duration was up to 90 weeks in schizophrenia and schizophreniform psychoses, compared with only 19 weeks in bipolar disorder (Yung and McGorry, 1996).

Period of depression. In the prodromal and residual phases of an acute psychotic episode, a period of depression (Werry et al., 1991; Yung and McGorry, 1996) has frequently been described.

Comorbid Features

Transient early symptoms of autism are often reported, with motor stereotypies such as hand flapping, head banging, and hand flicking the most prominent. Disruptive behavior disorders including attention-deficit/hyperactivity disorder (ADHD), oppositional-defiant disorder (ODD), and conduct disorder (CD) are commonly reported even prior to the diagnosis of PS (Alaghband-Rad et al., 1995). Other associated conditions include motor skills disorder and academic skills disorder (termed in DSM-IV TR as developmental coordination disorder and learning disorder, respectively). As a result, special education placement is required in up to 65% of these children (Alaghband-Rad et al., 1995; McClellan et al., 1999).

Prodromal Symptoms of PS

Recognizing the prodromal features of PS is important to quickly establish the diagnosis for the following reasons:

- *Early antipsychotic intervention* may be associated with a better long-term outcome (Helgason, 1990; Wyatt, Damiani, and Henter, 1998; Gunduz et al., 1999; Schroder et al., 1999; McGorry, 2000). With the advent of the second-generation antipsychotics and their lower rate of certain side effects, early intervention has become more acceptable.
- *The deficit process* (negative symptoms) is usually present at the first psychotic episode (McGlashan and Johanssen, 1996). This may mean that the deficit process begins prior to the onset of illness as currently defined.
- *Severe distress for the family* often results from early presentation of psychosis, and family members usually request treatment, as well.

In an attempt to identify prodromal symptoms of PS, Alaghband-Rad et al. (1995) retrospectively examined the premorbid clinical characteristics of those diagnosed with schizophrenia using *DSM-III-R* criteria (APA, 1987). They found the following to be common: social withdrawal, impaired school performance, markedly peculiar behavior, impaired hygiene, blunted inappropriate affect, vagueness/poverty of speech, odd magical thinking or perceptions, and marked lack of initiative.

Currently, research efforts focus on the prospective examination of prodromal symptoms of PS (McGlashan, 1998; McGorry, 2000; Woods, Miller, and McGlashan, 2001). Theoretically, the term psychotic disorder includes schizophrenia and psychotic mood disorders. But a bias exists toward applying this term to schizophrenia, as reflected by the content of the screening instruments designed to identify early psychotic and prepsychotic features. McGlashan (1998) and McGorry (2000) have used any one of these three key criteria to identify the prodrome:

1. *Brief intermittent psychosis*: One or more positive symptoms of psychosis such as hallucinations, suspiciousness, or unusual

thought content (scores of greater than 3 or 4 on these items on the Brief Psychiatric Rating Scale—BPRS) in the last three months, for at least several minutes a day, once a month.

2. *Attenuated positive symptoms*: At least one of the symptoms of schizotypal disorder and one of the symptoms of psychosis such as hallucinations, suspiciousness, or unusual thought content in subdued form (lower scores of 1 or 2 on these items on BPRS) in the past year and present at least once per week in the last month.

3. *Genetic risk and recent deterioration*: Having a first-degree relative with a history of any psychotic disorder or schizotypal personality disorder and a drop of more than 30 points on global assessment of functioning (GAF) for at least one month.

Using these criteria, 43% converted to the full disorder over 24 months in McGorry's (2000) sample and 50% in McGlashan's (1998) sample.

There are two major differences between these two studies. McGorry (1998, 2000) focused on ages 16 to 30 years and included affective psychoses, whereas McGlashan (1998) included a wider age range (12 to 45 years) and excluded affective psychoses from the target group. The term ultra-high-risk subjects is favored over the term prodrome by McGorry (2000), as it does not imply inevitable progress into a disorder; the term prodrome is typically used by McGlashan (1998). None of these at-risk or prodromal studies include measures that can identify affective symptoms characteristic of PBD despite compelling evidence that psychosis is common in PBD (Joyce, 1984; Werry et al., 1991; Carlson et al., 1994; Geller et al., 1998; McClellan et al., 1999; Carlson et al., 2000).

RECOGNITION OF PEDIATRIC BIPOLAR DISORDER

As the phenomenology of PBD was clarified, phenotypic age-based differences became apparent (see Table 1). Prepubertal bipolar disorder is variably termed prepubertal and early-adolescent-onset bipolar disorder (PEA-BD) (Geller et al., 1998), atypical bipolar disorder, or juvenile bipolar disorder (Wozniak et al., 1995; Biederman et al., 1996). PEA-BD predominantly refers to subjects less than 12 years of age. Adolescent-onset bipolar disorder (AO-BD) is more classic in presentation (Lewinsohn et al., 1995; Strober et al., 1995; McClellan et al., 1999),

TABLE 1

AGE-BASED COMPARISON OF PEDIATRIC BIPOLAR DISORDER (PBD)

Features	Prepubertal and Early-Adolescent-Onset Bipolar Disorder (PEA-BD)	Adolescent-Onset Bipolar Disorder (AOBD)
Irritable mood	Prominent (up to 98%)	Less prominent (up to 22%)
Interepisode recovery	Low (0–16%)	Moderate (20–50%)
Episodic versus chronic	Chronic	Episodic
Cycling	Ultradian	Rapid
Mixed	20–85%	Up to 25%
Common comorbid disorders	Attention deficit/hyperactivity disorder, oppositional-defiant disorder	Substance abuse, anxiety disorders, posttraumatic stress disorder

resembling adult bipolar disorder (Goodwin and Jamison, 1990), and commonly refers to youth older than 12. There are, however, similarities across the life span in the incidence of critical symptoms that define bipolar disorder, such as elated mood, irritability, and psychotic features (Geller et al., in press).

Prepubertal and Early-Adolescent-Onset Bipolar Disorder

Compared to AO-BD, PEA-BD presents with atypical, partially formed symptom complexes; a chronic disabling course; greater cognitive difficulties (Wozniak et al., 1995); and ultradian cycling (cycling within a day) (Geller et al., 1998; Geller et al., press). Psychosis is seen in 16% to 60% (Wozniak et al., 1995; Geller et al., 1998) of patients with PEA-BD. For example, Geller et al. (1998; in press) found grandiose delusions in 55% of their prepubertal manic sample. They propose the presence of either grandiosity or elated mood as essential for the diagnosis of mania, as opposed to irritability or elated mood as necessary in DSM-IV-TR.

124

ADHD and ODD are the two most common comorbid conditions in PEA-BD (Wozniak et al., 1995; Biederman et al., 1996; Geller et al., 1998). Although there is a high rate of overlap in symptoms of ADHD and PBD, five symptoms clearly distinguish PEA-BD from ADHD. They are elated mood, grandiosity, racing thoughts/flight of ideas, sleep disturbance, and hypersexuality. Identification of the primary disorder, age-related idiosyncrasies, and common comorbid conditions will lead to more effective treatment.

Adolescent-Onset Bipolar Disorder

AO-BD is underdiagnosed because euphoria, depression, and irritability are minimized or overlooked in 50% to 75% of youth with this disorder (Joyce, 1984; Werry et al., 1991; Carlson et al., 2000). Mixed episodes, more commonly presented in PBD, are particularly difficult to diagnose. Youth who present with mixed symptoms of mania and depression are often misdiagnosed with psychosis not otherwise specified, drug-induced psychosis, schizoaffective disorder, schizophreniform disorder, or brief reactive psychosis (Carlson et al., 2000). Although the symptoms of psychosis were recognized, the affective symptoms were not formulated as acute mania by community clinicians writing the discharge summaries (Carlson et al., 1994). Carlson hypothesized that this could be due to the severity of psychosis camouflaging the affective symptoms. Similar results can be deduced from a recent NIMH study of childhood-onset schizophrenia (Calderoni et al., 2001). In that study, 33 of 215 patients referred with PS were found to have psychotic mood disorders on structured interviewing. Furthermore, the follow-up data indicate that none of the subjects rediagnosed with mood disorders developed a clinical course resembling schizophrenia.

Prodromal Symptoms of PBD

Data thus far have emphasized the primacy of affective symptoms compared with prepsychotic symptoms as prodromal to PBD. Two approaches have been taken to identify the prodromal symptoms for PBD: retrospective studies of psychiatrically hospitalized youth ultimately diagnosed as having bipolar disorder (Egeland et al., 2000) and prospective examination of offspring of patients diagnosed with bipolar disorder (Fergus, 1999; Chang, Steiner, and Ketter, 2000; Wals et al., 2001). Egeland et al. (2000) studied the symptoms documented prior to the first hospital admission for bipolar disorder in a group of Amish patients. They reported high rates of episodic changes in mood (depression and irritability) and periods of increased energy plus anger dyscontrol. No gender differences were found in the distribution of symptoms. Many of these children were reported to be exquisitely sensitive and hyperalert to the feelings of others, both peers and adults alike. Rapid extreme changes from quiet to bold, as well as loud and hostile behavior were noted in many. The investigators found that the frequency of symptoms increased between the ages of 13 and 15. The average interval between the appearance of the first symptoms and the onset of a documented episode of bipolar disorder was 9 to 12 years.

Chang et al. (2000), looking at an offspring sample of bipolar patients, showed an increased rate of depressed and irritable mood (mixed), lack of affect modulation, and rejection sensitivity. The prodromal symptom profile they described was very similar to that found in the Amish study.

Yung and McGorry (1996) explored prodromal symptoms using a retrospective interview in an older sample of 16- to 30-year-olds soon after recovery from the first episode of psychotic bipolar disorder and schizophrenia. They found that sleep disturbance (100%), change in sense of self/world (87.5%), irritability (75%), depressed mood (75%), increased energy (75%), and a deterioration in role functioning (62.5%) usually preceded an acute episode of the 16- to 30-year-olds' bipolar disorder. Prodromal symptoms of schizophrenia resembled that of bipolar disorder in terms of sleep disturbance, irritability, and depression. Increased energy, elated mood, impulsivity, and increased activity were prominent in the prodrome of bipolar disorder. In contrast, social withdrawal and poor motivation were common in the prodrome of schizophrenia.

Efforts were made to address the ultra-high-risk group that includes less well-formed, attenuated, or intermittent symptoms among prepsychotic patients leading to schizophrenia. But similar attempts were not made to include symptoms of affect dysregulation to identify ultra-high-risk symptoms of bipolar disorder. Most of the prospective studies on very early recognition of PBD focused on offspring samples alone, where there was a clear genetic risk factor. It may be meaningless to widen the net of studying affect dysregulation alone, because it is a common thread in many disorders (e.g., reactive attachment disorder, borderline personality disorder, intermittent explosive disorder, and ODD).

Following the model used in detecting early psychosis, targeting the ultra-high-risk population is possible by developing measures to identify core and associated symptoms of PBD, including subjects who do not meet the full criteria (e.g., bipolar disorder not otherwise specified), not interpreting psychotic symptoms as pathognomonic of schizophrenia, and including children with a genetic risk for bipolar disorder.

PS AND PBD: SIMILARITIES AND DIFFERENCES

The major areas of clinical overlap between PS and PBD are symptoms of psychosis and chronicity.

Psychosis

The most common overlapping symptom is psychosis. Although it is the central feature of PS and is commonly seen in PBD, psychosis is not essential to the diagnosis of PBD. Furthermore, the frequency and type of psychotic symptom can differentiate PS and PBD. For example, in one study involving adults, tangential speech, driveling, neologisms, and paraphasia were present in up to 8% of patients with mania and 45% with schizophrenia. By contrast, flight of ideas was more common in bipolar disorder (75%) than schizophrenia (52%). Regardless of the nature of the thought disorder, manic patients responded better to treatment than schizophrenic patients (Jampala, Taylor, and Abrams, 1989). In children, schizophrenialike formal thought disorder may also be present in PBD (Caplan et al., 2000; Ulloa, Birmaher, and Axelson, 2000). The most common diagnoses in children and adolescents experiencing hallucinations and/or delusions are major depression, bipolar disorder, and, less often, schizophrenia (Kumra, 2000; Ulloa et al., 2000). Auditory hallucinations are particularly common in youth with major depression predisposed to develop bipolar disorder (Chambers et al., 1982; Birmaher et al., 1996). Furthermore, the presence of psychosis in bipolar disorder adversely affects prognosis in adults (Tohen et al., 1990). For example, the probability of remaining in remission for at least six months was 66% for patients with psychotic features, compared with 88% for patients without psychotic features. Among those with psychotic features, the highest risk of relapse was 90% for mood-incongruent symptoms and 60% for mood-congruent symptoms (Tohen, Tsuang, and Goodwin, 1992).

Chronicity

The chronic course usually associated with schizophrenia is attributed to negative symptoms, poor premorbid functioning, persistent positive psychotic features, mood-incongruent delusions and hallucinations, and loosening of associations. Although psychotic symptoms can be similar in PS and PBD, it takes longer for psychosis to resolve in youth with PS than in those with PBD (Werry et al., 1991). Longitudinal course and level of functioning is traditionally considered to be critical in differentiating bipolar disorder from schizophrenia across the life span, with a poorer prognosis associated with schizophrenia (Goodwin and Jamison, 1990; Werry et al., 1991; McClellan et al., 1999; Carlson et al., 2000). However, recent findings indicate that chronic ultrarapid cycling is also an indicator of poor prognosis in PEA-BD despite the absence of negative symptoms. Thus, a one year follow-up study that looked at PEA-BD reported a 37.1% recovery defined by symptomatic and functional improvement, and a 38.3% relapse rate in one year (Geller et al., 2001). It is unclear if the poor prognosis was due to a lack of organized treatment for the study subjects or to the inherently malignant course of PEA-BD.

Psychotic features, mood symptoms, family history, course, and functional impairment in PS and PBD are compared in Table 2.

CONCLUSION

PS is characterized by mood-incongruent hallucinations and delusions, formal thought disorder, insidious onset, chronic course, and associated developmental delays and abnormalities. Although PS is a severe variant with relatively poor prognosis, it is continuous with adult-onset schizophrenia.

Findings in the last decade characterize PEA-BD by irritability, mixed mania and depression, ultradian cycling, and chronic course.

TABLE 2
DIFFERENTIATING FEATURES OF PEDIATRIC
SCHIZOPHRENIA AND BIPOLAR DISORDER

Features	Pediatric Schizophrenia (PS)	Pediatric Bipolar Disorder (PBD)
Delusions	> Incongruent[abcd]	> Congruent[gh]
Grandiose delusions	11%[d]	50%[h]
Hallucinations	80%[d]	23%[i]
Thought disorder	> Loosening of associations[abcd]	Pressure of speech[h]
Nonpsychotic	7%[e]	25%[e]
Mood symptoms	Depression in prodromal and residual phase[f]	Prominent irritability, elated mood, depression, and mixed[ihj]
Family history	Less homotypic[f]	More homotypic[f]
Chronic impairment	> 90%[e]	25–40%[ghk]
Episodic	Not episodic[e]	Adolescent-onset bipolar disorder: 20–50%[eg] Prepubertal and early-adolescent-onset bipolar disorder: 0–16%[hl]

[a]Kolvin, 1971
[b]Green et al., 1984
[c]Watkins, Asarnow, and Tanguay, 1988
[d]Russell, Bott, and Sammons, 1989
[e]McClellan et al., 1999
[f]Werry, McClellan, and Chard, 1991

[g]Carlson, Bromet, and Sievers, 2000
[h]Geller et al., in press
[i]Geller et al., 1995
[j]Strober et al., 1995
[k]Wozniak et al., 1995
[l]Findling et al., 2001

AO-BD appears to be more episodic and closely resembles the adult-variant of bipolar disorder.

Careful examination and follow-up of children and adolescents with prepsychotic and early psychotic features found that nearly half of them converted to a full psychotic disorder, primarily schizophrenia. By contrast, affective dysregulation and extreme irritability with depression are consistently noted in early stages of PBD. Despite the presence of psychotic features in early PBD and affective disturbance in early PS and the confusion in distinguishing these two disorders in their prodromal stage, the effort to screen for both disorders in tandem early in the course of illness has been absent.

Earlier clinical studies suggested that PBD was frequently misdiagnosed as PS. As Werry et al. (1991) point out, diagnostic fashions run in cycles. It is equally undesirable not to recognize schizophrenia and related disorders. Accurate diagnosis is critical in implementing highly effective, prophylactic mood-stabilizing or antipsychotic treatment to avoid unnecessary suffering and disability. It is possible to differentiate PS and PBD based on type of symptoms and course of the illness. The chances of correctly distinguishing PBD from PS are increased by a systematic acquisition of history and mental status examination, consistent use of clear diagnostic criteria, characterizing mood-congruent and mood-incongruent delusions and hallucinations, and determining the overall course and level of function (Carlson et al., 1994; Calderoni et al., 2001).

REFERENCES

Alaghband-Rad, J., McKenna, K., Gordon, C. T., Albus, K. E., Hamburger, S. D., Rumsey, J. M., Frazier, J. A., Lenane, M. C. & Rapoport, J. L. (1995), Childhood-onset schizophrenia: The severity of premorbid course. *J. Amer. Acad. Child & Adol. Psychiat.*, 34:1273–1283.

American Psychiatric Association. (1987), *Diagnostic and Statistical Manual of Mental Disorders, 3rd ed.,* Text Revision (*DSM-III-TR*). Washington, DC: American Psychiatric Association.

——— (2000), *Diagnostic and Statistical Manual of Mental Disorders, 4th ed.,* Text Revision (*DSM-IV-TR*). Washington, DC: American Psychiatric Association.

Andreasen, N. C. (1999), Understanding the causes of schizophrenia. *New England J. Med.,* 340:645–647.

Asarnow, R. F., Asamen, J., Granholm, E., Sherman, T., Watkins, J. M. & Williams, M. E. (1994), Cognitive/neuropsychological studies of children with a schizophrenic disorder. *Schizophrenia Bull.,* 20:647–669.

Biederman, J., Faraone, S., Mick, E., Wozniak, J., Chen, L., Ouellette, C., Marrs, A., Moore, P., Garcia, J., Mennin, D. & Lelon, E. (1996), Attention-deficit hyperactivity disorder and juvenile mania: An overlooked comorbidity? *J. Amer. Acad. Child & Adol. Psychiat.,* 35:997–1008.

Birmaher, B., Ryan, N. D., Brent, D. A., Williamson, D. E. & Kaufman, J. (1996), Childhood and adolescent depression: A review of the past ten years. Part II. *J. Amer. Acad. Child & Adol. Psychiat.,* 35:1575–1583.

Calderoni, D., Wudarsky, M., Bhangoo, R., Dell, M., Nicolson, R., Hamburger, S. D., Gochman, P., Lenane, M., Rapoport, J. L. & Leibenluft, E. (2001), Differentiating childhood-onset schizophrenia from psychotic mood disorders. *J. Amer. Acad. Child & Adol. Psychiat.,* 40:1190–1196.

Caplan, R. (1994), Thought disorder in children. *J. Amer. Acad. Child & Adol. Psychiat.,* 33:605–615.

——— Guthrie, D., Tang, B., Komo, S. & Asarnow, R. F. (2000), Thought disorder in childhood schizophrenia: Replication and update of concept. *J. Child & Adoles. Psychiat.,* 39(6):771–778.

Carlson, G. A., Bromet, E. J. & Sievers, S. (2000), Phenomenology and outcome of subjects with early- and adult-onset psychotic mania. *Amer. J. Psychiat.,* 157:213–219.

——— Fennig, S. & Bromet, E. J. (1994), The confusion between bipolar disorder and schizophrenia in youth: Where does it stand in the 1990s? *J. Amer. Acad. Child & Adol. Psychiat.,* 33:453–460.

Chambers, W. J., Puig-Antich, J., Tabrizi, M. A. & Davies, M. (1982), Psychotic symptoms in prepubertal major depressive disorder. *Arch. Gen. Psychiat.,* 39:921–927.

Chang, K. D., Steiner, H. & Ketter, T. A. (2000), Psychiatric phenomenology of child and adolescent bipolar offspring. *J. Amer. Acad. Child & Adol. Psychiat.,* 39:453–460.

Egeland, J. A., Hostetter, A. M., Pauls, D. L. & Sussex, J. N. (2000), Prodromal symptoms before onset of manic-depressive disorder suggested by first hospital admission histories. *J. Amer. Acad. Child & Adol. Psychiat.,* 39:1245–1252.

Fergus, E. L. (1999), Offspring study of pediatric bipolar disorder. Poster presented at annual meeting of American Academy of Child and Adolescent Psychiatry, San Francisco, CA.

Findling, R. L., Gracious, B. L., McNamara, N. K., Youngstrom, E. A., Demeter, C. A., Branicky, L. A. & Calabrese, J. R. (2001), Rapid, continuous cycling and psychiatric comorbidity in pediatric bipolar I disorder. *Bipolar Disorders,* 3:202–210.

131

Frazier, J. A., Giedd, J. N., Hamburger, S. D., Albus, K. E., Kaysen, D., Vaituzis, A. C., Rajapakse, J. C., Lenane, M. C., McKenna, K., Jacobsen, L. K., Gordon, C. T., Breier, A. & Rapoport, J. L. (1996), Brain anatomic magnetic resonance imaging in childhood-onset schizophrenia. *Arch. Gen. Psychiat.,* 53:617–624.

Geller, B., Craney, J. L., Bolhofner, K., DelBello, M. P., Williams, M. & Zimerman, B. (2001), One-year recovery and relapse rates of children with a prepubertal and early adolescent bipolar disorder phenotype. *Amer. J. Psychiat.,* 158:303–305.

———— Sun, K., Zimerman, B., Luby, J., Frazier, J. & Williams, M. (1995), Complex and rapid-cycling in bipolar children and adolescents: A preliminary study. *J. Affective Disorders,* 34:259–268.

———— Williams, M., Zimerman, B., Frazier, J., Beringer, L. & Warner, K. (1998), Prepubertal and early adolescent bipolarity differentiate from ADHD by manic symptoms, grandiose delusions, ultra-rapid or ultradian cycling. *J. Affective Disorders,* 51:81–91.

———— Zimmerman, B., Williams, M., DelBello, M. P., Bolhofner, K., Craney, J. L., Frazier, J., Beringer, L. & Nickelsburg, M. J. (in press), *DSM-IV* mania symptoms in a prepubertal and early adolescent bipolar disorder phenotype compared to attention-deficit hyperactivity and normal controls. *J. Child Adolesc. Psychopharmacology.*

Goodwin, F. K. & Jamison, K. R., eds. (1990), *Manic-depressive illness.* New York: Oxford University Press.

Green, W. H., Campbell, M., Hardesty, A. S., Grega, D. M., Padron-Gayol, M., Shell, J. & Erlenmeyer-Kimling, L. (1984), A comparison of schizophrenia and autistic children. *J. Amer. Acad. Child & Adol. Psychiat.,* 23:399–409.

Gunduz, H., Alvir, J., Woerner, M., Robinson, D. & Lieberman, J. A. (1999), The impact of duration of untreated psychosis symptoms on treatment response of delusions and hallucinations. *Schizophrenia Res.,* 36:18.

Helgason, L. (1990), Twenty years' follow-up of first psychiatric presentation for schizophrenia: What could have been prevented? *Acta Psychiatrica Scandinavia,* 81:231–235.

Hollis, C. (1995), Child and adolescent (juvenile-onset) schizophrenia: A case control study of premorbid development impairments. *Brit. J. Psychiat.,* 166:489–495.

Jacobsen, L. K. & Rapoport, J. L. (1998), Research update: Childhood-onset schizophrenia: Implication of clinical and neurobiological research. *J. Child Psychol. Psychiat.,* 39:101–113.

Jampala, V. C., Taylor, M. A. & Abrams, R. (1989), The diagnostic implications of formal thought disorder in mania and schizophrenia: A reassessment. *Amer. J. Psychiat.,* 146:459–463.

Joyce, P. (1984), Age of onset in bipolar affective disorder and misdiagnosis as schizophrenia. *Psychol. Med.,* 14:145–149.

Kolvin, I. (1971), Studies in the childhood psychoses I. Diagnostic criteria and classification. *Brit. J. Psychiat.,* 118:381–384.

Kumra, S. (2000), The diagnosis and treatment of children and adolescents with schizophrenia: "My mind is playing tricks on me." *Child & Adol. Psychiat. Clinic of N. Amer.,* 9:183–199.

Kydd, R. R. & Werry, J. S. (1982), Schizophrenia in children under 16 years. *J. Autism Devel. Disorders,* 12:343–357.

Lewinsohn, P. M., Klein, D. N. & Seeley, J. R. (1995), Bipolar disorders in a community sample of older adolescents: Prevalence, phenomenology, comorbidity, and course. *J. Amer. Acad. Child & Adol. Psychiat.,* 34:454–463.

McClellan, J., McCurry, C., Snell, J. & DuBose, A. (1999), Early-onset psychotic disorders: Course and outcome over a 2-year period. *J. Amer. Acad. Child & Adol. Psychiat.,* 38:1380–1388.

McGlashan, T. H. (1996), Early detection and intervention with schizophrenia. *Schizophrenia Bull.,* 22:197–398.

——— (1998), Early detection and intervention with schizophrenia: Rationale and research. *Brit. J. Psychiat. Suppl.,* 172:3–6.

——— & Johanssen, J. O. (1996), Early detection and intervention with schizophrenia: Rationale. *Schizophrenia Bull.,* 22:201–222.

McGorry, P. (1998), Preventive strategies in early psychosis: Verging on reality. *Brit. J. Psychiat. Suppl.,* 172:1–2.

——— (2000), The nature of schizophrenia: Signposts to prevention. *Australian & New Zealand J. Psychiat.,* 34(Suppl.):S14–S21.

Murray, C. J. L. & Lopez, A. D. (1996), *The Global Burden of Disease.* Boston: Harvard University Press.

Russell, A. T., Bott, L. & Sammons, C. (1989), The phenomenology of schizophrenia occurring in childhood. *J. Amer. Acad. Child & Adol. Psychiat.,* 28:399–407.

Schroder, J., Bachmann, S., Weimer, D., Demisch, S., Hoffmann, J., Resch, F. & Mundt, C. (1999), Duration of untreated psychosis is associated with a poor treatment response in schizophrenia. *Schizophrenia Res.,* 36:9–10.

Strober, M., Schmidt-Lackner, S., Freeman, R., Bower, S., Lampert, C. & DeAntonio, M. (1995), Recovery and relapse in adolescents with bipolar affective illness: A five-year naturalistic, prospective follow-up. *J. Amer. Acad. Child & Adol. Psychiat.,* 34:724–731.

Tohen, M., Tsuang, M. T. & Goodwin, D. C. (1992), Prediction of outcome in mania by mood-congruent or mood-incongruent psychotic features. *Amer. J. Psychiat.,* 149:1580–1584.

——— Walternaux, C. M., Tsuang, M. T. & Hunt, A. T. (1990), Four-year follow-up of twenty-four first-episode manic patients. *J. Affective Disorders,* 19:79–86.

Ulloa, R., Birmaher, B. & Axelson, D. (2000), Psychosis in pediatric mood and anxiety disorders clinic: Phenomenology and correlates. *J. Amer. Acad. Child & Adol. Psychiat.,* 39:337–345.

Volkmar, F. R. (1996), Childhood and adolescent psychosis: A review of the past 10 years. *J. Amer. Acad. Child & Adol. Psychiat.,* 35:843–851.

Wals, M., Hillegers, M. H., Reichart, C. G., Ormel, J., Nolen, W. A. & Verhulst, F. C. (2001), Prevalence of psychopathology in children of a bipolar parent. *J. Amer. Acad. Child & Adol. Psychiat.,* 40(9):1094–1102.

Watkins, J. M., Asarnow, R. F. & Tanguay, P. E. (1988), Symptom development in childhood onset schizophrenia. *J. Child Psychol. Psychiat.,* 29:865–878.

Werry, J. S., McClellan, J. M. & Chard, L. (1991), Childhood and adolescent schizophrenic, bipolar, and schizoaffective disorders: a clinical and outcome study. *J. Amer. Acad. Child & Adol. Psychiat.,* 34:867–876.

Woods, S. W., Miller, T. J. & McGlashan, T. H. (2001), The "prodromal" patient: Both symptomatic and at-risk. *CNS Spectrums,* 6:223–232.

Wozniak, J., Biederman, J., Kiely, K., Ablon, S., Faraone, S. V., Mundy, E. & Mennin, D. (1995), Mania-like symptoms suggestive of childhood-onset bipolar disorder in clinically referred children. *J. Amer. Acad. Child & Adol. Psychiat.,* 34:867–876.

Wyatt, R. J., Damiani, L. M. & Henter, I. D. (1998), First-episode schizophrenia. Early intervention and medication discontinuation in the context of course and treatment. *Brit. J. Psychiat. Suppl.,* 172:77–83.

Yung, A. R. & McGorry, P. D. (1996), The initial prodrome in psychosis: Descriptive and qualitative aspects. *Australian & New Zealand J. Psychiat.,* 30:587–599.

PART III

SPECIAL SECTION ON TRAUMA AND ADOLESCENCE

INTRODUCTION TO SPECIAL SECTION

THE COMMITTEE ON ADOLESCENCE OF THE GROUP
FOR THE ADVANCEMENT OF PSYCHIATRY

Members of the GAP Committee on Adolescence who contributed to this special section include: Daniel F. Becker, Melita Daley, Monica R. Green, Robert L. Hendren, Lois T. Flaherty (Committee Chair), Warren J. Gadpaille, Gordon Harper, Robert A. King, Patricia Lester, Silvio J. Onesti, Mary Schwab-Stone, and Susan W. Wong.

The Group for the Advancement of Psychiatry (GAP) is an organization of some 300 psychiatrists dedicated to shaping psychiatric thinking, public programs, and clinical practice in mental health. It was founded in 1946 by a group of physicians whose wartime experiences had brought them to realize the urgency of greater public awareness of the need for new programs in mental health for the people of the United States. Since its beginnings under the dynamic leadership of the late Dr. William C. Menninger, GAP has been influential in shaping psychiatric thinking, public programs, and clinical practice in mental health. It continues today to pioneer in exploring issues and ideas on the frontiers of psychiatry and in applying psychiatric insights into the general medical, social, and interpersonal problems of our times. Its objectives are to analyze significant data in psychiatry and human relations, reevaluate old concepts, develop new ones, and apply this knowledge for the advancement of mental health. Membership in GAP is by invitation only. Each member belongs to a committee that is working in his or her area of special interest and expertise. The 25 committees meet regularly, select their own topics for exploration, invite participation by expert consultants from other disciplines, collect and evaluate data, and present the resulting work to the entire GAP membership for further and rigorous scrutiny before publication.

The GAP Committee on Adolescence, which came into being in 1969, has over the years included many distinguished ASAP members, among them Lois Flaherty, Clarice Kestenbaum, Richard Marohn, Derek Miller, Michael Kalogerakis, Joseph Noshpitz, Vivian Rakoff, and Harvey Horowitz.

Since its inception, the Committee on Adolescence of the Group for the Advancement of Psychiatry has concerned itself with the process of adolescence. Its first report (1968) examined normal adolescent development and its impact on the individual and on society as a whole. Its second report (1978) focused on the transfer of power and authority from established adults to developing adolescents. The third (1986) and fourth (1996) reports began the consideration of how situations that have immediate biological psychological and social consequences for the individual and society also put the adolescent process itself at risk. In the 1986 report, we stated,

Adolescence, even under the best of circumstances, is a stressful phase of life. Nevertheless, most adolescents negotiate this difficult period without serious harmful behavior. The ability to do so requires adequate developmental preparations, contributed to by appropriate biological, cognitive, emotional, familial, and societal influences. Conditions that compromise the developmental preparation for adolescence render the individual at far greater risk for a range of behaviors that constitute crises with potentially damaging consequences [p. xviii].

In this special section, we have focused our attention on how adolescents respond to stress, given their preparation (adequate or inadequate) to deal with it. These chapters consider the relationship of stress to trauma, trauma to injury, and injury to subsequent repair, psychopathology, or developmental impairment. They explore the questions of when and why stress becomes traumatic; what protects the individual and what makes the individual vulnerable; when a trauma becomes injurious; what internal and external factors support repair; what factors prevent repair and lead to psychopathology; what, above all, is the impact of stress, trauma, injury, repair, and psychopathology on adolescent development.

What do we mean when we state that stress has become traumatic? Krugman (1987) notes that, to use the construct of trauma fully, the definition of a traumatic event must be specific and the impact of the trauma as it radiates through all levels of the biopsychosocial system must be elaborated. One definition is implied by van der Kolk (1987): "The book considers the impact of experiences that overwhelm both psychological and biological coping mechanisms" (p. xii). Regarding outcome, he noted that long-term adjustments will be affected by the severity of the stressor and the individual's genetic predisposition, developmental phase, social support system, prior traumatizations, and preexisting personality.

It is understood that the biopsychosocial system of adolescents during their transition from childhood dependency to adult responsibility continually adjusts to the stress produced by their biological maturation, psychological perception, and social expectation. To that and additional stress, the adolescent responds according to the meaning of the situation within the adolescent's intellectual and emotional capacity to understand it, bear it, and cope with it. How the adolescent succeeds or fails will be manifested from the spectrum of adolescent response: from violence or detachment to engagement and mastery. The response will influence the adolescent's capacity to address and master future developmental tasks and stressful situations that must be dealt with one way or another.

Adolescents throughout the world have a high probability of being exposed to potentially traumatic events. This occurs in part by virtue of the unique features of adolescence, such as increased risk-taking behavior and involvement in activities outside the protective orbit of the family, and in part it is due to imposed or chosen social roles such as military combat or gang activity.

Trauma during the adolescent years comes at a vulnerable period as young people move beyond the protection of their families. Although most teenagers negotiate their adolescent years without serious harmful behavior, adolescence—even under the best of circumstances—is a stressful phase of life (GAP, 1986; 1996). Young people's successful coping with the stresses of adolescence is based on certain essential cognitive, emotional, familial, societal and cultural prerequisites. When these are lacking the adolescent's developmental preparation is compromised, placing the a youngster is then at far greater risk for a range of behaviors with potentially damaging consequences (GAP, 1986; 1996).

DSM-IV describes posttraumatic stress disorder (PTSD) as a specific group of serious symptoms following experiences that meet the above criteria. In this section, PTSD refers only to the full symptom complex defined by *DSM-IV*; posttraumatic symptoms (PTS) refer to the broader range of pathological consequences not subsumed under PTSD. PTSD and PTS are not the only consequences of traumatic events: There may be no clinically significant consequences, or other psychiatrically impairing or disabling conditions may result. This section will attempt to portray the enormous range of responses and extent to which individual vulnerability and risk factors play a role.

Trauma can stunt or derail emotional growth and result in the development of specific psychopathological syndromes. Acute and chronic posttraumatic disorders are not the only, or necessarily the most debilitating, consequences of trauma. Other possible sequelae include anxiety and depression, substance abuse, suicide, violent behavior, and enduring maladaptive personality patterns of thinking and feeling. Without successful intervention, these problems continue into adulthood.

Adolescents who have experienced trauma in childhood are at high risk for repetitively experiencing subsequent trauma with ever-more-pernicious outcomes. However, not all victims of trauma show noxious sequelae. The following vignettes illustrate how disparate the outcomes of trauma can be.

Vignette 1

The body of an 11-year-old boy is found in the woods near an area where he had been selling candy door-to-door to raise money for school activities. Police detectives remember that in the neighborhood near the woods where the body was found lives a 15-year-old boy who had been cooperating with the investigation of a man who had seduced and sexually victimized him. In the days prior to the murder, however, the teenager has suddenly stopped talking with the detectives, has smashed surveillance equipment that was placed in his home, has become uncommunicative with his parents, and has refused to attend therapy sessions. The youth is arrested and charged with murdering the younger boy (*New York Times*, October 2, 1997).

Vignette 2

Another 15-year-old witnesses the hanging of a child in a Nazi death camp. After surviving a year of brutalization and being haunted by memories of horror, he goes on to become an eloquent spokesperson against genocide, winning a Nobel peace prize (Wiesel, 1960).

140

Both of these adolescents were victims of trauma, but the outcomes for them were radically different. Why? Why does trauma affect some persons differently than others? Are there unique aspects of adolescence that make the impact of trauma différent for this period than for other phases of life? To what extent is traumatization of adolescents a public health problem? How does trauma experienced during childhood affect adolescent development? What is the effect of trauma on personality development? What are risk and protective factors? Are there important gender differences in response to trauma? Is sexual trauma uniquely different from other kinds of trauma? Are there some kinds of traumatization that irreparably damage individuals?

Methodology of Literature Review

The primary method used was the collection of references by individual committee members, each of whom focused on specific areas of their own research and expertise. A consensus process was used to identify studies that used standardized methods of data collection, identified sampling methods, and specified age and demographic characteristics of the study population. In addition, Medline searches were done using the words trauma and adolescence, as well as various subcategories such as disasters and abuse to retrieve articles published between 1980 and 2001 pertaining to the topic. We particularly attempted to find studies that compared adolescents' traumatic exposure and their responses to those of other age groups, both younger and older; unfortunately, these are relatively rare. The studies cited in the chapters in this section represent the current body of knowledge with respect to trauma and adolescents.

Organization of the Special Section

This section includes three chapters by the GAP Committee on Adolescence—"The Nature and Scope of Trauma," "The Impact of Trauma," and "Issues of Identification, Intervention, and Social Policy." In addition, three other chapters are included, by authors who were or are members of the committee: "Cross-Cultural and Gender Considerations of Trauma," "The Neurobiological Effects of Trauma," and "Interventions for Traumatized Adolescents." Although these latter chapters reflect input from all members of the committee, they are primarily the work of their authors. Finally, a chapter is included on "Late Adolescence and Combat PTSD" by Max Sugar, which discusses developmental aspects of the vulnerability of young soldiers to PTSD and other problems and is solely the author's work.

REFERENCES

Group for the Advancement of Psychiatry. (1968), *Normal Adolescence: Its Dynamics and Impact*, GAP Report No. 68. New York: Scribner.

———— (1978), *Power and Authority in Adolescence: The Origins and Resolutions of Intergenerational Conflict*, GAP Report No. 101. New York: Mental Health Materials Center.

———— (1986), *Crises of Adolescence: Teenage Pregnancy Impact on Adolescent Development*. GAP Report No. 118. New York: Brunner/Mazel.

———— (1996), *Adolescent Suicide*. GAP Report No. 140. Washington, DC: American Psychiatric Association.

Krugman, S. (1987), Trauma in the family: Perspectives on the intergenerational transmission of violence. In: *Psychological Trauma*, ed. B. A. van der Kolk. Washington, DC: American Psychiatric Press.

New York Times, October 2, 1997, 15-year-old held in young fundraiser's slaying. p. 1.

van der Kolk, B. A., ed. (1987), *Psychological Trauma*. Washington, DC: American Psychiatric Press.

Wiesel, E. (1960), *Night*. New York: Hill & Wang.

6 TRAUMA AND ADOLESCENCE I

THE NATURE AND SCOPE OF TRAUMA

THE COMMITTEE ON ADOLESCENCE OF THE GROUP
FOR THE ADVANCEMENT OF PSYCHIATRY

Members of the GAP Committee on Adolescence who contributed to this paper include: Daniel F. Becker, Melita Daley, Warren J. Gadpaille, Monica R. Green, Lois T. Flaherty (Committee Chair), Gordon Harper, Robert L. Hendren, Robert A. King, Patricia Lester, Silvio J. Onesti, Mary Schwab-Stone, and Susan W. Wong.

THE NATURE OF TRAUMA

The origin of the word trauma is the Greek word for wound. "Trauma" refers to both the experience of being hurt by an external noxious agent and the body's response to that hurt. This dual meaning is apt for psychological trauma, because it reflects the notion of an external cause as well as an inner subjective experience.

In psychological terms, "trauma" is used to refer to an event causing injury to the mind, as well as to describe mental injury. Just as physical trauma wounds and causes injury that may or may not heal, the impact of psychological trauma may or may not be mastered. The term traumatic stress is the one most commonly used in the recent scientific literature. This reflects an understanding of traumatic experience as a subset of stress.

Popular culture tends to focus on the event and not the individual response, but it is the nature of the response that is most important in understanding the effects of trauma on an individual's immediate and subsequent psychological functioning. It is the subjective psychological experience that is the crucial aspect of psychic trauma. In this sense, it could perhaps be said that trauma is in the eye of the beholder; trauma exerts its effects through the prism of meaning.

Given the centrality of subjective experience in defining a stress as traumatic, it is not surprising that the precise boundaries of trauma are difficult to specify. On one hand, some stress is probably a necessary condition for emotional growth. Normative stresses, such as weaning, brief parental absences, and the beginning of school or day care, are most often growth-promoting and foster normal development. On the other hand, there are events that overwhelm the child's coping capacity and are likely to have noxious effects on nearly everyone, such as assault, violent death of a parent, concentration-camp experiences, or extended combat—though even under conditions of extreme stress such as these, there are individual differences in how people react to stress. Between these extremes are events that have only the potential to be traumatic; in these situations, individual vulnerability and the presence or absence of social supports play a determinative role in shaping outcome.

DSM *Definitions of Trauma*

Attempts by the American Psychiatric Association (APA) to define trauma reflect the difficulties with boundaries. Posttraumatic stress disorder (PTSD) entered the psychiatric nomenclature in 1980 with *DSM-III*. The definition of a traumatic event, both in this manual and its revision, *DSM-III-R* (APA, 1987), was an event occurring outside the range of usual human experience. The *DSM-IV* (APA, 2000) broadened the definition of traumatic experience, listing two essential criteria: "1) The person experienced, witnessed, or was confronted with an event or events that involved actual or threatened death or serious injury, or a threat to the physical integrity of self or others, and 2) The person's response involved intense fear, helplessness, or horror" (pp. 467–468).

However, even the broader *DSM-IV* definition may not be inclusive enough with respect to adolescents. Events described by teenagers as traumatic (that is, "a terrible experience that most people never go through") may include such things as a parent's being sent to prison or a parent's revelation of a past suicide attempt. These events may be just as devastating in terms of sequelae for some youngsters as events more commonly considered to constitute severe trauma, such as rape (Giaconia et al., 1995).

Traumatic stresses may be categorized as acute versus chronic and early versus late in terms of the age at which they occur. Early childhood traumas, which are frequently reactivated in adolescence, are of particular significance. Table 1 summarizes the kinds of exposures that have been reported to produce traumatic responses in children and adolescents.

THE SCOPE OF TRAUMA

General Risk of Experiencing Trauma

Although conceptually a broad definition of trauma seems most valid, most epidemiological research has used the more restrictive definitions

TABLE 1

TYPOLOGY OF REPORTED TRAUMATIC EXPOSURES
IN CHILDREN AND ADOLESCENTS[1]

- **Small- and large-scale natural and technological disasters** (earthquake, flood, fire, tornado, hurricane, lightning strike, cyclone, nuclear reactor accident)
- **Accidents**
  Transportation calamities (train, airplane, ship, automobile)
  Severe accidental injury (burns, hit-and-run accidents, accidental shooting)
- **Intra- and extrafamilial violence**
  Kidnapping and hostage situations
  Community violence (gang violence, sniper attacks)
  Political, racial, or religious-related violence (terrorism, war, atrocities, torture)
  Massive catastrophic trauma (concentration camp)
  Witnessing rape, murder, interspousal violence, and suicidal behavior
  Sexual molestation, incest, exploitation, physical abuse
- **Life-threatening illnesses and life-endangering medical procedures**

---

[1]Reprinted from Pynoos, R. (1993), Traumatic stress and developmental psychopathology in children and adolescents. In: *American Psychiatric Press Review of Psychiatry,* Vol. 12, ed. J. M. Oldham, M. B. Riba, & A. Tasman. Washington, DC: American Psychiatric Press, p. 208. Used with permission.

contained in the *DSM*. Epidemiological studies of community populations in peacetime have shown that the likelihood of experiencing at least one traumatic event outside the range of normal experience (the *DSM-III-R* definition) by adulthood is fairly high. Breslau et al. (1997) found a lifetime prevalence of 62%; Kessler et al. (1995) found that 61% of men and 51% of women have had traumatic experiences. Adolescents, too, have a substantial risk for experiencing trauma. Giaconia and colleagues (1995) found that over 40% of adolescents in a large community sample had at least one traumatic experience by the age of 18. Two-thirds of a sample of teenagers in a Florida working-class community studied after a very destructive hurricane had experienced at least one prior traumatic or violent event (Garrison et al., 1995). An exposure rate of over 80% was found in a nonclinical sample of college students (Vrana and Lauterbach, 1994). The most common severe trauma for females involves assault; for males, it involves accidents.

Thus, traumatic events are very common. What about these events that makes them have the potential to cause harm is the next question to be considered.

Specific Risk Situations

Natural disasters. Earthquakes, fires, floods, hurricanes and severe storms occur throughout the world, causing death, injury, and property damage. These calamities are single events that might seem to involve fewer of the compounding variables present in so many other kinds of trauma. However, as is the case with war-related traumas, natural disasters also involve many kinds of stress and loss, including destruction of homes and schools, personal injuries, deaths of family members and friends, witnessing death and injury, and loss of social supports through destruction or disruption of community institutions (Garrison et al., 1995; Goenjian et al., 1995). Studies of disasters have attempted to quantify reactions to disaster in terms of external and internal variables. Duration and intensity of the event, proximity to the event, level of exposure, and emotional closeness to the victims have all been found to mediate effects (Pynoos, Steinberg, and Wraith, 1995). It is not necessary for children and adolescents to be direct victims of a disaster to experience traumatic effects (March et al., 1997).

Studying adolescents' responses to Hurricane Hugo, Garrison and colleagues (1993) found rates of PTSD between 1.5% and 6.2%

146

(depending on gender and ethnicity) one year later but noted that 20% still had symptoms of reexperiencing, and 18% had hyperarousal symptoms. These findings were similar to those found after Hurricane Andrew (Garrison et al., 1995); although only 3.0% of male adolescents and 9.5% of females met criteria for PTSD six months after the hurricane, most had some posttraumatic symptoms. In addition to gender, ethnicity played a role in response, with higher rates of symptoms in black and Hispanic adolescents than in white teens. Other aggravating factors were prior traumatic experience and comorbid psychiatric disorders. In contrast to the relatively low rates of morbidity in adolescents, about half of the adults studied after Hurricane Hugo met criteria for new-onset PTSD, other anxiety disorders, or depression (David et al., 1996).

The Armenian earthquake in 1988 resulted in around 25,000 deaths, almost two-thirds of which were children and adolescents. Trauma-related symptoms were widespread amid young survivors. Mean scores on the Child Posttraumatic Stress Disorder Index were in the severe range for children living near the epicenter of the earthquake, with lower levels for those who were farther away (Goenjian et al., 1995). This study did not distinguish adolescents' reactions from those of children or adults. The authors did note that PTSD was present in 91% of the children and adolescents seen for mental health treatment soon after the earthquake.

Asarnow and colleagues (1999) evaluated the effects of a Los Angeles earthquake on children and adolescents with preexisting depression who had already been recruited into a study of depression. One year after the earthquake, 28% had mild to moderate posttraumatic symptoms.

Man-made disasters. Man-made disasters include plane crashes, ship sinkings, and motor vehicle accidents—as well as building collapses, fires, and floods resulting from faulty construction. Although similar to natural disasters in terms of the havoc they cause, the effects of these accidents are complicated by the survivors' awareness that human agency is involved. A well-studied example of such calamities is the Buffalo Creek disaster of 1972, a community-destroying flood caused by the collapse of a mining company dam. Children, adolescents, and adults were studied two years after the disaster and then reassessed 15 years later (Green et al., 1991, 1994). At the time of the first assessment,

PTSD symptoms were present in 32% of children and adolescents and differed qualitatively across different age groups. As assessed by structured diagnostic interviews, the prevalence decreased to 7% at the second assessment. However, a small group of survivors who had been children and adolescents at the time of the flood were given more intensive interviews using psychodynamic approaches (Honig et al., 1993, 1999). Not only were more symptoms elicited in this group, but investigators found enduring defensive patterns of denial and psychogenic amnesia, as well as sequelae such as survivor guilt, obsessive feelings of responsibility, persistent rage toward the perceived perpetrators of the flood, preoccupation with thoughts of death, and counterphobic behavior. These psychodynamically oriented investigators hypothesized that they were observing the evolution of traumatically induced coping mechanisms into enduring personality traits.

A group of investigators evaluated fourth- to ninth-grade students attending schools in an area where there had been an industrial fire that killed 25 people and seriously injured 56 (March et al., 1997); widespread safety violations were found at the site of the fire. None of the students was in the building at the time of the fire, but some were exposed to it by going to the scene and/or by having a friend or relative who died or was injured. About 20% of the students showed either PTSD or posttraumatic symptoms nine months after the fire; depression and anxiety were also noted, as well as an increase in teacher-reported disruptive behavior. The presence of posttraumatic symptomatology was correlated with level of traumatic exposure (those who witnessed the fire and also knew someone who was killed or injured had the worst outcome). This study did not find age-related effects, possibly because the age range of the subjects was relatively narrow (10 to 16 years).

The impact of the sinking of the British cruise ship Jupiter on a group of 217 survivors who were adolescents at the time of the disaster was studied over a several-year period following the event, by Yule and associates (2000). They found an incidence of PTSD of over 50% (compared to 3.4% in a matched group of controls) during the five- to eight-year follow-up period; in 90% of those who developed PTSD, the onset was within six months of the disaster. A third of those who developed PTSD recovered within a year, but a third continued to be symptomatic five to eight years after the disaster. Levels of distress remained high relative to those in the control subjects, even in those who had recovered from PTSD.

War. Exposure to severe trauma engendered by wars and political conflicts is widespread among all age groups, all over the world. Among the consequences of these events are forced emigrations (refugees). These conflicts affect children and adolescents in many ways similar to the effects of natural disasters, including lack of adequate food, clothing, shelter, and medical care, as well as the losses of their families, homes, and communities.

Data gathered by the United Nations (United Nations Children's Fund, 1996) indicates that during the decade of the 1990s, more than 20 million children were displaced, 2 million killed, 1 million orphaned, 6 million seriously injured or disabled, and 12 million made homeless because of wars. The United Nations has estimated that over 300,000 children (defined as under age 18) are active combatants around the world. Most of these are adolescent boys, but girls also participate in armies.

Although the adverse psychological consequences of prolonged, armed conflict have been described since the time of the American Civil War, it was not until World War II that investigators began to record the effects of war on children and adolescents (Jensen and Shaw, 1993; Terr, 1996). Within the past two decades, increasing interest in the effects of traumatic exposure upon children (Terr, 1991)—perhaps along with increasing public awareness of the pervasiveness and chronicity of armed conflict throughout the world—has resulted in a wider array of studies of the impact of war on children and adolescents (e.g., Kinzie et al., 1986; Weine, Becker, McGlashan, Vojvoda, et al., 1995; Laor et al., 1996; see Jensen and Shaw, 1993).

Whereas some research has suggested little effect of age on traumatic response (Pynoos et al., 1987), other studies have discerned differential effects of traumatic exposure according to age and developmental stage (Terr, 1988; Sack et al., 1994; Weine, Becker, McGlashan, Laub, et al., 1995; Weine et al., 1998; see Pfefferbaum, 1997). Beyond considerations of developmental vulnerability or resiliency, there are additional reasons to think that adolescents may have different experiences of war trauma than those of younger children. Although younger children are more likely to be protected indoors during periods of fighting or occupation, adolescents may become directly involved in military or other resistance activities—and may be killed or imprisoned as potential combatants or abducted or raped by occupying forces (Pynoos et al., 1995). Nonetheless, there are relatively few studies of the effects of war trauma specifically on adolescents.

Those investigations that have been done on the response of adolescents to war-related trauma have tended to focus on refugee populations. Kinzie and colleagues (1986) studied Cambodian adolescent refugees in the United States who had suffered severe trauma in Khmer concentration camps as children. At the time of evaluation, approximately six years after the trauma exposure, half suffered from PTSD. A follow-up study three years later revealed a similar frequency of the PTSD diagnosis (Kinzie et al., 1989). Sack and colleagues (1993), reporting on a six-year follow-up evaluation during young adulthood, found persistence of the PTSD diagnosis—albeit with attenuation of symptom frequency and intensity, and with indications of good functional capacity. In a second epidemiologic study of Cambodian refugee youths and their parents from two different U.S. communities, Sack et al. (1994) found that PTSD could be diagnosed in only about one-fifth of adolescents and young adults (ages 13 to 25 years) who had been exposed to genocidal trauma about a dozen years previously. These data also indicated lower rates of PTSD in the index subjects than in their parents (Sack et al., 1994). For the parents—but not for the youths—there was an association between PTSD diagnosis and impaired functional capacity (Sack, Clarke, Kinney, et al., 1995). Finally, PTSD—and, to a lesser extent, major depression—were found to cluster across the two generations; this finding was apparently unrelated to potential mediating environmental variables, such as trauma exposure, shared living arrangements, or socioeconomic status (Sack, Clarke, and Seeley, 1995). In addition to these studies of Cambodian refugees in the United States, Mollica and colleagues (1997) evaluated Cambodian adolescent refugees in camps along the Thai border. A dose-effect relationship was found between traumatic exposure and psychiatric symptoms, though not between traumatic exposure and social functioning.

Weine, Becker, McGlashan, Vojvoda, et al. (1995) evaluated Bosnian adolescent refugees from the war in Bosnia-Herzegovina within the first year after their resettlement in the United States. These adolescent survivors of ethnic cleansing had typically been separated from their fathers and other adult male family members—who were sent to concentration camps—and, along with the remainder of their families, spent months fleeing capture by Serbian forces or being held in occupied territories. Their traumatic experiences included exposure to killing and other acts of violence, disappearance of loved ones without explanation, prolonged separation from family members, destruction of home and other property, detainment in refugee camps, deprivation of food and water, and forced emigration. Most were eventually reunited with their families, some of which were given the opportunity to emigrate to the United States or elsewhere. These investigators found that only 25% of the adolescent refugees met diagnostic criteria for PTSD, and fewer met criteria for a depressive disorder. A one-year follow-up revealed a rate of PTSD diagnosis that was lower still (Becker et al., 1999). At baseline and at one-year follow-up, PTSD rates in the adolescents were lower than those in the adults drawn from the same overall study group (Weine, Becker, McGlashan, Laub, et al., 1995; Weine et al., 1998). Social functioning was uniformly high. At both evaluation points, PTSD rates in these Bosnian adolescent refugees were much lower than those reported in the studies of Cambodian adolescent refugees (Kinzie et al., 1986, 1989; Sack et al., 1993). Perhaps, the authors speculated, the Bosnian adolescent refugees may have benefited from being able to remain within their families and having an easier acculturation to the United States than the Cambodian adolescents. With respect to the comparison of Bosnian adolescents to their parents, they observed that the adolescents in their study group may have been more resilient and more resistant to the pathological effects of trauma. These investigators also found indications that the adolescents who were most resilient were those whose parents had good courses with regard to psychiatric symptoms and social functioning, and those who had experienced helpful family, peer, and community environments (Becker et al., 1999).

These few studies of the psychological effects of war-related trauma upon adolescents suggest several considerations for those who may conduct further research in this area and for those who provide clinical care to these individuals. First, the proximity of adolescents to war-related traumatic events—as well as the duration of exposure and the intensity of traumatic experience—may affect psychological response (Becker et al., 1999; Jensen and Shaw, 1993; Mollica et al., 1997; Weine, Becker, McGlashan, Vojvoda, et al., 1995). Second, adolescents are likely to be influenced in their response to such trauma by family, peer, community, and cultural environments during and after the traumatic experience (Becker et al., 1999; Sack, Clarke, and Seeley, 1995; Weine, Becker, McGlashan, Vojvoda, et al., 1995). Third, the general finding that trauma-exposed adolescents are less symptomatic and demonstrate better social functioning than their adult counterparts may point to a relative resilience conferred by this particular stage of development (Becker et al., 1999; Sack et al., 1994; Sack, Clarke, Kinney, et al., 1995; Weine, Becker, McGlashan, Laub, et al., 1995). It should be noted, though, that acute or delayed symptoms of PTSD and depression, or impaired social functioning, may not be the only possible pathological effects of war-related trauma. Though still lacking adequate longitudinal data, we may speculate that early resilience could come at the cost of later psychiatric disorders, distorted defensive structures, the exaggeration of normal developmental anxieties (Jensen and Shaw, 1993), or difficulties with separation from family of origin and with the consolidation of identity (Weine, Becker, McGlashan, Laub, et al., 1995; Weine et al., 1997).

Finally, it is worth considering the possible effects of massive psychic trauma upon adolescents as they move into adult societal roles. History has demonstrated that, in many areas of the world, ethnic conflict and violence persist with unrelenting momentum. Children who grow up in a culture of mistrust, fear, or hatred—and for whom adolescent development culminates with the experience of genocidal trauma—may thereby be less likely to contribute to an ethos of multicultural tolerance as adults. They may also be more likely to perpetuate the cycle of organized violence between people of differing ethnic affiliations (Weine, 1999).

Urban violence.   Over the past decade, the research literature in the various fields related to child health and welfare has amply documented the alarming extent to which urban American youth are exposed to a range of potentially traumatic experiences. In major urban centers, large proportions of surveyed youth report witnessing violent incidents and being the victims of attacks. Jenkins and Bell (1994) found that 66% of students from a southside Chicago high school reported having witnessed a shooting, 45% had seen someone killed, and 27% had been victims of violence. Similarly high rates of Detroit adolescents reported violence exposure; 42% said they had witnessed a shooting or knifing and 22% had witnessed a murder (Schubiner, Scott, and Tzelepis, 1993). Reported rates of weapon carrying and fear of being harmed are also quite high among urban youth (Centers for Disease Control, 1993; Schubiner et al., 1993), suggesting the intuitive link between

152

exposure, the experience of trauma, and a range of psychological adaptations including behaviors that perpetuate the use of violent means to solve the problems of social living.

The high rates of exposure to violence revealed in these studies have stimulated investigations aimed at documenting the psychological consequences at different developmental stages. Richters and Martinez (1993) examined exposure to violence for 165 children ages 6 to 10 years from a low-income, moderately violent area of Washington, D.C. Of the first and second grade students, 19% had been victimized by some form of violence and 61% had witnessed violence to someone else; for the fifth- and sixth-grade students, rates of victimization and exposure were even higher (32% and 72%, respectively). Both self-reported victimization and exposure to violence in the community were related to distress symptoms (Martinez and Richters, 1993). Using a similar study design, Osofsky and colleagues (1993) also found high rates of violence exposure in 53 fifth-grade children in a New Orleans–area housing project. Mothers of 26% of the children reported that their children had seen shootings, 49% had seen woundings, and over 70% had seen weapons used. Witnessing community violence was significantly associated with reports of stress symptoms. These findings suggest that many urban youngsters enter adolescence having already been affected by significant violence exposure; the residue of their prior exposure will interact with the complicated forces of this stage of development.

Studies of inner city youth also demonstrate links between violence exposure and symptoms of depression (Freeman, Mokros, and Poznanski, 1993) and PTSD (Fitzpatrick and Boldizar, 1993). In a study of depressive symptomatology in 223 children ages 6 to 12 years, Freeman et al. (1993) found that 57 (25%) of their subjects spontaneously reported exposure to at least one traumatic event occurring to themselves or to a relative or friend. Children reporting such exposure had significantly more depressive symptoms than those who did not report traumatic exposure. In a study of 221 nonrandomly selected, low-income, inner-city African American youths, Fitzpatrick and Boldizar (1993) found that close to 85% had witnessed at least one violent act and that 43.4% reported having witnessed a murder. Having been directly victimized and having witnessed violence were strong predictors of PTSD symptomatology.

The tendency to use violence is another potential consequence of exposure to violence. DuRant et al. (1994) examined relationships between self-reported exposure to violence and the use of violence by 225 African American adolescents from housing projects in the Augusta, Georgia, area. Self-reported use of violence was positively associated with exposure to violence/victimization, family conflict, hopelessness, depression, and severity of corporal punishment. Having used violence was also significantly related to diminished sense of purpose in life and to lower expectation of being alive at age 25.

Current understanding of the psychological cost of community violence has relied heavily on the work of researchers and clinicians working with children exposed to acute trauma (Terr, 1983; Pynoos et al., 1987; Garbarino, Kostelny, and Dubrow, 1991; Terr, 1991; Garbarino et al., 1992). However, as Lorion and Saltzman (1993) note, the reactions of children who grow up in violent communities have more in common with the chronic adaptations of children living in war zones, where violence is chronic and pervasive in the environment. These include symptoms of anxiety, helplessness, futurelessness, numbness, and difficulty concentrating, as well as a syndrome of desensitization to threat, high levels of risk-taking, and participation in dangerous activities (Garbarino et al., 1992; Lorion and Saltzman, 1993).

Life-threatening illnesses and invasive medical procedures. These constitute another large category of trauma. Advances in medical care have increased the numbers of children and adolescents who survive what were formerly fatal conditions. However, the interventions associated with such life-saving care can be traumatic. Invasive medical procedures, surgery that can be disfiguring, and drugs with highly toxic side effects are all part of the contemporary medical armamentarium. In addition to the stress of the treatments themselves, survivors of such treatments often face the possibility of recurrences of illness, and they may experience sequelae such as infertility. Thus, these youngsters experience both acute and enduring stressors. Posttraumatic sequelae have been documented in child and adolescent cancer survivors (Stuber and Nader, 1995) and in victims of accidental injuries (Daviss et al., 2000) and burns (Stoddard et al., 1989).

Child maltreatment. Child maltreatment, like other forms of traumatic stress, can produce a variety of problems, including posttraumatic stress reactions. Compared with other age groups, teenagers are at relatively high risk for both physical and sexual abuse. Nearly 40% of all confirmed reports of child sexual abuse in the United States in 1997 occurred in children who were over age 11; over 17,000, or 35% of the total confirmed reports of physical abuse, occurred in this age group (U.S. Department of Health and Human Services, 1999). Some of these incidents represent new onset of victimization during adolescence, whereas others involve continuing or recurrent abuse that began earlier in life.

Prevalence rates for sexual abuse have been estimated as between 10% and 25% for females and 2% and 10% for males (Fergusson, Lynskey, and Horwood 1996). Most of these cases do not involve sexual intercourse. In a large New Zealand sample, Fergusson, Lynskey, et al. (1996) found rates for all types of sexual abuse to be comparable to the published estimates—17% for females and 3% for males. However, for severe sexual abuse, involving intercourse, they found much lower rates—5.6% for females and less than 1.4% for males. Their findings were based on self-report data—generally considered to be the most reliable, owing to frequent nonreporting of such occurrences—generated from interviews with subjects who had reached the age of 18 and who had been part of a large prospective study since birth.

Although parents tend to use physical punishment less with teenagers than with younger children, almost half of adults who responded in a large national survey reported having been disciplined in this fashion during their adolescent years (Straus and Kantor, 1994). In this study, corporal punishment during adolescence was found to be a risk factor for serious adult problems, including depression, suicide, alcohol abuse, and spousal and child abuse.

Histories of physical and/or sexual abuse are especially common among psychiatrically hospitalized adolescents, especially those with suicidal behavior, substance abuse, and major depressive disorder (Koltek, Wilkes, and Atkinson, 1998; Winegar and Lipschitz, 1999). Abuse histories are also prevalent among teenage runaways, with rates up to 86% having been found (Janus et al., 1995). A high prevalence of PTSD has been found in these groups when specific assessments have been done for this disorder.

Differential effects of abuse on adolescents as opposed to children have not been well studied. Tebbutt et al. (1997) studied child and adolescent victims of sexual abuse five years after the abuse. They found that the adolescents tended to show more depression, and the

155

children, more behavioral problems. They hypothesized that this difference was due to the age of their subjects at the time that they were assessed, since behavior problems in general are more common in children, and depression, in adolescents.

Abuse does not usually occur in isolation from other factors that place children at risk, making it difficult to separate the effects of abuse from those of other noxious influences. However, studies attempting to correct for confounding factors (such as parental conflict, parent–child relationship problems, and parental adjustment problems) have been able to demonstrate that abuse exerts effects over and above these other risk factors.

Brown et al. (1999) found specific effects of childhood abuse in a large random sample studied from childhood into young adulthood, using information from child protective services as well as self-reports. Using statistical methods to differentiate the specific effects of abuse from other factors, they found that more than one-third of youths who had been sexually abused as children suffered from depression and/or suicidal behavior. Being physically or sexually abused as a child increased the chance of being depressed or suicidal as an adolescent or adult by 300% to 400%. The association between repeated suicide attempts and sexual abuse was particularly strong, and adolescence was the period of highest risk for repeated suicide attempts.

Fergusson, Horwood, and Lynskey (1996) found that, in a birth cohort of over 1000 New Zealand children, those reporting sexual abuse prior to age 16 were more likely to have current major depression, anxiety disorder, conduct disorder, substance abuse disorder, and suicidal behaviors, at age 18. There was a relationship between the severity of the abuse and likelihood of disorder; the highest rates of psychiatric illness were found in those whose abuse included attempted or completed sexual intercourse, over 60% of whom had developed major depression.

Using the psychological autopsy method to study completed suicides, Brent and colleagues (1999) found a significant association between a lifetime history of abuse and suicide in adolescents. This association was particularly strong in the case of youngsters under age 16, 42% of whom had been abused and 11% of whom were being abused at the time of their deaths.

Physical abuse is more likely to be followed by depression, anxiety, or behavioral disturbances than by posttraumatic syndromes that meet *DSM* criteria. Pelcovitz and colleagues (1994) have noted, "Victims of adolescent physical abuse often live in an environment that is so dominated by violence that they are exposed to an ongoing process rather than a discrete 'event' " (p. 306). They add that, for these youngsters, abuse is not outside the range of their usual experience. These investigators found no PTSD but reported significant prevalence rates of major depression (40%), conduct disorder (16%), and oppositional-defiant disorder (20%) in a sample of adolescents with histories of physical abuse.

Bullying and harassment are unfortunately common experiences for many children and adolescents and can have far-reaching consequences (Nansel et al., 2001). About 4% of U.S. school students aged 12 to 18 say they are afraid of being attacked or harmed at school or on the way to and from school, and 13% report being targets of hate-related language (Kaufman et al., 2001). Youngsters who are different from the majority by virtue of race, ethnicity, or physical appearance are the most likely to be bullied. Gay and lesbian youth are frequently targeted (Drescher, 1998). Reactions to bullying and harassment are similar to reactions to other kinds of violence and abuse, ranging from depression and suicide to violent retaliation.

SUMMARY

Natural and man-made disasters, war and urban trauma, and child maltreatment are all frequently associated with multiple stressors. Despite the methodological difficulties inherent in studying these diverse forms of traumatic experience, similar posttraumatic responses have been found in people from many different cultures. Although adolescents as a group have been less extensively studied than adults, there is sufficient evidence that they are affected in similar ways by traumatic stress. The next chapter will explore the psychological effects of trauma during this vulnerable period of development.

REFERENCES

American Psychiatric Association (1987), *Diagnostic and Statistical Manual of Mental Disorders,* 3rd ed., Revised (*DSM-III-R*). Washington, DC: American Psychiatric Association.

——— (2000), *Diagnostic and Statistical Manual of Mental Disorders,* 4th ed. Text Revision (*DSM-IV-TR*). Washington, DC: American Psychiatric Association.

Asarnow, J., Glynn, S., Pynoos, R. S., Nahum, J., Guthrie, D., Cantwell, D. P. & Franklin, B. (1999), When the earth stops shaking: Earthquake sequelae among children diagnosed for pre-earthquake psychopathology. *J. Amer. Acad. Child & Adol. Psychiat.,* 38:1016–1023.

Becker, D. F., Weine, S. M., Vojvoda, D. & McGlashan, T. H. (1999), PTSD symptoms in adolescent survivors of "ethnic cleansing": Results from a 1-year follow-up study. *J. Amer. Acad. Child & Adol. Psychiat.,* 38:775–781.

Brent, D. A., Baugher, M., Bridge, J., Chen, T. & Chiappetta, L. (1999), Age and sex-related risk factors for adolescent suicide. *J. Amer. Acad. Child & Adol. Psychiat.,* 38:1497–1505.

Breslau, N., Davis, G. C., Andreski, P., Peterson, E. L. & Schultz, L. R. (1997), Sex differences in posttraumatic stress disorder. *Arch. Gen. Psychiat.,* 54:1044–1048.

Brown, J., Cohen, P., Johnson, J. G. & Smailes, E. M. (1999), Childhood abuse and neglect: Specificity of effects on adolescent and young adult depression and suicidality. *J. Amer. Acad. Child & Adol. Psychiat.,* 38:1490–1496.

Centers for Disease Control (1993), Violence-related attitudes and behaviors of high school students—New York City, 1992. *Morbidity and Mortality Weekly Report,* 42:773–777.

David, D., Mellman, T. A., Mendoza, L. M., Kulick-Bell, R., Ironson, G. & Schneiderman, N. (1996), Psychiatric morbidity following Hurricane Andrew. *J. Traumatic Stress,* 9:607–612.

Daviss, W. B., Mooney, D., Racusin, R., Ford, J. D., Fleischer, A. & McHugo, G. J. (2000), Predicting posttraumatic stress after hospitalization for pediatric injury. *J. Amer. Acad. Child & Adol. Psychiat.,* 39:576–583.

Drescher, J. (1998), *Psychoanalytic Therapy and the Gay Man.* Hillsdale, NJ: The Analytic Press.

DuRant, R. H., Cadenhead, C., Pendergast, R. A., Slavens, G. & Linder, W. C. (1994), Factors associated with the use of violence among urban black adolescents. *Amer. J. Public Health,* 84:612–622.

Fergusson, D. M., Horwood, J. & Lynskey, M. T. (1996), Childhood sexual abuse and psychiatric disorder in young adulthood: II. Psychiatric outcomes of childhood sexual abuse. *J. Amer. Acad. Child & Adol. Psychiat.*, 35:1365–1374.

———— Lynskey, M. T. & Horwood, J. (1996), Childhood sexual abuse and psychiatric disorder in young adulthood: I. Prevalence of sexual abuse and factors associated with sexual abuse. *J. Amer. Acad. Child & Adol. Psychiat.*, 35:1355–1364.

Fitzpatrick, K. M. & Boldizar, J. P. (1993), The prevalence and consequences of exposure to violence among African-American youth. *J. Amer. Acad. Child & Adol. Psychiat.*, 32:424–430.

Freeman, L. N., Mokros, H. & Poznanski, E. O. (1993), Violent events reported by normal urban school-aged children: Characteristics and depression correlates. *J. Amer. Acad. Child & Adol. Psychiat.*, 32:419–423.

Garbarino, J., Dubrow, N., Kostelny, K. & Pardo, C. (1992), *Children in Danger: Coping with the Consequences of Community Violence.* San Francisco: Jossey-Bass.

———— Kostelny, K. & Dubrow, N. (1991), What children can tell us about living in danger. *Amer. Psychol.*, 46:376–383.

Garrison, C. Z., Bryant, E. S., Addy, C. L., Spurrier, P. G., Freedy, J. R. & Kilpatrick, D. G. (1995), Posttraumatic stress disorder in adolescents after Hurricane Andrew. *J. Amer. Acad. Child & Adol. Psychiat.*, 34: 1193–1201.

———— Weinrich, M. W., Hardin, S. B., Weinrich, S. & Wang, L. (1993), Posttraumatic stress disorder in adolescents after a hurricane. *Amer. J. Epidemiol.*, 138:522–530.

Giaconia, R. M., Reinherz, H. Z., Silverman, B. A., Pakiz, B., Frost, A. K. & Cohen, E. (1995), Traumas and posttraumatic stress disorder in a community population of older adolescents. *J. Amer. Acad. Child & Adol. Psychiat.*, 34:1369–1380.

Goenjian, A., Pynoos, R. S., Steinberg, A. M., Najarian, L. M., Asarnow, J. R., Karayan, I., Ghurabi, M. & Fairbanks, L. A. (1995), Psychiatric comorbidity in children after the 1988 earthquake in Armenia. *J. Amer. Acad. Child & Adol. Psychiat.*, 34:1174–1184.

Green, B. L., Grace, M. C., Vary, M. G., Kramer, T. L., Gleser, G. C. & Leonard, A. C. (1994), Children of disaster in the second decade: A 17-year follow-up of Buffalo Creek. *J. Amer. Acad. Child & Adol. Psychiat.*, 33:71–79.

———— Korol, M., Grace, M., Vary, M. G., Leonard, A. C., Gleser, G. C. & Smitson-Cohen, S. (1991), Children and disaster: Age, gender and parental effects on PTSD symptoms. *J. Amer. Acad. Child & Adol. Psychiat.,* 30:945–951.

Honig, R. G., Grace, M. C., Lindy, J. D., Newman, C. J. & Titchener, J. L. (1993), Portraits of survival: A 20-year follow-up of the Buffalo Creek flood. *Psychoanal. Study of the Child,* 48:327–355. New Haven, CT: Yale University Press.

———— ———— ———— ———— ———— (1999), Assessing long-term effects of trauma: Diagnosing symptoms of avoidance and numbing. *Amer. J. Psychiat.,* 156:483–485.

Janus, M. D., Archambault, F. X., Brown, S. W. & Welsh, L. A. (1995), Physical abuse in Canadian runaway adolescents. *Child Abuse Negl.,* 19:433–47.

Jenkins, E. J. & Bell, C. C. (1994), Violence among inner city high school students and posttraumatic stress disorder. In: *Anxiety Disorders in African Americans,* ed. S. Friedman. New York: Springer.

Jensen, P. S. & Shaw, J. (1993), Children as victims of war: Current knowledge and future research needs. *J. Amer. Acad. Child & Adol. Psychiat.,* 32:697–708.

Kaufman, P., Chen, X., Choy, S. P., Peter, K., Ruddy, S. A., Miler, A. K., Fleury, J. K., Chandler, K. A., Planty, M. G. & Rand, M. R. (2001), *Indicators of School Crime and Safety: 2001.* NCES 2002-113/NCJ-190075. Washington, DC: U.S. Departments of Education and Justice.

Kessler, R. C., Sonnega, A., Bromet, E., Hughes, M. & Nelson, C. B. (1995), Posttraumatic stress disorder in the national comorbidity survey. *Arch. Gen. Psychiat.,* 52:1048–1060.

Kinzie, J. D., Sack, W., Angell, R., Clarke, G. & Ben, R. (1989), A three-year follow-up of Cambodian young people traumatized as children. *J. Amer. Acad. Child & Adol. Psychiat.,* 28:501–504.

———— ———— ———— Manson, S. & Rath, B. (1986), The psychiatric effects of massive trauma on Cambodian children, I: The children. *J. Amer. Acad. Child & Adol. Psychiat.,* 25:370–376.

Koltek, M., Wilkes, T. C. & Atkinson, M. (1998), The prevalence of posttraumatic stress disorder in an adolescent inpatient unit. *Can. J. Psychiat.,* 43:64–68.

Laor, N., Wolmer, L., Mayes, L. C., Golomb, A., Siverberg, D. S., Weizman, R. & Cohen, D. J. (1996), Israeli preschoolers under Scud missile attacks: A developmental perspective on risk-modifying factors. *Arch. Gen. Psychiat.,* 53:416–423.

Lorion, R. P. & Saltzman, W. (1993), Children's exposure to community violence: Following a path from concern to research to action. *Psychiatry,* 56:55–65.

March, J. S., Amaya-Jackson, L., Terry, R. & Costanzo, P. (1997), Posttraumatic symptomatology in children and adolescents after an industrial fire. *J. Amer. Acad. Child & Adol. Psychiat.,* 36:1080–1088.

Martinez, P. & Richters, J. E. (1993), The NIMH community violence project: II. Children's distress symptoms associated with violence exposure. *Psychiatry,* 56:22–35.

Mollica, R. F., Poole, C., Son, L., Murray, C. C. & Tor, S. (1997), Effects of war trauma on Cambodian refugee adolescents' functional health and mental health status. *J. Amer. Acad. Child & Adol. Psychiat.,* 36:1098–1106.

Nansel, T. R., Overpeck, M., Pilla, R. S., Ruan, W. J., Simons-Morton, B. & Scheidt, P. (2001), Bullying behaviors among U.S. youth: Prevalence and association with psychosocial adjustment. *J. Amer. Med. Assn.,* 285:2094–2100.

Osofsky, J. D., Wewers, S., Hann, D. M. & Fick, A. C. (1993), Chronic community violence: What is happening to our children? *Psychiatry,* 56:36–45.

Pelcovitz, D., Kaplan, S., Goldenberg, B., Mandel, F., Lehane, J. & Guarrera, J. (1994), Post-traumatic stress disorder in physically abused adolescents. *J. Amer. Acad. Child & Adol. Psychiat.,* 33:305–312.

Pfefferbaum, B. (1997), Posttraumatic stress disorder in children: A review of the past 10 years. *J. Amer. Acad. Child & Adol. Psychiat.,* 36:1503–1511.

Pynoos, R. (1993), Traumatic stress and developmental psychopathology in children and adolescents. In: *American Psychiatric Press Review of Psychiatry,* Vol. 12, ed. J. M. Oldham, M. B. Riba & A. Tasman. Washington, DC: American Psychiatric Press, pp. 205–238.

———— Frederick, C., Nader, K., Arroyo, W., Steinberg, A., Eth, S., Nunez, F. & Fairbanks, L. (1987), Life threat and posttraumatic stress in school-age children. *Arch. Gen. Psychiat.,* 44:1057–1063.

———— Steinberg, A. M. & Wraith, R. (1995), A developmental model of childhood traumatic stress. In: *Developmental Psychopathology,* Vol. 2, ed. D. Cicchetti & D. J. Cohen. New York: Wiley, pp. 72–95.

Richters, J. E. & Martinez, P. (1993), The NIMH community violence project: I. Children as victims of and witnesses to violence. *Psychiatry,* 56:7–21.

Sack, W. H., Clarke, G., Him, C., Dickason, D., Goff, B., Lanham, K. & Kinzie, J. D. (1993), A 6-year follow-up study of Cambodian refugee adolescents traumatized as children. *J. Amer. Acad. Child & Adol. Psychiat.,* 32:431–437.

―――― ―――― Kinney, R., Belestos, G., Him, C. & Seeley, J. (1995), The Khmer adolescent project: II. Functional capacities in two generations of Cambodian refugees. *J. Nerv. Ment. Dis.,* 183:177–181.

―――― ―――― & Seeley, J. (1995), Posttraumatic stress disorder across two generations of Cambodian refugees. *J. Amer. Acad. Child & Adol. Psychiat.,* 34:1160–1166.

―――― McSharry, S., Clarke, G. N., Kinney, R., Seeley, J. & Lewinsohn, P. (1994), The Khmer adolescent project: I. Epidemiologic findings in two generations of Cambodian refugees. *J. Nerv. Ment. Dis.,* 182:387–395.

Schubiner, H., Scott, R. & Tzelepis, A. (1993), Exposure to violence among inner-city youth. *J. Adol. Health,* 14:214–219.

Straus, M. A. & Kantor, G. K. (1994), Corporal punishment of adolescents by parents: A risk factor in the epidemiology of depression, suicide, alcohol abuse, child abuse, and wife beating. *Adolescence,* 29:543–561.

Stoddard, F. J., Norman, D. K., Murphy, J. M. & Beardslee, W. R. (1989), Psychiatric outcome of burned children and adolescents. *J. Amer. Acad. Child & Adol. Psychiat.,* 28:589–595.

Stuber, M. L. & Nader, K. O. (1995), Psychiatric sequelae in adolescent bone marrow transplantation survivors. *J. Psychother. Pract. Res.,* 4:1–4.

Tebbutt, J., Swanston, H., Oates, R. K. & O'Toole, B. I. (1997), Five years after child sexual abuse: Persisting dysfunction and problems of prediction. *J. Amer. Acad. Child & Adol. Psychiat.,* 36:330–339.

Terr, L. C. (1983), Chowchilla revisited: the effects of psychic trauma four years after a school-bus kidnapping. *Amer. J. Psychiat.,* 140:1543–1550.

―――― (1988), What happens to early memories of trauma? A study of twenty children under age five at the time of documented traumatic events. *J. Amer. Acad. Child & Adol. Psychiat.,* 27:96–104.

―――― (1991), Childhood traumas: An outline and overview. *Amer. J. Psychiat.,* 148:10–20.

———— (1996), Acute responses to external events and posttraumatic stress disorder. In: *Child and Adolescent Psychiatry*, 2nd ed., ed. M. Lewis. Baltimore: Williams & Wilkins, pp. 753–763.

United Nations Children's Fund (1996), *State of the World's Children*, Oxford: Oxford University Press, p. 13.

U.S. Department of Health and Human Services, Administration on Children, Youth and Families (1999), *Child Maltreatment 1997: Reports from the States to the National Child abuse and Neglect Data System*. Washington, DC: U.S. Government Printing Office.

Vrana, S. & Lauterbach, D. (1994), Prevalence of traumatic events and post-traumatic psychological symptoms in a nonclinical sample of college students. *J. Traumatic Stress*, 7:289–302.

Weine, S. M. (1999), *When History Is a Nightmare: Lives and Memories of Ethnic Cleansing in Bosnia-Herzegovina*. New Brunswick, NJ: Rutgers University Press.

———— Becker, D. F., McGlashan, T. H., Laub, D., Lazrove, S., Vojvoda, D. & Hyman, L. (1995), Psychiatric consequences of ethnic cleansing: Clinical assessments and trauma testimonies of newly resettled Bosnian refugees. *Amer. J. Psychiat.*, 152:536–542.

———— ———— ———— Vojvoda, D., Hartman, S. & Robbins, J. P. (1995), Adolescent survivors of "ethnic cleansing": Observations on the first year in America. *J. Amer. Acad. Child & Adol. Psychiat.*, 34:1153–1159.

———— Vojvoda, D., Becker, D. F., McGlashan, T. H., Hodzic, E., Laub, D., Hyman, L., Sawyer, M. & Lazrove, S. (1998), PTSD symptoms in Bosnian refugees 1 year after resettlement in the United States. *Amer. J. Psychiat.*, 155:562–564.

———— ———— Hartman, S. & Hyman, L. (1997), A family survives genocide. *Psychiatry*, 60:24–39.

Winegar, R. K. & Lipschitz, D. S. (1999), Agreement between hospitalized adolescents' self-reports of maltreatment and witnessed home violence and clinician reports and medical records. *Compr. Psychiat.*, 40:347–352.

Yule, W., Bolton, D., Udwin, O., Boyle, S., O'Ryan, D. & Nurrish, J. (2000), The long-term psychological effects of a disaster experienced in adolescence: I: The incidence and course of PTSD. *J. Child Psychol. Psychiat.*, 41:503–511.

7 TRAUMA AND ADOLESCENCE II

THE IMPACT OF TRAUMA

THE COMMITTEE ON ADOLESCENCE OF THE GROUP
FOR THE ADVANCEMENT OF PSYCHIATRY

Members of the GAP Committee on Adolescence who contributed to this special section include: Daniel F. Becker, Melita Daley, Monica R. Green, Robert L. Hendren, Lois T. Flaherty (Committee Chair), Warren J. Gadpaille, Gordon Harper, Robert A. King, Patricia Lester, Silvio J. Onesti, Mary Schwab-Stone, and Susan W. Wong.

NORMAL ADOLESCENT DEVELOPMENT AND VULNERABILITY TO TRAUMA

An understanding of normal adolescent development is crucial to the understanding of the impact of trauma in this age group. The developmental tasks of adolescence include

1. Coping with the physical changes of puberty
2. Mastering an upsurge of sexual and aggressive impulses
3. Developing autonomy from parents
4. Forging sustaining ties with peers and adults outside the family
5. Developing the capacity for intimacy with a romantic other
6. Establishing a durable sense of personal values
7. Consolidating a coherent identity (including gender, vocational, and ethnic roles
8. Achieving a sense of competency and industry in work or school
9. Planning realistically for eventual economic self-sufficiency.

These normative developmental challenges also pose potential areas of vulnerability for the adolescent, especially for the adolescent exposed to trauma. Overwhelming physical danger (experienced or witnessed) undermines fantasies of physical omnipotence and the adolescent's tentative moves towards autonomy from parental care and supervision. Sexual or aggressive trauma may either overstimulate the adolescent's own aggression (through stimulating defensive sadistic retaliatory anger) or by rendering dangerous the whole arena of sexual arousal or assertiveness. Feelings of mistrust, self-doubt, guilt, shame, or anxiety erode self-esteem, impede peer relations, interfere with academic or vocational functioning, and corrode a stable sense of identity.

Not only are adolescents particularly vulnerable to trauma during this developmental phase, they can react at this time to earlier traumatic events. The meaning to the adolescent of trauma experienced earlier can change; in effect, the trauma may be experienced anew. As an adolescent realizes the meaning of incest experienced during childhood, the memories of such experiences may take on different qualities and produce different responses. A previous exposure to trauma during childhood can have a variety of significant effects on adolescents. Early childhood traumas are frequently reactivated in adolescence, leading to the reemergence of problems that were thought to have been resolved. Moreover, in North American societies, the period of early adolescence is particularly stressful, involving as it does a number of developmental transitions (puberty, entrance into high school) that are accompanied by increased expectations and for which social support is limited (Dryfoos, 1998). Finally, adolescents have a tendency to take risks that expose them to trauma, with dangerous risk-taking behavior during adolescence more likely if there is a history of early abuse (Trickett, 1997). On the positive side, adolescents have potentially greater resources for protecting themselves. They have increased physical strength and increased ability to anticipate consequences and to develop plans for avoiding or escaping the threat of danger. Compared to younger children, they also have the availability of peers and adults outside the family as sources of aid and support.

The more advanced cognitive and emotional development of adolescents enhances their ability to appreciate and understand what they experience and have previously experienced. This may have both protective and risk-enhancing effects.

Studies of the Impact of Trauma During the Adolescent Years

Adolescents' responses to trauma, compared with those of younger children and adults, have not been well studied. Many of the studies that have included adolescents have lumped together their responses with those of younger children. However, a few studies, including those of combat trauma, disasters, and rape, have shown differential effects on adolescents consistent with the existence of particular vulnerabilities of this age. Adolescents who fought in Vietnam were more prone to develop posttraumatic stress disorder (PTSD) than were older soldiers; van der Kolk (1985) hypothesized that this was due to the intensity of their attachment to their combat buddies and the consequent magnitude of the loss that the young soldiers experienced when their friends were killed.

Comparing older and younger victims of sexual assault, Davidson and colleagues (1996) found the greatest likelihood of later suicide attempts in those who were assaulted prior to age 16. Similarly, Breslau et al. (1997) found that women who experienced trauma of any kind prior to age 15 were more vulnerable to developing PTSD as a sequel than were those whose trauma occurred at a later age. Two years after the Buffalo Creek disaster, adolescents were found to have higher levels of distress than younger children (Green et al., 1991). A major component of this tragedy was a loss of community as well as a sense of betrayal by the mining company whose negligence led to the disaster. These may have been particularly traumatic stresses for the adolescents, for whom normative development meant a social orientation outside their families and a confrontation with the imperfections of adult authority.

A few studies have indicate that adolescents may be less vulnerable than children or adults to certain kinds of trauma. Studies of Holocaust survivors indicate that the most devastating effects were on those who were infants during this massive trauma (Kestenbaum and Brenner, 1996); adolescents who survived did relatively well, faring better than adult survivors. The separations and deprivation of parental care, which all young victims experienced, were most damaging for the youngest children; most older children and adolescents had at least a residue of earlier healthy development to sustain them. Resourcefulness, group cohesiveness, a sense of invulnerability, rebelliousness, and a willingness to take risks were psychologically protective and actually enhanced the likelihood of adolescents' survival. Similar findings emerged from Weine and colleagues' (1995, 1998) studies of Bosnian survivors of ethnic cleansing, which indicated that adolescents were less traumatized than were adults. In their sample, however, younger survivors tended to experience less torture and other extreme conditions than did adults.

The importance of the subjective experience, which is influenced by developmental level, is underscored by the work of Rothe, Castillo-Matos, and Busquets (2002), who found that Cuban teenagers in a refugee camp rated the conditions of their confinement more stressful than the horrors they had witnessed in their failed sea crossings.

Traumatic experience colors the way in which adolescents work on the developmental task of coming to terms with an imperfect world. Terr and colleagues (1997) studied the reactions of children and adolescents after the 1986 Challenger spacecraft explosion, widely witnessed on television in schools, and of particular significance because a teacher was among the crew, all of whom were killed. Over the 14 months following the disaster, adolescents developed increasingly negative attitudes toward institutions, God, and the future of the world. These changes in their thinking were the most salient features of their responses, in contrast to children, who responded mainly in terms of symptoms.

Children and adolescents living near the site of a faulty nuclear-waste reactor manifested interactive effects of age and gender relative to developing posttraumatic responses secondary to the threat of radioactive environmental contamination (Korol, Green, and Gleser, 1999). Younger boys and adolescent girls were the most prone to developing symptoms. Knowing more about the reactor and radioactivity had a protective effect for boys but not for girls, who were more symptomatic the more knowledgeable they said they were.

BEHAVIORAL AND EMOTIONAL REACTIONS ASSOCIATED WITH TRAUMA

Range of Responses

Most adolescents who experience trauma, even severe trauma, do not develop PTSD. The work of Brent and colleagues (1992, 1996), who

168

studied friends of adolescent suicide victims, is instructive. These researchers looked for both immediate and delayed effects of exposure to this kind of trauma. During the first six months after the event, 5.4% of the survivor group studied developed PTSD; 8% met criteria for PTSD at three-year follow-up (Brent et al., 1992, 1996). Much more prevalent among this group were depression and anxiety disorders; approximately half developed diagnosable psychiatric disorders soon after learning of the suicide, and the same percentage showed residual disorders three years later.

Even within the spectrum of *DSM-IV*-defined criteria, there is a range of posttraumatic responses short of full PTSD. Evidence from community samples suggests that partial syndromes are much more common than PTSD in the general population and also following a specific stressor such as a natural disaster. Like the full PTSD syndrome, these subsyndromal conditions can be associated with significant impairment.

Adolescents who do develop posttraumatic responses show symptoms of avoidance, reexperiencing, and arousal that parallel those in adults who meet *DSM* posttraumatic stress disorder criteria (American Psychiatric Association, APA, 2000). Trauma-specific fears, depression and anxiety, and belligerence are also common. Even though a complete PTSD syndrome may not be present, a youngster can experience significant distress and impairment. Other disorders may ensue following trauma, even in the absence of posttraumatic reactions.

The long-term impact of experiencing trauma during the adolescent period may include increased sensitivity to loss and an increased vulnerability to anxiety and depression. More severe responses include various forms of dissociation, ranging from chronic psychic numbing to dissociative identity disorders and problems with relationships. The presence of comorbid trauma-related psychopathology along with depression, conduct disorder, or substance abuse markedly complicates treatment of the adolescent.

The following vignettes demonstrate two very different outcomes of early trauma on later adolescent development. In the first, a young woman presents with a victim identity and complex and evolving psychopathology. Although she experiences some symptomatic improvement with multimodal treatment, the persistent impact of early physical and sexual abuse can be seen in the derailment of the developmental tasks of adolescence. In the second vignette, a teenage girl in residential treatment initiates mastery of the developmental tasks of adolescence despite a history of early trauma. She also demonstrates an attachment to painful feelings as a source of identity.

Vignette 1. Ileana was a 16-year-old Hispanic female when she presented with a suicide attempt; at that time, she already had a history of numerous psychiatric hospitalizations for depression and suicidal behavior. Between the ages of 4 and 13, she had experienced severe physical and sexual abuse. She reported feeling chronically depressed and suicidal, having flashbacks and nightmares about the abuse almost every night, hearing a voice when she was upset, and having mood swings when she felt "hyper." She described accusatory voices, and the content of her talk was themes of hopelessness and despair. She spoke in great detail about her previous suicide attempts and failed treatment.

She was treated with clonidine .05 mg bid, chlorpromazine 75 mg hs and 25 mg PRN, and bupropion 150 mg per day. During the course of her hospitalization, her depression improved, but she continued to have a high level of anxiety and a very fixed view of herself as irreparably damaged victim and incurably mentally ill person. Her anxiety increased when she was presented with the possibility of going to a foster home instead of returning home or going to an institutional placement; this seemed related to conflict about her attachment to her family (notwithstanding the abuse) and her role as a severely dysfunctional person.

The hospital discharge diagnosis was severe depression and PTSD; the auditory hallucinations were thought to be mood congruent and possibly associated with depression but considered alternatively as a possible component of PTSD.

Over the course of the next two years, Ileana received placement in a therapeutic foster home, special education support at school, individual psychotherapy, and medication management. She was able to form a relationship with her foster parents and outpatient therapist. She was compliant in taking medications (bupropion and valproate) and did not abuse substances. Eventually, she began to experience success and to see herself in a more positive way, to the point of being able to acknowledge positive things about herself and take pleasure in her accomplishments. She required a great deal of support from all who worked with her and had to be hospitalized briefly twice. As she approached her 18th birthday, her anxiety increased. She remained unconvinced that she would ever be successful and still occasionally referred to herself as "psycho," "wacko," or "schizo." She continued to struggle with guilt about leaving her very dysfunctional family. She was not able to form lasting friendships with others her age, preferentially seeking the company of adults and making great demands on her foster parents. She remained unable to make productive use of leisure time and did not believe she would live to be an adult.

Ileana was moderately obese, and her attention to her appearance varied markedly from one day to the next. She would go out of her way to dress in attention-getting costumes one day and appear disheveled and unkempt another. She was withdrawn and uncooperative at times and made teasing comments about killing herself. She repeatedly talked about inability to be alone, feelings of emptiness, extreme mood swings in which she went from being suicidally depressed to feeling hyper. She described hearing a voice of an imaginary person called Freddie who gave her advice but also criticized her. Depressive symptoms and anxiety symptoms continued. She continued to have frequent nightmares about past sexual abuse. She never evidenced disordered thinking or any other signs suggestive of a schizophrenic illness.

Ileana's preoccupation with abandonment, her unstable self-image, her impulsivity, affective instability, and recurrent suicidal behavior—all borderline personality features—had become more prominent. Features suggestive of dissociative identity disorder included her lack of memory for periods of time, comments by observers that her speech and manner were markedly different at times, and her hallucinations. Her continued nightmares about sexual abuse and sense that she had no future were posttraumatic stress symptoms.

Vignette 2. Sarah, a 16-year-old girl, was living in a residential treatment program where she had been placed by child protective services because of sexual abuse by her stepfather. Before her removal from home, Sarah had attempted suicide by overdose. After coming to the residential program, she had persistent difficulties with adjustment, despite beginning individual and group therapy. She experienced decreased concentration with difficulty at school, distractibility, insomnia, nightmares, depressed mood, low self-esteem, guilt, daily tearfulness, hypervigilance, and pervasive anxiety. She also reported flashbacks of sexual abuse by her stepfather, a voice calling her name during quiet times alone, and infrequent visions of a dark figure trying to harm her.

At times, Sarah was a thoughtful girl who was reflective on her mental states; on difficult days, she was fearful of others' intentions, feeling empty and alone. The residential program had a high turnover in residents due to runaways; the unexpected departure of her peers escalated Sarah's anxiety and mistrust.

Because of her persistent distress, Sarah had a trial of paroxetine. Initially, she reported some decrease in anxiety and improved mood, but then she abruptly stated she no longer wanted to take medications. She reported that all she knew about herself was her depression: "If you take away my sadness, then I won't be me." Over the next few months, her symptoms worsened. Her schoolwork deteriorated, and she had difficulty engaging in therapy. During regular meetings with the psychiatrist, she continued to refuse medications but began to explore her feelings about her family, as well as her uncertainty about the program. She made an agreement with the psychiatrist that they would work together as a team, and that unless her symptoms increased, she would continue off medications, given her preference. Following this, Sarah inquired whether there was a medication that might help her focus on schoolwork, as she felt she had difficulty paying attention in class. She felt that a medicine that also helped her mood would be acceptable but that she did not want this to be the primary reason for taking medication. She started on bupropion and continued her individual therapy. Her depression and anxiety improved, as did her school performance. Except for periods of heightened distress, as such as her first therapy session with her family, her posttraumatic symptoms continued to improve over a 12-month period. Sarah had been able to develop ongoing, reliable relationships with her therapist and other staff members and had been able to exert control over the course and type of treatment. At her request, she was tapered off bupropion slowly and continued to have minimal symptoms. She finished high school, began working, and moved into a more independent living situation.

SPECIFIC POSTTRAUMATIC SYNDROMES

Adolescents exposed to trauma may manifest evidence of excessive autonomic arousal, including hyperarousal, increased startle response, and hyperactivity and irritability. Aggressive responses to minor provocations experienced as threats may ensue, thus paving a pathway from trauma to violence. In addition, they may retaliate with physical force or weapons in lethal ways (Osofsky et al., 1993; Steiner, Garcia, and Matthews, 1997; Lewis et al., 1997; GAP, this volume).

Difficulty concentrating, another common symptom, has obvious implications for youngsters in school or at work. Hyperactivity and inattentiveness, in addition to being responses to traumatic stress, are also cardinal symptoms of attention-deficit/hyperactivity disorder. These manifestations of posttraumatic response can be mistaken for ADHD. ADHD was actually the most common disorder found in a group of children and adolescents with confirmed sexual abuse histories (McLeer et al., 1994). Glod and Teicher (1996) found elevated activity levels in children with histories of abuse, of whom 21% met criteria for ADHD, though these investigators note that the question of whether such symptoms truly constitute ADHD remains unanswered. This and other work has raised important questions about the nature of the relationship between ADHD and PTSD. It is unclear whether there is an ADHD subtype that occurs in association with PTSD or whether many children who have trauma-related psychopathology are misdiagnosed as having ADHD. The significance of this controversy regarding adolescents is not clear. In theory at least, because the diagnosis of ADHD depends on onset of symptoms prior to age seven, it should be easier to distinguish ADHD from PTSD-related attentional and behavioral symptoms experienced after age seven. The difficulty, of course, comes when an adolescent presents with a history of repeated trauma as well as attention and behavior problems beginning in childhood.

Reexperiencing of intrusive recollections, or flashbacks, is the most specific trauma-related symptom. Avoidance is generally manifested by staying away from situations or places that trigger recollections of the traumatic event. In adolescents, this symptom may be manifested by school refusal and may be mistakenly treated as truancy.

Sleep disturbances include nightmares and fear of falling asleep. These are accompanied by electroencephalographic changes, including high REM density, shortened REM latency, and impaired sleep efficiency (Lester, Wong, and Hendren, this volume).

Dissociative Symptoms

Psychic numbing is a term used to describe a kind of detachment and withdrawal from all aspects of life, including one's feeling states, outside interests, and relationships. It is a type of dissociative symptom. People with psychic numbing lack the capacity to feel strong emotions, especially of love and tenderness. For adolescents, this inability interferes with the crucial developmental task of developing a capacity for intimacy. Constricted affect, apathy, and decline in functioning are additional components of this symptom, which may also resemble depression.

Trauma may also result in a spectrum of dissociative phenomena— ranging from feelings of unreality though trance and fugue states, depersonalization, amnesia, hysterical hallucinations, or even (at one extreme) "alters" of multiple personality phenomena. These interfere not only with day-to-day functioning, but also with emotional growth and maturation. Dissociative disorders also pose diagnostic challenges, being frequently confused with psychotic or organic mental conditions (Kluft, 1985; Silberg, 1996). This is particularly likely when alters are experienced as hallucinations, as in the case of Ileana described in Vignette 1.

Effects on Cognitive Functioning

Denial and avoidance of thought. Denial is common in the immediate aftermath of a disaster, especially one for which continued physical evidence is not present. Such was the case after the Challenger disaster, which happened quickly and left no visible evidence (Terr et al., 1997). Half of those who were present at the lift off and 80% of those who watched it on television initially denied the reality of the disaster. Continuing massive denial, linked to ongoing psychic numbing, is a response associated with an extended period of traumatization (Terr, 1991).

Attribution of responsibility for current and previous events. Self-blame is common after trauma. This may range from the abused child or adolescent's belief that she deserves the abuse, to a youth's conviction that he could have done more to prevent a disaster, or a child's feeling that she should not have survived when others died. Guilt over the perception that one is responsible for trauma is an important contributor to psychopathology. This is the probable reason that the friends of suicide victims (studied by Brent et al., 1996) who had the worst outcomes were those who had foreknowledge of their friends' plans.

Futurelessness. Particularly salient for adolescents is a sense of futurelessness. In our culture, this has been found in many inner-city teenagers who have been exposed to community violence. Futurelessness may be mistaken for the hopelessness that often accompanies depression. Rather than being a belief that things will never get better, however, it is a conviction that one will not live very long. In teenagers, it means the sometimes self-fulfilling belief that one will not survive into adulthood. Given that this belief is strongly reinforced by the high risks of violent death for many inner-city youngsters, it can be difficult to identify as part of a posttraumatic syndrome. The consequences of futurelessness for youth have not been formally studied. However, it is not hard to see that a teenager who does not expect to live very long has little reason to pursue personal or vocational goals.

Paranormal experiences. A belief in omens (certain events that could have served as warnings) was described by Terr (1991) as a characteristic feature of Type I or sudden, unexpected trauma. These beliefs result from a search for understanding why the trauma occurred and how it might have been avoided. Omens are linked to a sense of guilt and responsibility for the trauma.

The experience of a ghostly presence, or an actual hallucination, is also fairly common in adolescents after trauma. At least one such experience was reported by 42% of adolescents (compared to only 18% of children) after the Challenger disaster (Terr et al., 1997).

Intervention fantasies. Pynoos (1996) has described how adolescents are better able than children to envision changing traumatic events, owing to their maturity and greater appreciation of circumstances. Intervention fantasies are ways of coping with the sense of helplessness engendered by trauma; these include imagining how one could have altered fate by acting on the precipitating events, interrupting the traumatic action, reversing the consequences, and preventing future trauma. Teenagers also think about taking revenge: "They can imagine themselves or peers taking direct action, sometimes reckless or endangering, while maintaining a sense of narcissistic invulnerability" (p. 196). These revenge fantasies may remain just fantasies and may be expressed through constructive actions such as artistic endeavors—or, more ominously, they may be actualized, with the teenager enacting the role of an adolescent hero (or antihero, in the case of some recent school shootings in response to perceived harassment). In the latter case, the adolescent's fantasies of omnipotence, together with a failure to appreciate the degree of danger, can lead to rash and destructive actions. Cognitive appraisal of danger may be impaired following trauma. According to Pynoos (1996), "Mental modification in the form of spatial misrepresentation of threat may, if incorporated into an evolving mental schema, increase the risk of further victimization" (p. 198).

Decision-making ability is crucial as teens decide whether to act on revenge fantasies or to stay away from potentially dangerous situations believed to have placed them in danger—a behavioral outcome that can resemble phobic avoidance. A young person's ability to appraise risks realistically, to think through the consequences of behavior, and to mentally rehearse various scenarios are all important. The degree to which an adolescent has the ability to think of alternative modes of action and employ adaptive problem-solving skills will be important determinants of behavioral outcomes.

Memory. Memories can be condensed into a single event or depicted by image. The cause of the remembered event can be misattributed to the self instead of to the environmental agent. Memory of traumatic events appears to be fundamentally different from usual memory. Normal memories are integrated into a narrative that has affects as well as meaning associated with it—the story of what happened. However, traumatic experiences are recalled in terms of "memory anchor points" rather than as a sequence of events that make up an episode (Pynoos, 1996). These fragmented memories include various aspects of the trauma, such as interactions with others that were significant (the expression on an attacker's face, for example). Each of these anchor points is associated with a set of feelings, perceptions, and meanings. Because the memories are fragmented, they are not organized into a coherent narrative, and it is difficult for the adolescent to make sense out of what has happened.

This aspect of traumatic memory has important clinical implications. Youngsters can be helped enormously by assistance in processing traumatic memories. This assistance can come from parents, teachers and other supportive adults, peers, or therapists. If parents and other adults have also been traumatized, it will be difficult for them to assist their children in this process.

Repressed and recovered memory. The issue of repressed memory has attracted considerable controversy in recent years. It pertains to the absence over a period of time of conscious recall of traumatic events, with the apparent recovery of those memories much later. Typically, a traumatic event that has occurred in childhood is discovered through memory in adulthood, often in the context of therapy. The notion of recovered memory is rooted in the early observations of Freud and Breuer that patients suffering from hysteria were unable to remember important aspects of the trauma that had engendered their symptoms until they were hypnotized (Freud, 1893). Freud later came to believe that in many cases the reconstituted purported recollection had not in fact occurred, but instead represented wishful, but conflicted, fantasies.

Controversy has arisen over whether memories that are recovered in the course of therapy pertain to real or imaginary events. Critics of the validity of recovered memories have coined the term false memory syndrome to describe the imagined recollection of events that never took place, but that a person believes have happened. Therapists have been alleged to have planted memories of abuse in suggestible patients.

Experimental research on memory supports the idea that suggestible individuals (adults as well as children) can be made to believe that they remember fictitious events (Hyman and Pentland, 1992; Hyman, Troy, and Billings, 1995). Such pseudomemories can be facilitated by the use of repeated suggestion and imagery. But it is unclear whether conditions of laboratory research apply to actual life, and because traumatic memories are processed in a very different way from ordinary memories, they may be less malleable.

The findings of Chu and colleagues (1999), who studied a group of women on an inpatient unit for trauma-related disorders, suggest that although in some cases pseudomemories of abuse may have been precipitated by therapists, in most cases the memories had appeared outside therapy and were corroborated by external sources. They found that many patients had partial or complete amnesia for the abuse, along with dissociative disorders. Terr (1988, 1991) has noted that, in contrast to single traumatic events, which are usually followed by vivid memories, chronic recurring trauma such as that entailed in abuse is frequently accompanied by a variety of defenses, including dissociative amnesia.

Awareness of the possibility of distortions of memory and actual falsification in response to suggestion should serve as a reminder to therapists to avoid imposing their own reconstructions on patients' personal histories and should give them pause before prematurely concluding that trauma has occurred.

Effects on Character and Identity Development

Perhaps the most salient aspect of trauma for adolescent development is the sudden loss of innocence and sense of invulnerability that accompanies traumatic experience. In addition, the experience of symptoms and functional impairment threatens the young person's sense of competence and self esteem. One can imagine the sense of shame felt by the young Cuban refugees described by Rothe et al. (2002) who lost bowel and bladder control during their confinement in a refugee camp.

The development of a victim identity is another possible consequence of trauma and is particularly likely if chronic PTSD develops. Scrignar (1984) has conceptualized three phases in the clinical course of PTSD: 1) an immediate reaction; 2) a continuing state of acute PTSD in vulnerable individuals, with persistent symptoms and a preoccupation with the trauma; and 3) a chronic state, accompanied by demoralization and depression, in which the person's life centers around his or her disability and symptoms. Adolescents who enter this third stage may develop a rigid victim or survivor identity that prematurely forecloses the process of healthier adolescent identity formation. The role of victim may lead to the quest for special treatment and secondary gain.

Another adverse consequence may be a personality organized around a sense of grievance or the seeking of revenge. The psychological outcome may involve overuse of externalization of personal responsibility—an individual blames his subsequent behavior or difficulties on his having experienced trauma. This may be the outcome for those who experience trauma during adolescence, as well for as those who have a residue of trauma experienced during childhood. The implication of this understanding is that an important aim of therapy should be replacing the identity of being a victim with the coalescence of the identity of a developing adolescent (Green, this volume).

Krystal (1978) noted that character features of passivity and helplessness are possible outcomes of severe traumatization, commenting, "Among the lasting characterological changes following massive psychic traumatization are patterns of accepting a defeated inferior position and function for life" (p. 107).

Moral development may be affected in complex ways. Basic beliefs about ethical behavior are called into question when societal institutions are shattered. Adolescents in concentration camps had to steal food and otherwise engage in rule-breaking behavior to help themselves and others to survive, and they were faced with the challenge of developing new kinds of moral reasoning (Kestenbaum and Brenner, 1996). In some cases this could lead to more advanced moral development, as Goenjian and colleagues (1999) found when they compared a group of 13-year-old and 16-year-old adolescent survivors of the 1998 Armenian earthquake to other Armenian teens living in an unaffected town. Those who were directly exposed to the trauma of the earthquake were more likely to evidence a consolidation of more mature moral values, to understand that there are admixtures of good and bad, and to use autonomous decision making—all associated with an integrated stage of moral development not usually seen until late adolescence. This was as true of the 13-year-olds as it was of the 16-year-olds. The researchers hypothesized that the necessity of making difficult moral decisions had stimulated the adolescent survivors' thinking beyond simply relying on what they had been taught or feeling confused—both characteristic of earlier stages of moral development.

COMORBIDITY

The range of potential responses following traumatic stress is enormous and includes virtually the full range of psychopathological syndromes. Comorbidity is common; a likely reason for this is the extensive overlap between some of the symptoms of PTSD and those associated with other disorders, most notably the depressive and anxiety disorders (Kessler et al., 1995).

General Issues

Numerous epidemiological studies as well as research on clinical samples of adults have demonstrated that comorbidity with PTSD is extremely common, especially if the PTSD is chronic. Comorbidity generally increases the level of impairment and is thought to worsen prognosis as well. Findings in adolescents have been similar. The frequency with which this disorder and other affective disorders occur together raises many questions. Are affective disorders in trauma victims different from those arising without a context of trauma? Do they represent a final common pathway toward which trauma-induced psychopathology is one route, or are they phenotypes whose underlying pathogenesis is fundamentally different? Do these disorders simply occur coincidentally in some individuals, or does the presence of one predispose a person to develop the other? Yet another possibility is that various vulnerability or background factors (for example, poverty or parental substance abuse) may predispose children to both exposure to trauma (with all its sequelae) and to other forms of pathology (for example, conduct disorder, depression, and anxiety).

Although comorbid conditions are frequently cotemporaneous with PTSD in adults, in adolescents the tendency is for comorbid conditions to emerge later in the aftermath of trauma, suggesting that the trauma has set in motion processes that lead to the development of other illnesses.

The fact that there is some overlap in the symptom criteria for PTSD and other disorders, especially those for the mood and anxiety disorders, has raised the question as to whether comorbidity may be an artifact of current diagnostic classification systems (Kessler et al., 1995; Yehuda and McFarlane, 1995). However, even when diagnostically ambiguous symptoms are ignored, enough symptoms are left to fulfill criteria for more than one diagnosis, and patterns of comorbidity remain.

Anxiety and Depression

Posttraumatic syndromes, including acute stress reactions and acute and chronic forms of PTSD as defined by *DSM*, actually are less common following traumatic stress than are anxiety and depression. Trauma can involve many kinds of loss—of family members or friends, of schools and teachers, of communities. Thus, grief reactions, sometimes including severe depression, are frequently part of the traumatic stress response. This admixture is exemplified in the high rates of comorbid depressive symptoms and posttraumatic stress symptoms found in children who lost their relatives during a severe earthquake in 1988 in Armenia (Goenjian et al., 1995). As would be expected, those who experienced traumatic loss of significant people suffered from grief reactions and depression in addition to PTSD.

The onset and severity of depressive symptoms is enhanced by the persistence of symptoms of posttraumatic stress (Pfeffer et al., 1997). Furthermore, bereavement may be complicated by posttraumatic symptoms. Although this is understandable in cases of the violent death of a loved one, it has also been found that parental death in and of itself can engender symptoms commonly associated with PTSD (Harris, 1991; Stoppelbein and Greening, 2000). The terms traumatic grief and complicated bereavement have been used to describe a condition that includes elements of both grief and posttraumatic stress disorder (Prigerson et al., 1999).

Anxiety disorders, including panic disorder, agoraphobia and obsessive-compulsive disorder, have been found in adults with histories of physical or sexual abuse (Stein et al., 1996). Selective mutism has been described (Jacobsen, 1995). The clinical impression that obsessive-compulsive disorder can be a sequel of traumatic stress has been confirmed (de Silva and Marks, 1999). Intrusive thoughts and images may take on an obsessional quality. Idiosyncratic rituals or superstitious behaviors intended to avert recurrent danger may resemble more classical compulsions. A possible neurobiological correlate has been proposed (Dinn, Harris, and Raynard, 1999) to involve enhanced responsiveness of the basal ganglia-orbitofrontal neural circuits as a result of traumatically induced cognitive changes during childhood.

Substance Abuse

Substance abuse is prevalent among adult clinical populations with PTSD, and it has been especially well documented among Vietnam War veterans. The association of adolescent substance abuse and a history of physical and sexual abuse has also been well established. The strength of this association has been confirmed by large-scale surveys showing that abuse of alcohol and other substances is prevalent among adolescents who have been maltreated, especially if they have posttraumatic stress disorder (Bensley et al., 1999; Grilo et al., 1999; Kilpatrick et al., 2000). Many teens in substance abuse treatment programs have histories of maltreatment. Deykin and Buka (1997) found current prevalence rates of PTSD of 40% for females and 12% for males (approximately five times the rates in community samples) in adolescents aged 15 to 19 in seven publicly funded Massachusetts treatment facilities.

Because the use of substances usually involves a high-risk lifestyle, people who abuse substances are, in turn, much more likely to experience trauma. An interesting gender difference is that trauma generally precedes substance abuse in females but follows it in males.

Somatic Symptoms

The original conceptualization of hysteria was a condition characterized by the conversion of the distress of psychological trauma into physical symptoms. Our current classification system places physical symptoms without underlying medical causes under the rubric of somatoform disorders. This category includes several diagnoses, such as somatization, conversion, pain disorders, and hypochondriasis. A link between trauma and somatoform disorders is strongly supported by research on adolescents (Hubbard et al., 1995) as well as on adults (Lowenstein, 1990; Rogers et al., 1996). Among adolescents, pseudoseizures in particular have been linked to a history of sexual abuse (Wyllie et al., 1999).

An association between physical complaints and childhood trauma, especially sexual abuse, among patients seen in general medical settings is increasingly being recognized (Barsky et al., 1994; Leroi et al., 1995; Leserman et al., 1998). Symptoms of abdominal and chronic pelvic pain are particularly common among abuse victims.

Brief Psychotic Reactions

Brief psychotic reactions can occur in children and adolescents as well as adults following trauma (Volkmar, 1996; APA, 2000). Typical symptoms include auditory hallucinations, for example, hearing the voice of a dead person. These symptoms may be difficult to distinguish from intrusive reexperiencing symptoms, although they are different phenomena. Adding diagnostic complexity, such symptoms are sometimes indicative of comorbid psychotic disorders such as schizophrenia, bipolar disorder, or substance-induced psychosis. Cultural influences may play a role, as trauma-related psychotic reactions are most prevalent in the United States among ethnic minorities, and, worldwide, in developing countries.

The presence of psychotic reactions is unrelated to the severity of PTSD symptoms but is associated with overall severity of psychopathology, including the presence of violent behavior. Finally, posttraumatic symptoms can occur as a reaction to a psychotic episode, which is itself a terrifying experience (Shaw, McFarlane, and Bookless, 1997).

Disruptive Behavior Disorders and Antisocial Behavior

Neglect and/or physical abuse during childhood have been found to be associated with conduct disorders in adolescence (Pelkovitz et al., 1994). Not only physical abuse during childhood, but also verbal abuse, has been linked to personality disorders in adulthood (Johnson et al., 1999, 2001). The mechanisms by which these links operate have been hypothesized to involve failures in attachment as well as learned patterns of behavior. The role played by posttraumatic reactions is unclear.

One study looked at trauma in children and adolescents with ADHD and found that, although the risk of experiencing trauma or suffering from PTSD was not increased in youngsters with ADHD over that of normal controls, those with ADHD who did experience trauma had severe psychosocial dysfunction relative to those with ADHD, but without trauma exposure (Wozniak et al., 1999).

Steiner and colleagues (Steiner et al., 1997; Cauffman et al., 1998) have also studied incarcerated juvenile offenders and found that full and partial posttraumatic stress disorders are prevalent in both male and female offenders. They noted that symptoms of traumatization might be particularly difficult to recognize in delinquent adolescents, who are reluctant to acknowledge them due to a sense of shame about what they experience as being crazy. Some of the trauma exposure these youngsters experienced was due to their violent lifestyles as teenagers, but much was related to growing up in violent families and communities.

Although most abused children do not become violent, and not all violent people were abused as children, it appears that there is a subset of vulnerable children in whom being abused is a precursor for violent behavior (Rivera and Widom, 1990; Meyers et al., 1995). In a similar way, sexual abuse is a risk factor for later sexual offending (Skuse et al., 1998).

Suicide

Adolescence is a time of particular vulnerability to suicide (GAP, 1997). Stressful life events, or triggering factors, are frequent in the period immediately preceding an adolescent's suicide or suicide attempt. Typically, these stresses involve interpersonal conflicts, separations, and rejections. But it is accumulated lifetime stresses, such as separations from parents, physical and sexual abuse, family discord and violence, that create a vulnerability to triggering events. This kind of accumulation of stress constitutes "a profound mediator of suicidal behavior rather than a discrete triggering factor" (Pfeffer, 1996, p. 329).

Part of the vulnerability to suicide created by stress may be understood in terms of the meaning of traumatization, especially abuse, to the child or adolescent victim. Particularly salient are the sense of powerlessness, low self-esteem, and stigmatization that follow trauma.

Teen Pregnancy

The risk of pregnancy during adolescence is increased among teenagers who have been sexually abused (Stevens-Simon and Reichert, 1994). It is likely that the unprotected sexual activity that results in pregnancy is the consequence of a complex array of trauma-related factors, including problems with affect regulation and impulse control, low self-esteem, and lack of hope for the future. In addition, sexual promiscuity may represent a defensive reaction of turning passive into active (Sugar, 1983). The following vignette depicts an adolescent girl who experiences a cascade of adverse experiences, any one of which would have been stressful enough to impair development and result in severe disability. She makes attempts at restoration through a pathological attachment and early pregnancy. This case illustrates the kind of multiple layers of trauma that clinicians often hear about from patients with significant impairment.

Vignette 3. Sonya, a 15-year-old girl, initially came to clinical attention when she presented to the emergency room accompanied by her foster mother after taking a serious overdose of steroids with the intention of ending her life. She reported being chronically depressed for years and feeling that she would rather be dead. The patient had a long-standing history of polycystic kidney disease and had had multiple hospitalizations for medical complications over the three years preceding her overdose. She stated she was fed up with her quality of life and could not go on.

At the age of three, Sonya witnessed the fatal shooting of her mother by her biological father. Her father was sentenced to life imprisonment for murder, and she and her two-year-old brother were placed in a foster family. She was sexually abused by her foster father from age 10 to age 14. Her foster mother did not believe her when she disclosed the abuse.

The patient went into kidney failure within the first few days after the overdose and then underwent a kidney transplant from her brother. She had some chronic rejection over the next few years but was overall medically stable.

Sonya became pregnant at age 18 and immediately was married to the child's father, with a subsequent chaotic relationship. Her pregnancy was complicated owing to her abdominal kidney, and she went into premature labor and delivered at 28 weeks. The baby had significant developmental delay, and Sonya had a great deal of difficulty coping. Sonya was divorced in a year and had little contact with the child's father thereafter. She suffered from ongoing depressive and anxiety symptoms and often felt suicidal.

RISK AND PROTECTIVE FACTORS

In general, there is a dose-response relationship between trauma and posttraumatic reactions (Pynoos et al., 1995; Goenjian, 1995). Significant mediating variables include proximity to the event, extent of destruction of resources, losses of significant others, and degree of immediate threat to life. Abuse of a child or adolescent—whether physical, sexual or psychological—by a trusted adult has been held to have a particularly noxious effect because it involves a betrayal of trust.

The response to trauma is dependent on an individual's vulnerability and resilience. Some events would be traumatic to anyone; other events may or may not be traumatic, depending on the social and cultural milieu and the individual's coping skills.

Continuation of symptoms beyond six months in adolescents has been linked to prior traumatic experience and psychiatric morbidity, female sex, and level of exposure (Garrison et al., 1993, 1995). These findings are similar to those in studies of young adults, in whom chronic PTSD (defined as greater than one year's duration), compared with PTSD of shorter duration, has been specifically associated with female sex, higher rates of comorbid anxiety and depressive disorders, and a family history of antisocial behavior (Breslau and Davis, 1992). Development of posttraumatic symptoms after an earthquake in a sample with preexisting depression was associated with resource loss, preexisting anxiety, and the use of cognitive coping styles (Asarnow et al., 1999).

It appears that different mechanisms are involved in acute stress reactions than those that operate in long-term responses; immediate reactions are fairly universal, whereas long-term responses are more likely to be influenced by coping skills and environmental and social supports.

Although mild forms of posttraumatic symptoms, with some impairment, are common after trauma, most victims do not develop severe posttraumatic symptoms, and only a minority go on to develop PTSD. Posttraumatic symptoms tend to peak soon after a single-event trauma and then decline rapidly over the next 12 months. In their study of adolescents six months after a hurricane, Garrison and colleagues (1995) found that, although most still had some posttraumatic symptoms, only 3.0% of males and 9.5% of females met criteria for PTSD.

Effects of Culture

The impact of trauma and the responses of individuals to trauma are shaped by the culture in which they live (see Gadpaille, this volume). People learn from their cultures what are considered to be stressful events and how they are expected to respond to such stressful events. In the Hurricane Andrew study (Garrison et al., 1995), ethnicity played a role in response, with higher rates of symptoms in black and Hispanic adolescents than in white teens, which could not be attributed to socioeconomic status alone.

It is likely that some events would be traumatic for any person, regardless of culture, but other events vary in their perceived severity depending on the their social meaning (Servan-Scheiber, Le Lin, and Birmaher, 1998). Socially constructed roles affect the meaning of trauma experienced, as well as the meaning of that perpetrated on others. A violent teen may be honored as a hero in revolutionary struggles or feared and emulated in an urban ghetto. Ideology and religion play an important role in defining the meaning of exposure to violence and danger. Violence experienced as part of a cohesive group or understood in an ideological context may less traumatic than violence experienced as random. For example, a young Palestinian male wounded in fighting Israeli soldiers is seen as a hero in a holy war in accordance with his understanding of Islam. Because of the strong appeal of ideology to adolescents, they are particularly prone to join in armed combat on the basis of perceived struggles for justice (United Nations Children's Fund, 1996). Cultural values and ethnic identity are transmitted from parents to children. The transmission of the cultural value that wrongs must be avenged, along with an identity of having been traumatized by an enemy, may help to explain how ethnic hatreds and violence persist over multiple generations (Odejide, Sanda, and Odejide, 1998).

The effects of combat trauma can be mitigated by the social status that accompanies the role of war hero or gang leader. In addition, a society can ameliorate the impact of trauma and facilitate an individual's resumption of normal functioning through group support and ritualized ways of coping (Gadpaille, this volume). Some cultures provide a cleansing and purification ritual for warriors returning from battle (Silver, 1994). The warrior's participation in killing others is thereby given absolution, which can heal the aftereffects of his own traumatization. In contrast, the individualism of modern Western society may lead to the expectation that individuals should cope with their emotional wounds by themselves, potentially resulting in an isolation that tends to compound the noxious effects of trauma.

Gender Differences

One of the most robust findings in the research literature is that trauma has gender-specific effects, with females more vulnerable to developing posttraumatic symptoms (Breslau et al., 1997). Although females are more likely to experience sexual trauma and males are more likely to experience serious accidents, the differences in type of events experienced does not account for the marked sex differences in symptom formation.

Gender differences in the response to trauma appear across all age groups. Females tend to respond with anxious or depressive reactions, and males with externalizing or disruptive behavior, including violent aggression (Heath, Bean, and Feinauer, 1996). The reasons for this are

187

unclear and may reflect differential socialization, biological predispositions toward symptom expression, or very likely a combination of these.

In the following vignette, a young male with a history of neglect and sexual abuse presents with a history of drug abuse, risk-taking behaviors, and physical aggression. During his residential treatment, he begins to embrace adolescent issues of his biological and psychological identity and consideration of future adult roles, which may be either fulfilled or derailed after he leaves treatment.

Vignette 4. Ken was a 16-year-old boy court-ordered into residential treatment after arrest for drug dealing and stealing. His history had been marked by multiple disruptions in caretaking. Before he was six, his stepfather sexually molested him. He was cared for intermittently by his mother, who was dependent on drugs. Largely unsupervised at home, he became part of a gang because the older males looked out for him. At age 11, he was one of the youngest members to be "jumped in" to the gang. He described several years of selling street drugs and proving himself by harming others. In the group home, he struggled with angry outbursts, depression, numbness, nightmares, bed-wetting, and a chronic sense of shame. He had a capacity to connect with others and proved himself a leader in the residential peer group. Over 15 months of treatment, Ken became more stable symptomatically, but he continued to struggle with violent thoughts. He reported fantasies of sinking a knife into other people. He was afraid that one day he would act on these feelings, stating that he missed the exciting sensation of harming others.

Ken was uncertain about his identity and struggled between images of himself as a helpless young boy, a gang member, and a teacher for children like himself. He made plans to graduate and attend college at age 18. However, he left the program early to move in with his girlfriend, who was six months pregnant. He was conflicted about changing his plans but felt that he needed to live up to his responsibilities of becoming a man.

Familial Transmission of Traumatic Effects

Studies of children of Holocaust survivors and war veterans reveal a high prevalence of posttraumatic stress symptoms among the offspring of those who have experienced severe traumatic stress reactions (Danieli, 1998). This is true even when the parents have not told their children about their own traumatic experiences. Transmission of symptoms has been postulated to occur on the basis of parental rearing practices and/or children's witnessing of parental symptoms. Research on nonhuman primates provides a possible explanation (Suomi and Levine, 1998). Monkeys who grow up in the wild are uniformly afraid of snakes, whereas monkeys bred in captivity do not have this fear unless they witness it in other monkeys. So powerful is the transmission process that captive monkeys become afraid of snakes after only a single exposure to the fear reactions of feral monkeys. These findings suggest how trauma responses could be transmitted from one generation to the next and why the effects of trauma can be far-reaching and go beyond a single generation.

Although young children's responses to trauma are very much influenced by the reactions of their parents, this is less true for adolescents. For example, Garrison et al. (1995) found that teenagers' responses to Hurricane Andrew were unrelated to their parents' symptomatology or exposure to this disaster. It is likely that adolescents' reactions are based more on their own cognitive appraisals of events than are the reactions of younger children.

Quality of Attachment as a Mediating Factor

Secure, supportive ties to family and peers serve as important protective factors in the face of potential trauma. They also serve as the basis of an underlying expectation that the world is predictably safe, that others are benign, and that dangers can be surmounted. Although trauma calls these assumptions into question, current and internalized perceptions of soothing and protective others influence the impact of trauma.

In young children, social referencing—the meaning of the caretaker's affective response—is a key determinant of response to uncertain or potentially threatening situations. Even in older children, parents' subjective response to a danger (e.g., air raids during the Blitz) may influence the child's resultant anxiety more than the degree of objective danger (Freud, 1973; Pynoos et al., 1995). Parents' physical presence in the traumatic situation, their affective reaction, coping style, and perceived efficacy influence the child's reaction. In the aftermath, the parents' continued physical and psychological availability is crucial,

189

as well as their ability to cope with their own upset, ability to tolerate the child's affect and assist in soothing the teen's upset, and ability to assist in his or her cognitive and emotional reappraisal. When there is parental conflict or agency in the trauma, or when the parents' own upset is intense, their capacity to mitigate the child's trauma is compromised.

An individual's attachment relationships influence the impact of trauma. Pathological attachment may arise out of experiences such as abuse and may predispose individuals to experience subsequent trauma. In turn, the experience of trauma has an impact on relationships; the essence of trauma is the undermining of secure attachment. Healthy attachment may be protective against activation or reactivation of traumatic experience. Attachment theory can inform our methods of intervention. For example, interpersonal therapy emphasizes reconnecting important relationships that have been disrupted (Mufson and Dorta, 2000).

In the following vignette, a girl suffering from early physical and sexual trauma and current physical abuse demonstrates some of the profound impact of early trauma on subsequent attachment relationships. Focused only on issues of survival and maintaining attachment, she has not yet been able to begin adolescent developmental tasks.

Vignette 5. A 14-year-old girl seen in outpatient psychotherapy, Jessica was first brought to treatment because of her grandmother's concerns about her behavior, specifically stealing, lying, and seductive dancing. Furthermore, her school was concerned about her poor school performance, including disruptive behavior, distractibility, and staring into space. Jessica experienced early physical and sexual abuse and repeated disrupted attachments during her childhood. Before she was three, her father was murdered, and her mother developed an addiction to street drugs. Jessica was molested at age three and then placed with extended family, who frequently locked her in a room by herself. She was removed at age six and placed in foster care, where a foster brother sexually abused her. She was rescued from foster care by her grandmother, who brought concerns about Jessica's hygiene to child protective services. From age eight until the time she entered treatment, she lived with her grandmother, who felt that Jessica was "bad like her mother" (obviously a self-fulfilling prophecy), although she was fond of Jessica and wanted her to do well in life. Now, at 14, Jessica had been in two prior outpatient therapies, both of which had ended abruptly when the providers moved away.

Initially, Jessica was quite solicitous with her therapist, trying to give her treasured belongings. As the therapy progressed, she shared fears of rejection and abandonment through art, rap songs, and doll play but was reluctant to talk directly about her feelings. She preferred to create worlds inhabited only by children who had many belongings as well as a punitive system of justice, with the older ones kicking and hitting the younger ones. She created images of children at sea, crying for help but drowning in the ocean. She developed more friends at school, and her grades improved somewhat. Her grandmother continued to bring in intermittent reports of her disobedience, such as talking in class and stealing candy at the corner store. At home, Jessica spent most of her time alone in her room listening to music, as her grandmother was tired at the end of the day and did not like to talk or go places. Jessica was reluctant to talk about her grandmother and focused primarily on the things her grandmother gave her. Neither Jessica nor her grandmother had ever reported any physical punishment as part of their relationship.

In her second year of therapy, Jessica was abruptly removed from the care of her grandmother when she told a classmate that she had been whipped repeatedly with an extension cord on her legs and back, showing him the welts on her legs. The classmate told a teacher, who reported the events to child protective services. When her therapist inquired why Jessica had not told any adult about the whippings, which were reportedly routine, she stated, "Because then you would have to follow that rule . . . the one that says you have to tell someone and I have to live somewhere else." Jessica's experience with caretaker losses had taught her that tolerating repeated injury was preferable to losing an important relationship.

In one study of Vietnam veterans, a prior history of good adolescent friendships was predictive of PTSD, whereas, paradoxically, a history of poor adolescent friendships was more likely in those who did not have PTSD. In addition, this study reported a number of patients with good premorbid adjustment, low childhood trauma, and good adolescent relationships who experienced prolonged trauma in Vietnam and who developed severe PTSD (Lindy, Grace, and Green, 1984). One possible explanation for this counterintuitive finding is that the soldiers with a history of close friendships had formed the most intense attachments to their buddies and were most traumatized by the losses they experienced in war. In addition, it is likely that there is a particular vulnerability to loss of friends during the late-adolescent period. (See section on

Normal Adolescent Development and Vulnerability to Trauma, this issue).

CONCLUSION

Trauma exerts its effects through a complex interplay of biological, psychological, and social factors. The outcome may be recovery or psychopathology. Table 1 illustrates in a schematic way the effects of mediating processes on the impact of trauma.

In order to understand the impact of traumatic experience on an individual adolescent, it is essential to understand the meaning of the experience for that youngster. This knowledge, in turn, requires an understanding of the teenager's developmental and social history as well as his or her cultural frame of reference.

Protective factors include a strong personal and family background. Therefore, understanding an individual's biological and psychological development in a sociocultural context is crucial to understanding the impact of trauma. Such understanding can guide clinical attempts to reduce the potentially harmful effects of trauma and to repair the pathological outcomes that may occur.

Not all teenagers who have experienced trauma will develop posttraumatic symptoms, and not all of those with symptoms will develop long-

TABLE 1

THE IMPACT OF TRAUMA

lasting psychopathology or impairment, let alone a full PTSD syndrome. At the same time, research studies have demonstrated that impairment is usually present when there is a history of exposure to severe trauma and some symptoms are present, even without the full syndrome. The challenge to the clinician is to understand the role that trauma exposure is playing in the overall functioning and symptom pattern of an individual teenager. The centrality of meaning to the experience of trauma makes it impossible to reduce to a symptom list the psychiatric disturbances that result from it. We cannot understand the sequelae to trauma simply in terms of psychiatric diagnoses.

It is important for mental health professionals to recognize the effects of trauma on adolescents and to understand the contribution of trauma to adolescent and adult psychopathology. Interventions to prevent and to treat pathological outcomes of trauma involve adolescents and their families, therapists, educational institutions, social institutions, and public policy. Appropriate intervention can literally be life-saving and can have an impact, not only on the adolescent's future, but on future generations. The human cost of failure to intervene is enormous.

REFERENCES

American Psychiatric Association (1987), *Diagnostic and Statistical Manual of Mental Disorders,* 3rd edition, revised (*DSM-III-R*). Washington, DC: American Psychiatric Association.

———— (2000), *Diagnostic and Statistical Manual of Mental Disorders,* 4th edition, Text Revision (*DSM-IV-TR*). Washington, DC: American Psychiatric Association.

Asarnow, J., Glynn, S., Pynoos, R. S., Nahum, J., Guthrie, D., Cantwell, D. P. & Franklin, B. (1999), When the earth stops shaking: Earthquake sequelae among children diagnosed for pre-earthquake psychopathology. *J. Amer. Acad. Child & Adol. Psychiat.,* 38:1016–1023.

Barsky, A. J., Wool, C., Barnett, M. C. & Cleary, P. D. (1994), Histories of childhood trauma in adult hypochondriacal patients. *Amer. J. Psychiat.,* 151:397–401.

Bensley, L. S., Spieker, S. J., Van Eenwyk, J. & Schoder, J. (1999), Self-reported abuse history and adolescent problem behaviors: II. Alcohol and drug use. *J. Adol. Health,* 24:173–180.

Brent, D. A., Moritz, G., Bridge, J., Perper, J. & Canobbio, R. (1996), Long-term impact of exposure to suicide: A three-year controlled follow-up. *J. Amer. Acad. Child & Adol. Psychiat.,* 35:646–653.

———— Perper, J., Moritz, G., Allman, C., Friend, A., Schweers, J., Roth, C., Balach, L. & Harrington, K. (1992), Psychiatric effects of exposure to suicide among the friends and acquaintances of adolescent suicide victims. *J. Amer. Acad. Child & Adol. Psychiat.,* 31:629–640.

Breslau, N. & Davis, G. C. (1992), Posttraumatic stress disorder in an urban population of young adults: Risk factors for chronicity. *Amer. J. Psychiat.,* 149:671–675.

———— Davis, G. C., Andreski, P., Peterson, E. L. & Schultz, L. R. (1997), Sex differences in posttraumatic stress disorder. *Arch. Gen. Psychiat.,* 54:1044–1048.

Cauffman, E., Feldman, S. S., Waterman, J. & Steiner, H. (1998), Posttraumatic stress disorder among female juvenile offenders. *J. Amer. Acad. Child & Adol. Psychiat.,* 37:1209–1216.

Chu, J. A., Frey, L. M., Ganzel, B. L. & Matthews, J. A. (1999), Memories of childhood abuse: Dissociation, amnesia, and corroboration. *Amer. J. Psychiat.,* 156:749–755.

Danieli, Y., ed. (1998), *International Handbook of Intergenerational Legacies of Trauma.* New York: Plenum Press.

Davidson, J. R., Hughes, D. C., George, L. K. & Blazer, D. G. (1996), The association of sexual assault and attempted suicide within the community. *Arch. Gen. Psychiat.,* 53:550–555.

de Silva, P. & Marks, M. (1999), The role of traumatic experiences in the genesis of obsessive-compulsive disorder. *Behav. Res. Ther.,* 37:941–951.

Deykin, E. V. & Buka, S. L. (1997), Prevalence and risk factors for posttraumatic stress disorder among chemically dependent adolescents. *Amer. J. Psychiat.,* 154:752–757.

Dinn, W. M., Harris, C. L. & Raynard, R. C. (1999), Posttraumatic obsessive-compulsive disorder: A three-factor model. *Psychiatry,* 62:313–324.

Dryfoos, J. G. (1998), *Safe Passage: Making It Through Adolescence in a Risky Society.* New York: Oxford University Press, 1998.

Freud, A. (1973), *Infants without Families: The Writings of Anna Freud,* Vol. 3. New York: International Universities Press.

Freud, S. (1893), On the psychical mechanisms of hysterical phenomena, *Standard Edition,* 3:25–39. London: Hogarth Press, 1953.

Garrison, C. Z., Bryant, E. S., Addy, C. L., Spurrier, P. G., Freedy, J. R. & Kilpatrick, D. G. (1995), Posttraumatic stress disorder in adolescents after Hurricane Andrew. *J. Amer. Acad. Child & Adol. Psychiat.*, 34:1193–1201.

———— Weinrich, M. W., Hardin, S. B., Weinrich, S. & Wang, L. (1993), Post-traumatic stress disorder in adolescents after a hurricane. *Amer. J. Epidemiol.*, 138:522–530.

Glod, C. A. & Teicher, M. H. (1996), Relationship between early abuse, posttraumatic stress disorder, and activity levels in prepubertal children. *J. Amer. Acad. Child & Adol. Psychiat.*, 35:1384–1393.

Goenjian, A., Pynoos, R. S., Steinberg, A. M., Najarian, L. M., Asarnow, J. R., Karayan, I., Ghurabi, M. & Fairbanks, L. A. (1995), Psychiatric comorbidity in children after the 1988 earthquake in Armenia. *J. Amer. Acad. Child & Adol. Psychiat.*, 34:1174–1184.

———— Stilwell, B. M., Steinberg, A. M., Fairbanks, L. A., Galvin, M. R., Karayan, I. & Pynoos, R. S. (1999), Moral development and psychopathological interference in conscience functioning among adolescents after trauma. *J. Amer. Acad. Child & Adol. Psychiat.*, 38:376–384.

Green, B. L., Korol, M., Grace, M., Vary, M. G., Leonard, A. C., Gleser, G. C. & Smitson-Cohen, S. (1991), Children and disaster: Age, gender and parental effects on PTSD symptoms. *J. Amer. Acad. Child & Adol. Psychiat.*, 30:945–951.

Grilo, C. M., Sanislow, C., Fehon, D. C., Martino, S. & McGlashan, T. H. (1999), Psychological and behavioral functioning in adolescent psychiatric inpatients who report histories of childhood abuse. *Amer. J. Psychiat.*, 156:538–543.

Group for the Advancement of Psychiatry. (1997), *Adolescent Suicide: Formulated by the Committee on Adolescence.* Washington, DC: American Psychiatric Press.

Harris, E. S. (1991), Adolescent bereavement following the death of a parent: An exploratory study. *Child Psychiat. Hum. Dev.*, 21:281.

Heath, V., Bean, R. & Feinauer, L. (1996), Severity of childhood sexual abuse. *Amer. J. Family Ther.*, 24:305–314.

Hubbard, J., Realmuto, G. M., Northwood, A. K. & Masten, A. S. (1995), Comorbidity of psychiatric diagnoses with posttraumatic stress disorder in survivors of childhood trauma. *J. Amer. Acad. Child & Adol. Psychiat.*, 34:1167–1173.

Hyman, I. E. & Pentland, J. (1992), The role of mental imagery in the creation of false childhood memories. *J. Memory and Language,* 35:101–117.

———— Troy, T. H. & Billings, F. J. (1995), False memories of childhood experiences. *Appl. Cogn. Psychol.,* 9:181–197.

Jacobsen, T. (1995), Case study—Is selective mutism a manifestation of dissociative identity disorder? *J. Amer. Acad. Child & Adol. Psychiat.,* 34:863–866.

Johnson, J. G., Cohen, P., Brown, J., Smailes, E. M. & Bernstein, D. P. (1999), Childhood maltreatment increases risk for personality disorders during early adulthood. *Arch. Gen. Psychiat.,* 56:600–606.

———— ———— Smailes, E. M., Skodol, A. E., Brown, J. & Oldham, J. M. (2001), Childhood verbal abuse and risk for personality disorders during adolescence and early adulthood. *Compr. Psychiat.,* 42:16–23.

Kessler, R. C., Sonnega, A., Bromet, E., Hughes, M. & Nelson, C. B. (1995), Posttraumatic stress disorder in the national comorbidity survey. *Arch. Gen. Psychiat.,* 52:1048–1060.

Kestenbaum, J. S. & Brenner, I. (1996), *The Last Witness: The Child Survivor of the Holocaust.* Washington, DC: American Psychiatric Press.

Kilpatrick, D. G., Acierno, R., Saunders, B., Resnick, H. S., Best, C. L. & Schnurr, P. P. (2000), Risk factors for adolescent substance abuse and dependence: Data from a national sample. *J. Consult. Clin. Psychol.,* 68:19–30.

Kluft, R. P. (1985), *Childhood Antecedents of Multiple Personality.* Washington, DC: American Psychiatric Press.

Korol, M., Green, B. L. & Gleser, G. C. (1999), Children's responses to a nuclear waste disaster: PTSD symptoms and outcome prediction. *J. Amer. Acad. Child & Adol. Psychiat.,* 38:368–375.

Krystal, H. (1978), Trauma and affects. *Psychoanal. Study of the Child,* 33:81–116. New Haven, CT: Yale University Press.

Leroi, A. M., Bernier, C., Watier, A., Hedmond, M., Goupil, G., Black, R., Denis, P. & Devroede, G. (1995), Prevalence of sexual abuse among patients with functional disorders of the lower gastrointestinal tract. *Int. J. Colorectal Dis.,* 10:200–206.

Leserman, J., Li, Z., Drossman, D. A. & Hu, Y. J. (1998), Selected symptoms associated with sexual and physical abuse history among female patients with gastrointestinal disorders: The impact on subsequent health care visits. *Psychol. Med.,* 28:417–425.

Lewis, D. O., Moy, E., Jackson, L. D., Aaronson, R., Restifo, N., Serra, S. & Simos, A. (1985), Biopsychosocial characteristics of children who later murder: A prospective study. *Amer. J. Psychiat.,* 142:1161b–1167b.

———— Yeager, C. A., Swica, Y., Pincus, J. H. & Lewis, M. (1997), Objective documentation of child abuse and dissociation in 12 murderers with dissociative identity disorder. *Amer. J. Psychiat.,* 154:1703–1710.

Lindy, J. D., Grace, M. C. & Green, B. L. (1984), Building a conceptual bridge between civilian trauma and war trauma: Preliminary psychological findings from a clinical sample of Vietnam veterans. In: *Post-Traumatic Stress Disorder: Psychological and Biological Sequelae,* ed. B. A. van der Kolk. Washington, DC: American Psychiatric Press, pp. 44–57.

Lowenstein, R. (1990), Somatiform disorders in victims of incest and child abuse. In: *Incest-Related Syndromes of Adult Psychopathology,* ed. R. P. Kluft. Washington, DC: American Psychiatric Press, pp. 75–107.

McLeer, S. V., Callaghan, M., Henry, D. & Wallen, J. (1994), Psychiatric disorders in sexually abused children. *J. Amer. Acad. Child & Adol. Psychiat.,* 33:313–319.

Meyers, W. C., Scott, K. S., Burgess, A. W. & Burgess, A. G. (1995), Psychopathology, biopsychosocial factors, crime characteristics, and classification of 25 homicidal youths. *J. Amer. Acad. Child & Adol. Psychiat.,* 34:1483–1489.

Mufson, L. & Dorta, K. P. (2000), Interpersonal psychotherapy for depressed adolescents: Theory, practice and research. *Adolescent Psychiatry,* 25:139–167. Hillsdale, NJ: The Analytic Press.

Odejide, A. O., Sanda, A. O. & Odejide, A. I. (1998), Intergenerational aspects of ethnic conflict in Africa: The Nigerian experience. In: *International Handbook of Intergenerational Legacies of Trauma,* ed. Y. Danieli. New York: Plenum Press.

Osofsky, J. D., Wewers, S., Hann, D. M. & Fick, A. C. (1993), Chronic community violence: What is happening to our children? *Psychiatry,* 56:36–45.

Pelcovitz, D., Kaplan, S., Goldenberg, B., Mandel, F., Lehane, J. & Guarrera, J. (1994), Post-traumatic stress disorder in physically abused adolescents. *J. Amer. Acad. Child & Adol. Psychiat.,* 33:305–312.

Pfeffer, C. R. (1996), Suicidal behavior as a response to stress. In: *Severe Stress and Mental Disturbance in Children,* ed. C. R. Pfeffer. Washington, DC: American Psychiatric Press, pp. 181–208.

———— Martins, P., Mann, J., Sunkenberg, M., Ice, A., Damore, J. P., Gallo, C., Karpenos, I. & Jiang, H. (1997), Child survivors of suicide:

Psychosocial characteristics. *J. Amer. Acad. Child & Adol. Psychiat.,* 36:65–74.

Prigerson, H. G., Shear, M. K., Jacobs, S. C., Reynolds, C. F. III, Maciejewski, P. K., Davidson, J. R., Rosenbeck, R., Pilkonis, P. A., Wortman, C. B., Williams, J. B., Widiger, T. A., Kupfer, D. J. & Zisook, S. (1999), Consensus criteria for traumatic grief: A preliminary empirical test. *Brit. J. Psychiat.,* 174:67–73.

Pynoos, R. S. (1996), Exposure to catastrophic violence and disaster in childhood. In: *Severe Stress and Mental Disturbance in Children,* ed. C. R. Pfeffer. Washington, DC: American Psychiatric Press, pp. 181–208.

———— Steinberg, A. M. & Wraith, R. (1995), A developmental model of childhood traumatic stress. In: *Developmental Psychopathology,* Vol. 2, ed. D. Cicchetti & D. J. Cohen. New York: Wiley, pp. 72–95.

Rivera, B. & Widom, C. S. (1990), Childhood victimization and violent offending. *Violence & Victims,* 5:19–35.

Rogers, M. P., Weinshenker, N. J., Warshaw, M. G., Goisman, R. M., Rodriguez-Villa, F. J., Fierman, E. J. & Keller, M. B. (1996), Prevalence of somatoform disorders in a large sample of patients with anxiety disorders. *Psychosomatics,* 37:17–22.

Rothe, E., Castillo-Matos, H. & Busquets, R. (2002), Posttraumatic stress disorder in Cuban adolescent refugees during camp confinement. *Adolescent Psychiatry,* 26:97–124. Hillsdale, NJ: The Analytic Press.

Scrignar, C. B. (1984), *Post-Traumatic Stress Disorder: Diagnosis, Treatment, and Legal Issues.* New York: Praeger.

Servan-Scheiber, D., Le Lin, B. & Birmaher, B. (1998), Prevalence of posttraumatic stress disorder and major depressive disorder in Tibetan refugee children. *J. Amer. Acad. Child & Adol. Psychiat.,* 37:874–879.

Shaw, K., McFarlane, A. & Bookless, C. (1997), The phenomenology of traumatic reactions to psychotic illness. *J. Nerv. Ment. Dis.,* 185:434–441.

Silberg, J. L. (1996), *The Dissociative Child.* Lutherville, MD: Sidran Press.

Silver, S. (1994), Lessons from Child of Water. *Amer. Indian & Alaska Native Mental Health Res.,* 6:1–22.

Skuse, D., Bentovim, A., Hodges, J., Stevenson, J., Andreou, C., Lanyado, M., New, M., Williams, B. & McMillan, D. (1998), Risk factors for development of sexually abusive behaviour in sexually victimised adolescent boys: a cross sectional study. *Brit. Med. J.,* 317:175–179.

Stein, M. B., Walker, J. R., Anderson, G., Hazen, A. L., Ross, C. A., Eldridge, G. & Forde, D. R. (1996), Childhood physical and sexual abuse in patients with anxiety disorders and in a community sample. *Amer. J. Psychiat.,* 153:275–277.

Steiner, H., Garcia, I. G. & Matthews, Z. (1997), Posttraumatic stress disorder in incarcerated juvenile delinquents. *J. Amer. Acad. Child & Adol. Psychiat.,* 36:356–365.

Stevens-Simon, C. & Reichert, S. (1994), Sexual abuse, adolescent pregnancy, and child abuse: A developmental approach to an intergenerational cycle. *Arch. Ped. Adol. Med.,* 148:23–27.

Stoppelbein, L. & Greening, L. (2000), Posttraumatic stress symptoms in parentally bereaved children and adolescents. *J. Amer. Acad. Child & Adol. Psychiat.,* 39:1112–1119.

Sugar, M. (1983), Sexual abuse of children and adolescents. *Adolescent Psychiatry.* 11:199–211. Hillsdale, NJ: The Analytic Press.

Suomi, S. J. & Levine, S. (1998), Psychobiology of intergenerational effects of trauma: Evidence from animal studies. In: *International Handbook of Multigenerational Legacies of Trauma,* ed. Y. Danieli. New York: Plenum Press, pp. 623–637.

Terr, L. C. (1988), What happens to early memories of trauma? A study of twenty children under age five at the time of documented traumatic events. *J. Amer. Acad. Child & Adol. Psychiat.,* 27:96–104.

————— (1991), Childhood traumas: An outline and overview. *Amer. J. Psychiat.,* 148:10–20.

————— Bloch, D. A., Michel, B. A., Shi, H., Reinhardt, J. A. & Metayer, S. (1997), Children's thinking in the wake of Challenger. *Amer. J. Psychiat.,* 154:744–751.

Trickett, P. K. (1997), Sexual and physical abuse and the development of social competence. In: *Developmental Psychopathology: Perspectives on Adjustment, Risk, and Disorder,* ed. S. S. Luthar, J. A. Burack, D. Cicchetti & J. R. Weisz. New York: Cambridge University Press, pp. 390–416.

United Nations Children's Fund (1996), *State of the World's Children.* Oxford: Oxford University Press, p. 13.

van der Kolk, B. A. (1985), Adolescent vulnerability to posttraumatic stress disorder. *Psychiatry,* 48:365–370.

Volkmar, F. R. (1996), Child and adolescent psychoses: A review of the past 10 years. *J. Amer. Acad. Child & Adol. Psychiat.,* 35:843–851.

Weine, S. M., Becker, D. F., McGlashan, T. H., Laub, D., Lazrove, S., Vojvoda, D. & Hyman, L. (1995), Psychiatric consequences of ethnic cleansing: Clinical assessments and trauma testimonies of newly resettled Bosnian refugees. *Amer. J. Psychiat.,* 152:536–542.

———— Vojvoda, D., Becker, D. F., McGlashan, T. H., Hodzic, E., Laub, D., Hyman, L., Sawyer, M. & Lazrove, S. (1998), PTSD symptoms in Bosnian refugees 1 year after resettlement in the United States. *Amer. J. Psychiat.,* 155:562–564.

Wozniak, J., Crawford, M. H., Biederman, J., Faraone, S. V., Spencer, T. J., Taylor, A. & Blier, H. K. (1999), Antecedents and complications of trauma in boys with ADHD: Findings from a longitudinal study. *J. Amer. Acad. Child & Adol. Psychiat.,* 38:48–55.

Wyllie, E., Glazer, J. P., Benbadis, S., Kotagal, P. & Wolgamuth, B. (1999), Psychiatric features of children and adolescents with pseudoseizures. *Arch. Pediatr. Adol. Med.,* 153:244–248.

Yehuda, R. & McFarlane, A. C. (1995), Conflict between current knowledge about posttraumatic stress disorder and its original conceptual basis. *Amer. J. Psychiat.,* 152:1705–1713.

8   TRAUMA AND ADOLESCENCE III

ISSUES OF IDENTIFICATION, INTERVENTION, AND SOCIAL POLICY

THE COMMITTEE ON ADOLESCENCE OF THE GROUP
FOR THE ADVANCEMENT OF PSYCHIATRY

Members of the GAP Committee on Adolescence who contributed to this special section include: Daniel F. Becker, Melita Daley, Monica R. Green, Robert L. Hendren, Lois T. Flaherty (Committee Chair), Warren J. Gadpaille, Gordon Harper, Robert A. King, Patricia Lester, Silvio J. Onesti, Mary Schwab-Stone, and Susan W. Wong.

Knowledge about the nature, scope, and impact of trauma in adolescence carries with it the imperative to identify those trauma-exposed adolescents who need psychiatric intervention and to provide appropriate assistance to them. To be effective, interventions should prevent long-term noxious effects as well as ameliorate the aftereffects of trauma in those who already show sequelae. A subsequent chapter in this special section deals with interventions. This chapter focuses on the issues involved in identification and intervention, including the need for appropriate training for psychiatrists and other mental health workers.

DIAGNOSTIC ISSUES AND ASSESSMENT

A key part of the enhanced understanding of trauma has been the recognition that there are specific sequelae in the form of symptoms and syndromes. We now have general agreement about posttraumatic symptoms as well as diagnostic criteria for syndromes. These standardized criteria have led to more systematic approaches to the evaluation of trauma victims. They have facilitated community surveys to determine the extent of exposure to trauma and its impact. Assessment methods and diagnostic criteria are still evolving. Although there is not yet a gold standard for assessment of trauma and its sequelae, work has been proceeding rapidly, and there are now many questionnaires and standardized interviews available. These standardized assessment tools have enabled much of the research in the past two decades, which has dramatically increased awareness of the extent to which adolescents in today's world are exposed to a wide range of potentially traumatic experiences.

Asking about Traumatic Experiences

Inquiry about trauma history should be made routinely as part of any comprehensive diagnostic assessment of an adolescent. Special care should be taken to ask about violence exposure, including abuse, in urban youth, runaways, and any teenager with a history of suicidal or delinquent behavior or substance abuse (Clark, Lesnick, and Hegeous, 1997; Steiner, Garcia, and Matthews, 1997). Victims of war and natural disasters should be asked about their experiences and their feelings about these experiences as well as about posttraumatic symptoms. Interviewers often shy away from asking about painful experiences, feeling that it will be too upsetting, but trauma victims are usually willing to talk about such experiences, and the experience of telling their stories can be helpful to them (Weine et al., 1995).

Assessment of Symptoms

The categorization and severity rating of symptoms is an important way of understanding the effects of trauma on individuals. The realization that a similar constellation of symptoms could be found in diverse populations exposed to various kinds of trauma, across different ethnic and cultural backgrounds and age groups, was a landmark in the history of psychiatric nosology. Such studies helped to establish the utility of symptom and behavioral profiles to make diagnoses providing the basis for much of the current research conducted on trauma. The recognition that various symptoms related to traumatic stress can be seen at all ages, even in young children, laid the foundation for much important research.

Although it is important to determine who meets criteria for posttraumatic stress disorder (PTSD) and other disorders, the presence of symptoms and constellations of symptoms that do not meet full criteria for a disorder in the literature also has clinical significance. Subsyndromal conditions, characterized by some but not all symptoms necessary for a diagnosis of PTSD, are common in trauma survivors and can be accompanied by significant impairment (Stein et al., 1997).

Assessing Traumatic Exposure

Another approach is to list a variety of kinds of experiences that would be traumatic for most people and to ask whether the teenager has experienced any of these. This kind of approach has been most developed with regard to violence exposure, for which researchers have developed a number of fairly simple instruments to use in both clinical and nonclinical populations. Support for the validity of this kind of assessment is provided by consistent findings that the level of symptoms and/or impairment is correlated with the degree of violence exposure. For example, Schwab-Stone and colleagues (1999) used a checklist, adapted from an earlier version (Richters and Martinez, 1993), to study the effects of violence exposure on urban youth. The checklist included the following categories: 1) seriously wounded, 2) shot or shot at, 3) attacked or stabbed with a knife, 4) threatened with serious bodily harm, 5) chased by gang or individuals, 6) beaten up or mugged. Questions about these experiences can be answered with yes or no and then the number of yes responses totaled to obtain a numerical score for quantifying violence exposure.

Generally, direct victimization is differentiated from witnessing violence. Thus, adolescents might be asked whether they have ever been beaten up or mugged (direct victimization) or seen someone else beaten up or mugged (witnessing). Some surveys query the relationship of the victim to the witness, under the assumption that witnessing violent victimization of a close friend or relative is worse than seeing a stranger being attacked.

War and genocide involve a complex array of experiences, which have been termed massive psychic trauma. This kind of trauma involves multiple losses, including loss of whole communities and individuals' sense of being a part of a community. One example of a way of assessing genocidal trauma is the Communal Traumatic Experiences

Inventory, a clinician-administered questionnaire that screens for 30 kinds of traumatic events commonly associated with ethnic cleansing. It was specifically developed by Weine and colleagues for their 1995 study of adolescent and adult Bosnian refugees who had been resettled in the United States.

Natural disasters also typically involve community disruption and loss of basic necessities of life in addition to the precipitating traumatic event. Goenjian et al. (1999) quantified the severity of trauma experienced by adolescents in a devastating earthquake. They used a scale in which researchers rated severity of trauma from one to five. Examples of very severe trauma included witnessing mutilation or death, hearing screams of torment, or being trapped or seriously injured. In addition, the investigators ranked the level of adversity experienced following the earthquake according to a five-point scale; severely adverse conditions included being frequently cold or hungry, being without adequate shelter, lacking transportation, and being physically ill.

Assessment of Impairment

Impairment is an important parameter of psychiatric disorder. The dimension of impairment includes both subjective distress and interference with functioning in work, school, or social roles. The presence of symptoms alone may not interfere with functioning, and thus (in theory, at least) a youngster who has experienced trauma may be symptomatic but not show impairment. On the other hand, an adolescent may appear on the surface to function well yet have significant impairment in areas of functioning that are less obvious to outside observers. An adolescent who is attending school and keeping up academically, who is refraining from using drugs or engaging in other high-risk behavior, but who is, at the same time, avoiding intimate relationships, may appear to be functioning well; yet this youngster is deficient in an important area of psychological functioning. In order to understand impairment, it is necessary to consider the normative developmental tasks of adolescence and whether a teenager is proceeding adequately in these various realms. A comprehensive assessment necessitates inquiry into all aspects of normal adolescent functioning.

Specific kinds of impairment related to trauma should, of course, be ascertained. These include such issues as difficulties with concentration, problems sleeping, and avoidance of going outside or to places where reexperiencing might occur. Somaticization, with various kinds of physical symptoms, is also common and should be inquired about, although it is not part of the *DSM* criteria.

Measurement of psychological defenses is potentially a very important aspect of assessment. Although this has traditionally been done clinically in the context of psychodynamic psychotherapy and psychoanalysis, attempts have been made to develop instruments that can be used for research studies. For example, Steiner et al. (1997) used two different measures of defenses and showed that more immature defenses predominated in adolescents with histories of violence exposure and that a distinct defensive profile differentiated adolescents who met full criteria for PTSD from those who had partial syndromes. Repression, denial, and splitting were higher in the partial posttraumatic stress group, suggesting that perhaps these defenses protected against the development of the full syndrome.

Assessment of Preexisting Conditions and Risk Factors

As discussed in the previous chapter, not all trauma victims develop significant symptoms or impairment, and many of those who do will recover without treatment. Thus, one of the goals of assessment is to determine who needs treatment. Assessment of risk and protective factors is a key component of the evaluation. Given the influence of premorbid functioning on outcome, information about school and social and family relationships prior to the trauma is crucial. These will influence the clinical course following the trauma and can help in the determination of how much outside support will be needed.

Assessment of premorbid and comorbid conditions. Comorbid psychiatric disorders can arise after traumatic experience or can be preexisting. This is true of PTSD as well as of anxiety, depression, and other conditions. Thus, it is important to ascertain whether any of these conditions existed prior to the trauma and whether there has been prior traumatization.

Premorbid psychiatric disorders, in addition to affecting the psychopathological outcomes of trauma, can also comprise risk factors for trauma itself. In other words, preexisting psychopathology can increase the likelihood of traumatic injury. One must consider, therefore, whether or not the trauma is related to the adolescent's behavior. Contrast, for example, the experience of being in an earthquake with that of being injured in a drive-by shooting while running the streets. In the latter case, preexisting psychopathology may have contributed to the event. Gerring and colleagues (1998) documented a 20% prevalence of preexisting attention-deficit/hyperactivity disorder among children and adolescents admitted to a program for victims of closed head injury.

Although many questions about the relationship between comorbid illnesses and PTSD remain, from a clinical perspective, comorbid conditions need to be assessed and treated appropriately. For this reason, an assessment should be comprehensive enough to identify all possible conditions and predisposing factors. A symptom-based approach, that is, one that specifically inquires about a wide range of symptoms, is most likely to uncover all psychopathology. This approach is in contrast to an approach that is limited to screening questions about various disorders, bypassing further inquiry if the initial response is negative.

Assessment of suicidal adolescents.   Because abuse is such a strong risk factor for depression and suicidality, clinicians should screen for abuse in cases of depression or suicidality and should keep in mind that adolescents with histories of sexual abuse and suicide attempts are at high risk for repeat attempts.

Assessing the Cultural Context

Essential areas to cover in this part of the evaluation include the following: 1) family functioning, strengths/weaknesses; 2) community/culture/religion; 3) quality of the adolescent's social network; and 4) prior history of child/family traumatic experience, either on the part of the family as a whole, or the child. The parents' involvement in the trauma and its aftermath are also important.

The practice parameters of the American Academy of Child and Adolescent Psychiatry (AACAP, 1997) for the assessment of children and adolescents emphasize the importance of "a full appreciation of the child and family's cultural context" (p. 9S) as part of a comprehensive evaluation. This appreciation is particularly important in the evaluation of trauma-related psychopathology. An understanding of an adolescent's community or neighborhood gives important information about the likelihood of exposure to trauma (such as urban violence), as well as the availability of resources (for example, recreational, academic, and faith-based institutions) that can potentially mitigate the effects of such adverse circumstances as poverty, poor housing, and high crime rates (GAP, this volume). As Gadpaille (this volume) points out, culture shapes the response to trauma.

Assessing Subjective Experience

Equally important to an appreciation of social and cultural context is an understanding of the adolescent's attitude towards this conduct. Does an urban teenager feel doomed to an early death because of the prevalence of urban violence? Does a suburban youngster surrounded by affluence and attending a school where only successful athletes seem to be valued feel alienated?

Assessment should also focus on the meaning of the traumatic exposure to the individual adolescent. The essence of a trauma is its impact on the individual. This impact, the experience of an event as traumatic, is dependent on the individual's perceptions of the event. These perceptions are a product of culture, individual perspective, and individual reactivity. Developmental level plays an important role; the age and developmental level of the adolescent at the time of the traumatic event, as well as at the present time, affect the impact of trauma. A meaningful understanding of an adolescent involves both the assessment of the effects of trauma experienced during childhood and the evaluation of the impact of traumatic experiences during adolescence itself.

Assessment Tools

Methods of assessment include the clinical interview and various structured assessment tools (AACAP, 1998). Although all have potential utility for screening and for evaluating the effectiveness of treatment, there is no gold standard for evaluating trauma-related psychopathology. A structured interview or questionnaire is not a substitute for a clinical interview, which is ideally a "comprehensive, detailed, and flexible inquiry within a context of empathic rapport" (AACAP, 1997, p. 13S). Such an interview will have greater sensitivity for detecting symptoms and defensive styles (Honig et al., 1993).

207

DSM-IV. *DSM-IV* represents the third iteration of diagnostic criteria for the trauma-related syndromes, which were first introduced in 1980 with *DSM-III.* In *DSM*, these syndromes are categorized as anxiety disorders (in contrast to the *International Classification of Diseases-*10th Revision (ICD-10, WHO, 1992), which considers them stress reactions). Acute stress disorder is a new category added to *DSM-IV* for a posttraumatic syndrome that lasts at least two days but no longer than four weeks. In addition to the symptom constellation of reexperiencing and avoidance, it includes three or more of the following dissociative symptoms occurring either during or after experiencing the distressing event: 1) a subjective sense of numbing, detachment, or absence of emotional responsiveness, 2) a reduction in awareness of one's surroundings (e.g., being in a daze), 3) derealization, 4) depersonalization, and 5) dissociative amnesia (i.e., inability to recall an important aspect of the trauma).

DSM provides a framework for clinicians to evaluate patients. The clinician can simply inquire about each of the listed symptoms in his or her own words and then note whether or not the symptom was endorsed. For these systems to be reliable, both the interviewer and the patient must understand the meaning of the questions. *DSM-IV* was designed so that it could be used as a structured assessment tool, and in fact the PTSD component of it has demonstrated good reliability and validity in adults.

Semistructured interviews. Semistructured interviews involve a set format and questions but allow the interviewer to deviate from this format or skip out if he or she feels it is necessary. Some reasons for skipping out might be to explain questions if it appears that the respondent does not understand them or to probe further, asking more questions if the answers are unclear or if the respondent answers no to a question but seems distressed about it. This kind of format resembles a clinical interview. Many of these instruments contain sections that cover PTSD symptoms and are based on the *DSM*. An example that has good interrater reliability and validity is the Schedule for Affective Disorders and Schizophrenia for School-Age Children—Present and Lifetime version (KSADS—PL), which, despite its name, is designed for use in adolescents up to age 17 as well as children (Kaufman et al., 1997). This instrument is designed for a comprehensive diagnostic assessment and has a PTSD module. Other interviews have been specifically developed for the assessment of PTSD, for example, the Clinician-Administered PTSD Scale for Children and Adolescents, *DSM-IV* version (Nader et al., 1996). Information about reliable and valid instruments for use in children and adolescents is shown in Table 1; further information is available at the National Center for Post-Traumatic Stress Disorder website, *http://www.ncptsd.org/treatment/assessment/child_measures.html.* All of these instruments have limitations; they are reviewed in the AACAP "Practice Parameters for the Assessment and Treatment of Children and Adolescents with Posttraumatic Stress Disorder" (1998).

Barriers to Assessment

For several reasons, trauma histories and posttraumatic symptomatology may be overlooked. Reluctance to acknowledge symptoms is common among certain groups of adolescents. Shame about acknowledging symptoms inhibits disclosure when a culture stigmatizes mental illness; it is especially difficult to acknowledge frightening phenomena such as reexperiencing symptoms or hallucinations, which may be seen as suggestive of insanity. Failure on the part of caretakers or professionals to acknowledge trauma-related problems is also a factor in underdiagnosis. In their study of Tibetan refugee children, Servan-Scheiber, Le Lin, and Birmaher (1998) found resistance on the part of caretakers to the idea that the children and adolescents might have been affected adversely by separation from their parents and a months-long journey through dangerous conditions to escape from Tibet. In addition, the children themselves often denied or minimized symptoms, despite displaying obvious signs of distress (Servan-Scheiber et al., 1998). Steiner and colleagues (1997) have drawn attention to the high and unrecognized prevalence of PTSD and posttraumatic symptoms in violent juvenile delinquents, who are similarly reluctant to acknowledge their symptoms. An additional factor in this group is that the presence of more obvious psychopathology may discourage further inquiry. None of the referrals of this group of incarcerated juvenile delinquents for psychiatric evaluations evidenced concerns that these adolescents might be experiencing trauma-related problems (Steiner et al., 1997). Adolescents with alcohol use disorders are a group in whom histories of trauma and trauma-related psychopathology are common but often overlooked (Clark et al., 1997).

209

TABLE 1

STRUCTURED ASSESSMENT TOOLS FOR TRAUMA IN CHILDREN AND ADOLESCENTS

Instrument	Domain Assessed	Format	Target Age Group	# of Items/ Ratings per Item	Times to Administer (in Minutes)	Allows Multiple Trauma	Corresponds to DSM Diagnostic Criteria	Published Psychometrics
Childhood PTSD Interview	PTSD	Interview	Not Specified	93/1	30–45	Yes	Yes	Yes
Children's Posttraumatic Stress Disorder Inventory	PTSD	Interview	7–18	43/1	15–20	No	Yes	Yes
Clinician Administered PTSD Scale for Children	PTSD	Interview	7–18	33/2	30–120	Up to 3	Yes	Yes
Dimensions of Stressful Events	Traumatic Events	Interview	Not Specified	24/varies	15–30	Yes	Yes	Yes
Parent Report of Child's Reaction to Stress	PTSD	Self-report	Not Specified	79/1	30–45	Yes	No	Yes

TABLE 1 (*continued*)
STRUCTURED ASSESSMENT TOOLS FOR TRAUMA IN CHILDREN AND ADOLESCENTS

Instrument	Domain Assessed	Format	Target Age Group	# of Items/ Ratings per Item	Times to Administer (in Minutes)	Allows Multiple Trauma	Corresponds to DSM Diagnostic Criteria	Published Psychometrics
PTSD Reaction Index*	PTSD+	Interview	6–17	20/1	15–20	No	Part	Yes
Trauma Symptom Checklist for Children	Post-traumatic Symptoms	Self-report	8–16	54/1	10–20	Yes	No	Yes
Traumatic Events Screening Inventory*	Traumatic Events	Interview	4 and up	18/varies	10–30	Yes	Yes	Yes
When Bad Things Happen Scale	PTSD*	Self-report	8–13	95/1	10–20	No	Yes	Yes

* = Parent version available

PTSD+ = Measure PTSD and other Posttraumatic symptoms

National Center for Post-Traumatic Stress Disorder, Department of Veterans Affairs, used with permission, information about specific instruments is available at the Center's Website: *http://www.ncptsd.org/treatment/assessment/child_measures.html*

Avoidance of situations and stimuli that are reminders of traumatic events is a posttraumatic symptom. This is a defense against painful reexperiencing. Avoidance can extend to not thinking about or talking about the traumatic event, thus interfering with disclosure. Steiner et al. (1997) found that subjects interviewed twice were more likely to give histories of trauma exposure and to report posttraumatic symptoms during the second interview than during the first. They hypothesized that the first interview may have evocatively served to loosen some of the defenses protecting against disclosure.

Patients often fail to make a connection between their symptoms and the traumatic events that triggered them; one should not conclude that a connection is absent because of an adolescent's lack of awareness of it. It is sometimes necessary to ask repeatedly about specific events or event categories. One should also ask about frightening or upsetting experiences. Asking, "What bothers you most now?" as well as "What is the worst thing that ever happened?" can help to identify continuing preoccupations with past traumatic stress (Stein et al., 1997). Finally, clinicians should keep in mind that the absence of PTSD symptoms does not mean that no trauma has occurred. As we have seen, the sequelae of trauma can include a wide variety of responses in addition to symptoms typically classified as part of the PTSD syndrome.

Considerations Regarding the Time Frame of the Assessment

Diagnosis is generally based on an evaluation done at a single point; thus, it is inevitably a snapshot of a condition that is not static and evolves over time. Even if multiple interviews are conducted and information is gathered from several sources, the duration of the assessment period is likely to be limited to a few weeks, at most. This limitation is particularly important to keep in mind with respect to adolescents, who may appear similar to adults in terms of their signs and symptoms but are moving rapidly on a developmental trajectory. They are in the midst of rapid and far-reaching changes and experience a variety of what have been termed crises of development. The experience of traumatic stress occurring in the midst of a developmental crisis may result in a clinical picture that appears more flamboyantly deranged than is actually the case. Youngsters whose development has not proceeded optimally in the past will be affected by trauma in different ways from those whose development had been unhindered. The challenge for the clinician is to be able to distinguish between what is part of a developmental process and what is the result of traumatic stress. Studies with the kind of longitudinal follow-up that would allow us to understand the developmental patterns of adolescents who have experienced trauma are badly needed.

How best to deal with the time between exposure to trauma and the onset of trauma-related psychopathology is an important methodological issue. Although it is generally accepted that there can be a delay of months or even years between a traumatic experience and the onset of clinically significant conditions, there is no general agreement what kind of time frame to apply in assessment. This will vary with the goal of the assessment (e.g., clinical services versus epidemiological survey). Some studies have assessed lifetime exposure, and others have assessed only exposure within the past year or even less. Studies of natural disasters such as floods or earthquakes seem to be easier methodologically, as the date of the index traumatic event can be easily ascertained. But even in these cases, the initial event is usually followed by a series of ongoing stressful experiences, such as absence of basic life necessities and dislocation from home, which vary in duration among survivors, so that there is not an easily definable time frame for the exposure.

Because there is a correlation between the number of events experienced and the severity of symptoms and impairment, it is important to gather information regarding all of the different kinds of trauma an adolescent may have experienced. A related issue is the frequency of events, that is, how often they occur. For example, a question might be asked as to how often a youngster has witnessed neighborhood violence in the past month.

The effects of these factors—total number of events, the severity of events, and the frequency of events in daily life—are cumulative, so that there is a kind of dose-response effect. The fact that each of these parameters can vary so much makes assessment of the impact of trauma particularly challenging.

Informants

As with the internalizing disorders (anxiety and depression), children's and adolescents' reports of posttraumatic symptoms are often different from their parents' perceptions. Parents consistently report lower levels

of internalizing symptoms in their offspring than do the children themselves (Pfefferbaum, 1997). For young children, this finding raises
questions about the accuracy of the children's reports, but for adolescents, it is more likely an indication of parental underestimation of
their children's distress. Reasons for this include the parents' own level
of distress, which may make it difficult to appreciate their children's
distress; teenagers' lack of communication with their parents about
feelings; and cultural prohibitions against expression of feelings of
vulnerability. Most studies have relied on adolescents' own reports
as a primary source of information, sometimes comparing them with
parents' reports. In view of the generally acknowledged tendency for
adolescents to under-report histories of trauma and feelings of vulnerability (AACAP, 1997) there seems little likelihood that information
obtained from them would falsely inflate the prevalence of traumatic
experience and posttraumatic symptoms.

Physiological Measures

Given an extensive knowledge base about the stress response on various
body functions, it may seem that a measurement of physiologic changes
would be a useful way of assessing the impact of trauma. Indeed, stress
responses have been studied in laboratory settings. For example, the
galvanic skin response has been used since the 1970s to gauge individual
responses to noxious stimuli in a controlled environment. Of course,
these experimental stimuli are not of the same order of magnitude as
traumatic experiences that occur in natural disasters or those suffered
during wars or criminal victimization.

Although there are no laboratory tests that could be used clinically
for diagnostic or treatment purposes, researchers such as Schwartz and
Perry (1994) have recommended that simple measures of physiologic
function, such as blood pressure and pulse, be obtained routinely,
especially in youngsters who are recent trauma victims, as these indices
are often elevated and their return to normal can provide one measure
of improvement.

Limitations of Current Diagnostic Systems

Many investigators have suggested that assessment must go beyond
the *DSM* criteria, which are mainly designed to assess a specific syn-

drome that arises in response to a single event. For example, Weine and colleagues (1995) have postulated that victims of massive, repetitive, or sustained psychic trauma have qualitatively and quantitatively different experiences from those who have experienced single events. These investigators found that, although symptoms of depression were common in Bosnian refugees, their symptoms did not meet criteria for major depressive disorder; the most common depressive diagnosis they were given was depression not otherwise specified. These researchers felt they might have been seeing a specific kind of trauma-related depression that is not adequately described in the current nomenclature. Evaluators who looked only for major depressive disorder as a comorbid condition would not have appreciated this pattern. Cultural differences in communication and language, as well as in symptom expression, must be taken into account. For example, in some cultures, mood and anxiety states are likely to be expressed predominantly in somatic terms.

ISSUES OF INTERVENTION AND PUBLIC POLICY

Pitfalls and Risks in Dealing with Trauma

A sensitivity to the meaning of the trauma to the young person, as distinct from an exclusive focus on symptom assessment, is crucial. Some have suggested that an excessive focus on diagnostic criteria and psychiatric disorders may exacerbate the central experience of trauma victims, which is the loss of trust and meaning and connection to others that they experience, and that such an approach is actually a disservice to them (Kleinman and Kleinman, 1991). A comprehensive approach to assessment that takes into account the likelihood of comorbid conditions, and an understanding of the societal context in which trauma occurs, can mitigate against such partial, unidimensional methods.

Ethical and legal aspects of disclosure. After information about trauma exposure has been obtained during the course of an assessment, the evaluator must decide how to proceed. Disclosure, although potentially therapeutic, is also anxiety provoking. When the disclosure takes place in the context of therapy, the increased distress can be managed therapeutically. In psychiatric evaluations, this is not always an option.

Few researchers seem to have dealt with the issue of what to do after information about trauma exposure has been obtained during the course of an assessment. In addition, the possibility that some kinds of covering over defenses may be protective against the development of full PTSD raises questions as to whether uncovering trauma and/or encouraging catharsis is always in the patient's best interest. Mental health professionals have an ethical obligation to facilitate treatment when it is indicated. They must also be knowledgeable about the legal requirements to report abuse.

Is there a culture of trauma? Given the high prevalence of trauma exposure in normal life, with an estimated lifetime exposure of 70% of people to direct involvement in traumatic events (Foa, 1999), trauma-exposure can almost be considered an expectable life event. As PTSD has entered public awareness, there has been criticism that the term is being overused and that people are being led to believe that any adversity must, of necessity, be traumatic.

Shepard (2001) has depicted the attempts to provide special treatment to Vietnam War veterans, to help them overcome the presumed traumatic impact of their military experience, as having backfired, postulating that these attempts have instead contributed to long-term disability. The focus on PTSD, he maintains, has resulted in labeling veterans as helpless victims. He points out that issues of individual vulnerability and preexisting psychopathology (especially character pathology) have been downplayed both as a result of pressures from veterans' advocacy groups and because of the guilt of society over sending them to an unpopular war.

Shepard (2001) is critical of psychotherapy in general and of a cultural value that promotes sharing of feelings as opposed to the military tradition of keeping a stiff upper lip and getting on with life. One implication of this view is that treatment programs that encourage survivors to talk about their traumatic experiences and symptoms may lead to permanent impairment by focusing on what is wrong with them and sending a message that they are damaged and incurable.

Although there is no question, as we have said, that a person's responses to trauma are shaped by the individual's unique ways of thinking and feeling as well as by the reactions of the social environment (see GAP, this volume; Gadpaille, this volume), it is unclear how far the findings about war veterans diagnosed with PTSD can be applied to adolescents. But the caveats about causing long-term impairment by unnecessary treatment or misguided attempts at treatment that could make things worse seem valid. Also, many war veterans are late adolescents during their combat experience (Sugar, this volume). Most adolescents will have some adverse experiences as they negotiate the uncertain terrain of this important period of life, but this does not mean that they should expect to be traumatized. They do not need therapy for every bad thing that happens, and not all need help other than the support of family and friends, even after events that are outside the usual range of experience. People who talk to others immediately after a traumatic incident have been described as conducting self-therapy (Foa et al., 2000) and may be able to recover without further intervention.

Weine, who, with colleagues, has worked with adolescents in Bosnia, has criticized what he has termed the exportation by American psychiatrists of the concept of PTSD to war-torn countries where it is not meaningful (Weine, 1999). He points out that in areas of the world that are ravaged by war over multiple generations, the term PTSD is not applicable as there is no "post" to the trauma. This caveat seems applicable as well to adolescents exposed to ongoing urban trauma and to those who have grown up in abusive environments. Nonetheless, the fact is that these youngsters do suffer from their noxious environments. The question really is how best to help them cope.

Cultural differences in the experience of trauma have implications for our interventions and for understanding developmental psychopathology (Gadpaille, this volume). We can extrapolate from the knowledge of how some societies facilitate recovery and reintegration of traumatized individuals. Greater use of support and therapy groups and a treatment approach that envisions recovery and healing as likely outcomes promote the goal of an individual's reentry into society as a well-functioning person. Individual psychotherapy can help adolescents understand how their own cultural and gender-based customs contribute to the shaping of their maladaptive responses to trauma and can assist them in finding more adaptive ways of coping. (For further discussion of interventions, see Green, this volume.)

Clearly we need to understand better the impact of trauma and ways in which social attitudes and institutions can ameliorate or exacerbate its effects. And we can all agree that diagnosis and understanding of a complex psychological condition cannot be reduced to a symptom checklist. It is clear, however, from the seminal studies of the effects of the Holocaust to more recent research on the impact of urban trauma, that psychological trauma can have devastating effects on individuals, causing lasting pain and suffering and crippling psychological functioning as much as the worst physical injuries. Just as in the 1960s the deterioration seen in hospitalized patients with chronic mental illness was blamed on institutionalization rather than seen as a possible outcome of the illness itself, the psychological impairment in people who have experienced trauma may be blamed on their treatment rather than viewed as a possible aftereffect of trauma. Although issues such as secondary gain from victimhood are important, they are only part of a complex picture involving severity of traumatic stress, individual vulnerability, and societal responses.

The Link between Trauma and Violence

The important contribution of trauma to violent and antisocial behavior in adolescence and adulthood is generally underestimated and not sufficiently appreciated (Meyers et al., 1995; Lewis et al., 1997; Steiner et al., 1997). It is certainly not reflected in public policy toward youthful offenders. Lewis and colleagues (1985) have documented the prevalence of extreme forms of childhood abuse in the lives of violent incarcerated juveniles. In addition to histories of abuse, multiple neuropsychiatric deficits were present in this population, including learning disabilities and evidence of brain damage, suggesting an accumulation of risk factors. Lewis and colleagues (1997) also found a significant number of adult murderers (14 out of 150 referred for psychiatric evaluations, including some who were on death row) who had experienced extreme forms of abuse as children and were currently suffering from dissociative disorders.

Effects of the Terrorism of September 11, 2001

In the United States, the impact of the September 11, 2001, terrorist attacks on the World Trade Center and Pentagon and subsequent threats to public safety significantly challenged the mental health community. In addition to the overwhelming impact on adolescents directly exposed to trauma and traumatic bereavement, adolescents and their families throughout the nation experienced various levels of stress and anxiety, as well as traumatic exposure through news coverage of these events.

218

There have also been a number of related social changes such as heightened public security and military mobilization in the face of ongoing terrorist threats. In the larger population, many groups of adolescents and their families are at increased risk for stress and impaired coping. These include those with underlying anxiety disorders, prior traumatic exposure, and/or insecure attachment, as well as those living within communities disproportionately affected by poverty, urban violence, and limited social services. Furthermore, adolescents with family members employed in high-risk professions (including emergency workers, mail-service employees, and airline staff) are at increased risk for stress. In the current environment, ongoing fears about personal safety may strain each individual's capacity to cope with stress. Adolescents without a cohesive family, group, or community may experience increased isolation. Others may experience heightened anxiety, fears, aggression, and high-risk behaviors (Pynoos, 2001).

Inadequate Resources

The increase in traumatic stress and public anxiety following the terrorist attacks resulted in an increased awareness of the importance of mental health treatment for psychological trauma throughout the country. These recent events have underscored the need to improve training for psychiatrists in a number of areas: 1) crisis management; 2) consultation to community groups, media organizations, and schools; 3) screening, assessment and treatment of traumatic stress and traumatic bereavement; and 4) posttrauma public policy and research issues.

The current infrastructure for child and adolescent mental health treatment in the United States is limited in its capacity to address both specialized treatment for traumatic stress and bereavement, as well as to handle the increased public anxiety. The lack of sufficient numbers of mental health professionals trained to work with children and adolescents, as well as other barriers to treatment, have been well documented (U.S. Public Health Service, 2000). In addition, changes in the field of psychiatry have compounded the problem.

Changes in Residency Training

Psychoanalysis and psychoanalytically oriented therapy were predominant modes of therapy in the United States from the early 1920s until the 1960s. These modes of treatment involve conceptualizations of the importance of early life experiences, especially traumatic experiences, in shaping adult functioning and personality. Beginning in the mid-1950s, the course of American psychiatry and psychoanalysis changed dramatically due to a number of factors, including the development of medications, new treatment modalities, and reduced funding for residency training. These changes have profoundly influenced how psychiatric residents are trained. Psychiatric training programs are facing significant problems in this era of managed care. There has been a general shift away from learning psychotherapeutic skills to a focus on psychotropic medications. This has affected the ability of a new generation of psychiatrists to respond effectively to trauma victims.

As a result of the deficiency of adequate psychotherapy training, many residents are feeling at a loss in terms of treating patients who have been traumatized by the tragic events of September 11th. The residents who serve as Fellows of the Group for the Advancement of Psychiatry are of the opinion that trainees around the United States are recognizing that their training has not equipped them to deal with situations requiring crisis intervention (GAP Fellows, personal communication, 2002). The educational challenges presented by September 11 have implications for a number of areas, including psychiatry residency training and ongoing continuing psychiatric education. It is of utmost importance that such skills be taught, because treatment of any sort does not necessarily come without risk of harm. Inadequate or inappropriate treatment can be just as harmful as no treatment.

CONCLUSION

Particular developmental considerations are involved in assessment of adolescents with regard to trauma, and sociocultural factors also may affect adolescents' responses. Clearly, the answers are not all in as to whether all adolescents who have been exposed to potentially traumatic events should be assessed. It seems reasonable that some screening be done in high-risk populations. Although standardized approaches have many limitations, they can be useful in screening populations and have the potential of aiding in decisions about who needs treatment. Psychiatric diagnostic evaluations of adolescents who present for treatment in clinical settings should routinely include an inquiry about trauma exposure as well as posttraumatic symptoms, because clinical populations have a high probability of trauma exposure and posttraumatic syndromes. Assessment for psychiatric disorders should be part of any trauma intervention program. In evaluating youngsters who are known to have been exposed to trauma, it is important to evaluate risk factors for adverse sequelae, including past history of psychiatric disorder, prior exposure to trauma, and current family environment. In all cases, assessments must be developmentally appropriate and culturally sensitive.

Separating the immediate acute effects of trauma from its long-term impact is an important conceptual step. The data support the notion that individual risk and protective factors, including social and cultural factors, are much more important determinants of long-term impact than of immediate responses. If there is a culture of trauma, it is likely the result of the social and cultural factors that come into play in the aftermath of acute traumatic experience. Interventions aimed at the period after the acute traumatic stress must take into account these factors and seek to minimize the development of a chronic victim identity. This challenge is perhaps nowhere more pressing than in the case of adolescents.

REFERENCES

American Academy of Child and Adolescent Psychiatry (1997), AACAP official action: Practice parameters for the psychiatric assessment of children and adolescents. *J. Amer. Acad. Child & Adol. Psychiat.,* 36(suppl.): 4S–20S.

———— (1998), Practice parameters for the assessment and treatment of children and adolescents with posttraumatic stress disorder. *J. Amer. Acad. Child & Adol. Psychiat.,* 37(10 suppl.): 4S–26S.

Clark, D. B., Lesnick, L. & Hegeous, A. M. (1997), Traumas and other adverse life events in adolescents with alcohol abuse and dependence. *J. Amer. Acad. Child & Adol. Psychiat.,* 36:1744–1751.

Foa, E. (1999), Exposure therapy can help patients with PTSD. *Clinical Psychiatry News,* October.

———— Keane, T. M. & Friedman, M. J. eds. (2000), *Effective Treatments for PTSD: Practice Guidelines from the International Society for Traumatic Stress Studies.* New York: Guilford Press.

Gerring, J. P., Brady, K. D., Chen, A., Vasa, R., Grados, M., Bandeen-Roche, K. J., Bryan, R. N. & Denckla, M. B. (1998), Premorbid prevalence of ADHD and development of secondary ADHD after closed head injury. *J. Amer. Acad. Child & Adol. Psychiat.,* 37:647–654.

Goenjian, A., Stilwell, B. M., Steinberg, A. M., Fairbanks, L. A., Galvin, M. R., Karayan, I. & Pynoos, R. S. (1999), Moral development and psychopathological interference in conscience functioning among adolescents after trauma. *J. Amer. Acad. Child & Adol. Psychiat.,* 38:376–384.

Honig, R. G., Grace, M. C., Lindy, J. D., Newman, C. J. & Titchener, J. L. (1993), Portraits of survival: A 20-year follow-up of the Buffalo Creek flood. *Psychoanal. Study of the Child,* 48:327–355. New Haven, CT: Yale University Press.

Kaufman, J., Birmaher, B., Brent, D., Rao, U., Flynn, C., Moreci, P., Williamson, D. & Ryan, N. (1997), Schedule for Affective Disorders and Schizophrenia for School-Age Children—Present and Lifetime Version (K-SADS-PL): Initial reliability and validity data. *J. Amer. Acad. Child & Adol. Psychiat.,* 36:980–988.

Kleinman, A. & Kleinman, J. (1991), Suffering and its professional transformation: Toward an ethnography of interpersonal experience. *Cult. Med. Psychiat.,* 15:275–301.

Lewis, D. O., Moy, E., Jackson, L. D., Aaronson, R., Restifo, N., Serra, S. & Simos, A. (1985), Biopsychosocial characteristics of children who later murder: A prospective study. *Amer. J. Psychiat.,* 142:1161b–1167b.

——— Yeager, C. A., Swica, Y., Pincus, J. H. & Lewis, M. (1997), Objective documentation of child abuse and dissociation in 12 murderers with dissociative identity disorder. *Amer. J. Psychiat.,* 154:1703–1710.

Meyers, W. C., Scott, K. S., Burgess, A. W. & Burgess, A. G. (1995), Psychopathology, biopsychosocial factors, crime characteristics, and classification of 25 homicidal youths. *J. Amer. Acad. Child & Adol. Psychiat.,* 34:1483–1489.

Nader, K. O., Kreigler, J. A., Blake, D. D., Pynoos, R. S., Newman, E. & Weather, F. W. (1996), *Clinician-Administered PTSD Scale for Children and Adolescents for DSM-IV.* Los Angeles: National Center for PTSD and UCLA Trauma Psychiatry Program, Department of Psychiatry, UCLA School of Medicine.

Pfefferbaum, B. (1997), Posttraumatic stress disorder in children: A review of the past 10 years. *J. Amer. Acad. Child & Adol. Psychiat.,* 36:1503–1511.

Pynoos, R. (2001), In the wake of September 11: Public mental health planning and the clinician. Presentation at Public Mental Health in the Mass Media, October 24, University of California, Los Angeles.

Richters, J. E. & Martinez, P. (1993), The NIMH community violence project: I. Children as victims of and witnesses to violence. *Psychiatry*, 56:7–21.

Schwab-Stone, M., Chen, C., Greenberger, E., Silver, D., Lichtman, J. & Voyce, C. (1999), No safe haven: II. The effects of violence exposure on urban youth. *J. Amer. Acad. Child & Adol. Psychiat.*, 38:359–367.

Schwartz, E. D. & Perry, B. D. (1994), The post-traumatic response in children and adolescents. *Psychiatr. Clin. North Amer.*, 17:311–326.

Servan-Scheiber, D., Le Lin, B. & Birmaher, B. (1998), Prevalence of posttraumatic stress disorder and major depressive disorder in Tibetan refugee children. *J. Amer. Acad. Child & Adol. Psychiat.*, 37:874–879.

Shepard, B. (2001), *A War of Nerves: Soldiers and Psychiatrists in the Twentieth Century*. Cambridge, MA: Harvard University Press.

Stein, M. B., Walker, J. R., Hazen, A. L. & Forde, D. R. (1997), Full and partial posttraumatic stress disorder: Findings from a community survey. *Amer. J. Psychiat.*, 154:1114–1119.

Steiner, H., Garcia, I. G. & Matthews, Z. (1997), Posttraumatic stress disorder in incarcerated juvenile delinquents. *J. Amer. Acad. Child & Adol. Psychiat.*, 36:356–365.

U.S. Public Health Service (2000), *Report of the Surgeon General's Conference on Children's Mental Health: A National Action Agenda* (Rep. No. 017-024-01659-4). Washington, DC: Department of Health and Human Services.

Weine, S. M. (1999), *When History Is a Nightmare: Lives and Memories of Ethnic Cleansing in Bosnia-Herzegovina*. New Brunswick, NJ: Rutgers University Press.

—— Becker, D. F., McGlashan, T. H., Laub, D., Lazrove, S., Vojvoda, D. & Hyman, L. (1995), Psychiatric consequences of ethnic cleansing: Clinical assessments and trauma testimonies of newly resettled Bosnian refugees. *Amer. J. Psychiat.*, 152:536–542.

World Health Organization (1992), *International Classification of Diseases, 10th Revision*. Geneva: World Health Organization.

9 CROSS-CULTURAL AND GENDER CONSIDERATIONS OF TRAUMA

WARREN J. GADPAILLE

This special section concerns itself primarily with individual instances of trauma in the developmental process of adolescence. However, to address broader cross-cultural and gender issues, one must also consider culturewide, potentially traumatic events that affect large segments of populations, and broad cultural attitudes and values that play a role in the nature and incidence of trauma and also influence the perception of and response to trauma. We must also note that, although our focus is on adolescents, just as in many other aspects of adolescence for which we might desire a cross-cultural perspective, there is a paucity of data pertaining specifically to that developmental stage. To gain any breadth of perspective, one must include information dealing with all age groups, in the hope that it will be helpful in throwing light on the adolescent experience.

A few statistics about the worldwide incidence of trauma and traumatic conditions help to illustrate the magnitude of the problem, without even touching on individual incidents of trauma. Between 1972 and 1992, natural disasters and other calamities killed approximately 3 million people worldwide and adversely affected about 8 hundred million. In 1994, 48 countries were at war or experiencing violent internal conflict. In the United States, 2 million people each year experience injuries and property damage from natural disasters alone, such as fire, floods, earthquakes, and severe storms (Meichenbaum, 1995).

Human torture and other forms of traumatic degradation are so widespread as to deserve special note. In 1983, the World Human Rights Guide estimated that only one-fifth of the world population could speak out freely without severe reprisals from their own governments. It was estimated in 1992 that about 14 million refugees existed. Various reports indicate that an enormous number had been tortured; the lowest estimate was 700,000 and the highest was 4,900,000 (Baker, 1992). These estimates do not count other populations of the tortured, such as nonrefugees, nonsurvivors, prisoners of war, and those who do not report it.

It has been suggested (Weisaeth, 1995) that man-made traumas are more damaging to mental health than are natural disasters. This is thought to be due to their greater unpredictability, uncontrollability, and culpability. It is much more difficult to know the low point: When is the worst over? How long will the torture last? How bad will the abuse get? When will we know the worst final consequences of a nuclear disaster?

CROSS-CULTURAL CONSIDERATIONS

The descriptive categories in this section are not exhaustive because of the relatively small amount of literature that could be found on this subject. These, and those in the sections that follow, are also not mutually exclusive, because any culture influences a number of aspects of trauma. They are arbitrary categories that facilitate discussion of the interaction of culture and the effects of trauma.

In this chapter, Native Americans (including Alaskan Indians) are seen as members of distinct, non-Western cultures. Some assume that they have been thoroughly assimilated into Western culture, but this is not true. Their acculturation into Western culture, when it occurred at all, is very recent, especially in the west and in Alaska. It is most often very tenuous, in part because of its recency and in part because it is forced upon them by Western culture dominance. Western culture is not a part of their bones or their spirit or their world view, and they usually remain strongly influenced by their traditional cultures.

In general, differences in response to and recovery from traumatic events are the result of complex interactions of individual or shared traits, the specific events themselves, and environmental or cultural factors.

Culturally Ascribed Meanings and Values

Cultures that believe in karma and reincarnation. These cultures foster an acceptance of what happens to one in life rather than a sense of personal determinism with some form of rebellion against it. This is characteristic, for example, of Buddhist cultures in general, including much of Southeast Asia with related philosophies. Buddhist philosophy, for example, emphasizes nonconfrontational interpersonal relations and an acceptance of things as they are; the concept of karma and reincarnation assume that one's present life circumstances are determined by one's deeds in previous lives. This results in a sense of fatalism and acceptance of suffering during torture. Cambodian Buddhists associate the word for torture, and torture itself, with these Buddhist concepts. There is a greater sense of personal guilt and a lesser sense that one can influence the events of one's life. These philosophies help to determine symptoms and responses to trauma (Morris and Silove, 1992; Friedman and Marsella, 1996).

A study of Cambodian child survivors of massive trauma (Kinzie et al., 1986) found that their cultural background helped to minimize overt symptoms and social consequences of any symptoms; symptoms were primarily private and subjective. There was no evidence of acting out, truancy, disruptive behavior, or alcohol or drug abuse. There was, however, a very high level of posttraumatic stress disorder (PTSD)—50%—and depression. American adolescents, in contrast, are more likely to respond to stress by acting out with antisocial and drug-seeking behavior.

Cultures that discourage the overt expression of emotion. This is also a characteristic of Buddhist cultures, and this cultural attitude can not only modify the nature and expression of inevitable responses to trauma, it can also intensify symptomatology. In another example, the traditional Armenian cultural value of outward appearance of prosperity emphasizes the importance that one's family appears good and healthy to others in the community (Koskov, 1991). There is an emphasis on not expressing feelings as adults and on teaching children not to do what comes naturally, which is to be openly emotive. An essential sign of outward prosperity is children's behavior and health. For either an adult or child to be ill or to request or require help is shameful. In Koskov's report of psychological intervention with families of child survivors of the 1988 Armenian earthquake, it was found that the parents increased their children's symptoms by interfering with the expression of their feelings associated with the disaster and by projecting their own unacceptable emotions and distress onto their children. When intervention was able to be helpful to the children despite these difficulties, the parents could receive vicarious benefit as their children improved.

Cultures that believe in witchcraft and similar supernatural influences. Many African, Asian, and Native American cultures, among many others, share such beliefs. These concepts can greatly exacerbate the psychological consequences of traumata that might not in other cultures be seen as overwhelming. An American Indian teenage girl suffered a broken leg that was medically uncomplicated by serious sequelae; this would not ordinarily be thought an event that lay beyond the range of usual human experience. But she belonged to a tribal group that believed in witchcraft, and she perceived the accident in the context of a curse laid on her family; she developed many symptoms of PTSD. Such beliefs also are often accompanied by tribal taboos against any discussion of witchcraft, especially with nontribal individuals; this heightens the sense of isolation and can interfere with seeking psychological help (Manson et al., 1996).

In China, Malaysia, and South Asia generally, there are illnesses unrecognized by Western medicine (but of great reality within some cultures) that are interpreted as evidence of black magic or action of malign spirits. *Koro* is the belief that the penis is shrinking into the body and will cause death. *Dhat* is the fear of loss of semen through the urine, also an ultimate cause of death; Ayurvedic philosophy holds that vital essence is most highly concentrated in semen. Mild and inconsequential illnesses may be terrifying if they are perceived as evidence of such malign influence and thought likely to lead to such dreaded consequences. These beliefs result in severe psychiatric and physical debilitation (even otherwise-unexplained death) in the sufferers (Kirmayer, 1996).

Cultures that emphasize widely extended meanings of family. Among many others, this is very common among Native American groups. In cultures with narrowly defined, biological families, PTSD in survivors is unusual following the death of relatively peripheral persons. In this case example, the native culture of the traumatized adolescent extended the concept of family far beyond mere blood relationship; family is a psychological construct deriving more from sharing a kindred spirit. For this girl, a brother who felt like a brother was no less a brother than a biological sibling. She was reacting to the death of a foster sibling several years following but caused by an accident that she had not witnessed, to whom she was not biologically related, who was not an age contemporary, and with whom she was not interpersonally involved. Nevertheless, her development of clinical PTSD symptoms was consistent with her cultural ideology (Manson et al., 1996).

Cultures that accept or require physically painful and/or seriously dangerous practices. This would include tattooing, scarification, piercing, and other nongenital body altering procedures such as footbinding, male circumcision and subincision, and female genital circumcision involving mild to severe genital tissue destruction. Any of these practices would serve for discussion in this context, but female circumcision is perhaps the most dramatic and widely studied and will serve as the somewhat extended illustrative example here. Female circumcision is a euphemism for many of the grossly destructive and medically harmful procedures it covers, but another common term, female genital mutilation, is considered demeaning and insulting in the cultures where it is practiced. Therefore, female circumcision will be used in this chapter.

The term female circumcision (FC) encompasses all degrees of destructive surgery, from the least destructive (excision of the clitoral hood) to pharaonic circumcision or infibulation: the removal of the clitoris, labia major, and minor; sewing together of the sides of the remaining pudendal tissue, leaving only a very small opening for urine and menstrual products; and binding the girl's legs together for several weeks so that the area heals with a permanent scar closure. Such drastic procedures may require reincision to permit intercourse and almost always to permit childbirth, with resuturing following delivery. It is typically performed on prepubescent children with nonsterile techniques by women of the village or group. It understandably produces immediate and long-term morbidity and mortality, painful intercourse, decreased or lost sexual pleasure, and psychopathology as well—although not inevitably (Gordon, 1991; Lane and Rubinstein, 1996).

FC is extremely widespread in Africa, the Near and Middle East, Southern Asia, and even in Western countries, usually among immigrants from the above areas (Joseph, 1996). It is estimated that at least 110 million women have been subjected to such procedures; currently, 6,000 per day are circumcised (Toubia, 1994; Lane and

Rubinstein, 1996). The degree of the surgery varies among cultural groups; one overall estimate is that 85% is limited to clitoral excision (Lane and Rubinstein, 1996) whereas in Somalia approximately 80% receive pharaonic circumcision (Gruenbaum, 1996; Morris, 1996). Prevalence of all procedures ranges from 5% in Uganda and Zaire to 98% in Somalia and Djibouti (Toubia, 1984).

It is commonly thought that FC is essentially an Islamic custom, but this is not true. Such genital surgeries predate recorded history and are probably of African origin; they are found in Egyptian mummies. Although most of the cultures in which FC is presently performed are Muslim, it must be assumed that the Muslims adapted to preexisting practice; it is virtually unknown in 80% of the Arab world (Gordon, 1991; Joseph, 1996). Most Islamic scholars oppose any but the most limited form of clitoral circumcision, because the Prophet and other religious authorities are in favor of preserving the sexual pleasure of both men and women (Berkey, 1996). Anything more than "light" female circumcision, less extensive than male circumcision, is expressly forbidden by the Koran (Winkel, 1995). Even these procedures are considered to be only recommended. Muslim leaders are not always scholars, however; in 1959, one of Egypt's most prominent religious leaders issued a formal opinion that FC is an Islamic duty incumbent upon all Muslims (Lane and Rubinstein, 1996).

Most researchers consider that these procedures were initiated by and served the interests of males: to insure and preserve virginity and fidelity by controlling unbridled female passion, to preserve family honor and patriarchal hereditary purity, and to provide greater sexual pleasure to the male by making the vaginal opening tighter (Berkey, 1996; Gruenbaum, 1996). Although these original reasons are still acknowledged, especially the latter and especially by women, there are now some cultures in which more men than women object to the procedure (Morris, 1996). In almost all instances worldwide, however, it is women who most favor even the extreme FC and most adamantly oppose its abolition (Gruenbaum, 1996; Joseph, 1996; Lane and Rubinstein, 1996; Morris, 1996). To gain any real understanding of the cultural place of such a dangerous and destructive procedure, one must recognize that in all known cultures, this custom is not only approved by women but also carried on through the agency of women. This is essentially violence perpetrated by women against female children.

It is women who are accountable in today's cultures for FC, and it is through women that change must occur. There are worldwide movements for its abolition, but they operate against great female opposition. Western feminist outrage often attempts to ride roughshod over indigenous cultural sensitivities, appears arrogant and patronizing, and can produce the opposite of the desired effect (Gruenbaum, 1996; Lane and Rubinstein, 1996). It was an occasion of such cultural insensitivity that caused the reactionary *fatwa* by the Egyptian Muslim leader just mentioned and the lifting of an earlier Egyptian legal ban against all such procedures. There are movements within the cultures in which FC is practiced to do away with all or at least the most drastic surgeries, but they represent at present a small minority of mainly well-educated women. It is expected that significant change will take generations, at least.

This is not an issue of only academic interest to Western psychiatrists and mental (or other) health workers. Refugees and immigrants from areas with strong advocacy for FC form sizable communities in many Western countries and are vociferous in their wish to continue the custom; laws in Western countries are not always unambiguous regarding the procedures (Winter, 1994). And students from these areas with concerns about or sequelae of FC are beginning to present themselves at health care facilities (Lane and Rubinstein, 1996; Morris, 1996; Wollard and Edwards, 1997).

One wonders what would impel cultures to maintain and even advocate practices that are or seem to be maladaptive. Although FC is clearly maladaptive with regard to the health and sexuality of female individuals, however, it does not appear to be maladaptive in terms of the survival of the group. One would assume that is has negative consequences on the fertility of women undergoing the most severe procedures, but the only study we are aware of refutes that idea. Gruenbaum (1996) found that women who had pharaonic infibulation had a higher birthrate than those with only clitoral circumcision. (Other reasons for continuance of the practice are discussed in the section of this chapter on cross-cultural differences in perceptions of trauma.)

Cultures that accept and/or value dissociative states. Such cultures comprise approximately 90% of the cultures of the world (Bourguignon, 1971). In these cultures, there are institutionalized and culturally patterned states of altered consciousness that are accepted and valued by the group. Hegeman (1995) describes how persons who exhibit such states are not isolated or stigmatized but are offered ritualized means to reidentify with and reenter the group, often with new and socially more valued identities. She postulates that trauma usually underlies dissociative states, regardless of culture, but also recognizes nontraumatic sources of dissociation. The cultural rituals permit the traumatized individual to contain and overcome the consequences of the trauma.

Traumatic parental sadism (from the viewpoint of the child) exists in many cultures. In Bali, mothers tease their just-weaning or just-weaned children by pretending to nurse a doll or by nursing another infant until the child is driven into a frenzy of despair, longing, and jealousy. When the intensity of frustration can no longer be tolerated, the child will suddenly go blank, enter a trance, and begin displaying ritualized hand movements he or she is already learning that will be part of the yearly trance dance rituals the whole village performs as part of its yearly pageants. This dance involves a malignant witch who has magical power to harm the villagers and depicts the controlled, stylized collective expression of dissociated rage and ultimate revenge against the witch, who represents the frustrating sadistic mother. The dance allows expression and mastery of the trauma (Hegeman, 1995).

Cultures that accept child/adult sexuality. When sexual interactions, including intercourse, between adults and children are sanctioned as a normal part of life and development, the interaction does not require or entail a coercive or violent and threatening adult and a frightened, traumatized child. Levett (1995) cites a South African community in which most girls, by age five or six, become sexually engaged with a series of older males, from brothers and fathers to other kin and neighbors. Women who had been part of this activity became indignant and angry when it was suggested that they were abused. Early pregnancy and having to leave school could be seen as conferring socioeconomic disadvantage. But to the women the sexual activity was part of normal behavior and learning and was not perceived as abusive or traumatic.

Cross-Cultural Differences in Personal Perceptions of and Responses to Trauma

In general, individuals' perception of and response to trauma follow culturally ascribed meanings and values. But there can be differences in the degree to which various groups identify with overall traditional cultural values. And in diverse cultural areas such as the United States, rape victims can have very differing perceptions of their trauma and different outcomes, depending on their subcultures' attitudes and supports.

The importance of family and community. The great importance of the (usually extended) family in many cultures can significantly modify the nature and response to trauma, depending on the availability of that family. In the Kinzie et al. (1986) study of the psychiatric effects of massive trauma on Cambodian children, it was found that the degree of emotional disturbance was not related to the amount of trauma, but to whether or not the child was reunited with a nuclear family member in the United States. In further studies of adolescent Cambodian refugees (Sack, Clarke, and Seeley, 1996; Sack, Seeley, and Clarke, 1997) it was found that previous war trauma was highly predictive of PTSD, whereas depression was more related to postsettlement trauma (the presence or absence of family). Depression in these samples decreased with time, but PTSD did not.

Degree of identity with traditional culture and cultural activities. The Exxon Valdez oil spill affected native Indian Alaskans more than nonnatives due to the role of subsistence activities in native culture. Because of the importance of such activities in the history and future of the culture, the prevalence of psychiatric disorders varied in terms of individuals' participation in subsistence activities and the strength of their cultural identity (Palinkas et al., 1993).

Acceptance of traumatic cultural practices. There is little evidence in anthropological literature that pubescent boys subjected to circumcision as part of puberty rites in Stone Age or near–Stone Age cultures are massively traumatized. Subjective fear and pain at the time are normal, but the rewards of acceptance into male adult society with the attendant rituals and privileges seem to compensate for the trauma.

Over the millennia, the cultures that practice female circumcision seem to have effected an almost total reversal in how the women perceive what happens to them as children. The vast majority of such women minimize the importance of the trauma and find in its consequences sources of pride, aesthetic and personal superiority, and cultural identity (Gruenbaum, 1996; Lane and Rubenstein, 1996; Morris, 1996). In these cultures, "girls grow up knowing that circumcision is essential if they are some day to be considered fit to marry, find a man willing to marry them, and raise a family" (Morris, 1996, p. 46). Pain is regarded as an essential part of life and a toughening experience in preparation for motherhood. Mothers would not think of leaving their daughters unmarriageable.

Women of these cultures often perceive that the labia and clitoris are ugly, masculine parts of girls, and that their removal results in smooth beauty and cleanliness (Gruenbaum, 1996; Morris, 1996). Women who have been pharaonically circumcised feel superior to and taunt those with lesser surgeries, to the extent that the latter girls sometimes ask to have the more destructive procedure performed (Gruenbaum, 1996). Although in most, if not all, instances their own sexual response is diminished or destroyed, their self-esteem is based more on pleasing their husbands, and almost universally they believe that the tight, infibulated vaginal opening is preferable because it pro-duces more friction and therefore greater pleasure for the man. They are contemptuous of noninfibulated women, believing their "gaping openings" to be incapable of giving men pleasure.

As indicated earlier, there is no real evidence that men remain the active proponents of this belief and the practice of FC. In the imaginary circumstance that all women of all these cultures suddenly give up FC, there might arise an outcry among the males to continue it. It is also possible that the belief in being able to provide superior male sexual pleasure is a millennia-long cultural delusion that men have no interest in female sexual pleasure and prefer sexually unresponsive partners.

Joseph (1996) offers a psychodynamic explanation to explain in part the persistence of FC. She postulates that the girl dissociates from intolerable pain and rage and thus seems to recover from it. But as an adult member of a cultural group in which all women deal with the same early trauma, she then has to traumatize her own daughters and the next generation in accord with the unconscious principle that trauma demands repetition. The woman's unconscious sadistic self is able to get rid of the memory and the inner pain by turning it outward and inflicting it on others.

Acceptance of blame and guilt. For traditional Cambodian men and women, the maintenance of sexual purity (virginity before marriage and fidelity afterwards) is the supreme value. Its loss is the ultimate shame for the woman, her husband, and her extended family, even her community. It makes no difference how that purity is lost, even if by rape; it is the loss that counts. The blame is hers, and she accepts the shame and guilt. The punishment is loss of everyone's respect, ostracism and isolation, even "justified" murder by her husband. If her rape occurred in isolation from her family and community (as in escape attempts from Vietnam or the Pol Pot regime, in a Thai work camp, or by pirates capturing boat people) she is further isolated, because her sense of guilt prevents her from revealing it and trying to get help.

This is a particular problem for Cambodian and Vietnamese female refugees, the vast majority of whom were raped and gang-raped over months and years, regardless of age, before they were able to escape. Even when resettled elsewhere, the cultural mores by which they were reared pose a major impediment to rehabilitative therapy, because they still tend to live and function in their own cultural groups and to deal with husbands or other males who share the same punitive values (Mollica and Son, 1989; Chester, 1992).

Identification with victims in warfare. During and following the Vietnam War, it was found that Native American and Alaskan Indian, Japanese American, and Hawaiian American soldiers faced a different set of trauma-inducing problems than did most Caucasian or even black American soldiers. The enemy—those they were supposed to kill—often looked like themselves and their friends, families, and neighbors. In addition, they were required to attack and kill nonwhite people by a white government that many of them had experienced as racist. Identification with the enemy made killing a much more personal thing, much more difficult to compartmentalize or distance oneself from. Traumatic responses were higher in this group (Manson, 1997).

Learned helplessness. Manson (1997) postulates that minorities in affluent Western countries who have often found it necessary to be dependent, perhaps most or all of their lives, on government subsistence programs develop a form of learned helplessness. This may compromise optimal development of coping skills with which to master acute traumatic experiences such as war.

Acceptance of witchcraft beliefs. As previously discussed, such beliefs can intensify the trauma associated with otherwise relatively minor occurrences. They can also moderate the trauma following major events.

In rural Tlaxcala, Mexico, sudden and unexpected deaths of infants and young children were relatively common at the time (early 1960s) that the data were collected for Fabrega and Nutini's (1994) study. When such a death occurs, an attack by the bloodsucking witch Tlahuelputchi is almost universally utilized as an explanation. Because many such deaths are due to some degree of maternal carelessness (overlaying the infant in the bed, maternal overfeeding and the infant's regurgitation during maternal sleep) as well as probably some instances of infanticide, this belief serves to externalize both the cause and the guilt and to mobilize intense kin and neighbor support. Some actual manipulation of the facts and evidence is often required, such as relocation of the baby's body, in order to conform with beliefs about the typical actions of the witch; such actions may not be fully and deliberately conscious. Although others in the community may express some suspicions, the spouse and other family members give firm support to the probably hallucinatory and dissociative evidence of the Tlahuelputchi. This is a highly emotionally expressive culture, and the mother often manifests dramatic psychological and somatic symptoms in the days or one or two weeks following the death. It is stated that she is usually "back to herself" in two or three weeks. Compared with the prolonged grief and traumatic symptomatology following one's child's death in some cultures, this relatively rapid recovery is doubtless facilitated by the externalizing belief system.

Differing views of child–adult sexual activity. Unlike the South African community described earlier, the dominant view in the United States is that sexual interaction between an adult and a child below the age of consent is always against the child's best interests and is always considered damaging. Whether or not this perception is invariably correct (see section on greater or lesser trauma from sexual violence), it sets the stage for severe trauma. Neither children nor adults in the U.S. culture have any accepted and internalized belief system that such behavior is normal or natural. Thus, children are often or usually harmed by the actions of an adult from whom they expect nonsexual attention that they are generally reared to label wrong and bad. Similarly, in this culture, adults perceive no positive cultural sanctions for such activity and can only cajole, coerce, threaten, and/or brutally physically harm any child with whom they engage sexually. Even if the child initially felt no trauma (perhaps kindness and cajolery were the routes to sexual involvement), the law or other adults will make it traumatic by labeling it so and via the legal procedures in which the child will become enmeshed. This discussion in no way condones child rape or other vicious and violent sexual acts that would be equally traumatic in permissive societies. It merely illustrates that this culture's mores play a role in manufacturing the trauma of child/adult sexuality.

Different perceptions of what constitutes the trauma of torture. Because of widely disparate cultural attitudes about what is shameful or degrading, events that would be benign in some cultures become horrific in others. Organizations or governments that set about torturing those of their own cultures make use of such idiosyncrasies. In Iran, part of the torture of male prisoners is the practice of showing them the dead bodies of executed prisoners. However, it is not the dead body per se that is intolerable; it requires the exposure of the dead prisoners' genitals to intimidate them and to be perceived as a sexual assault. For a very religious Iranian woman to have her headscarf removed, exposing her hair to a foreign male, is very sexually degrading. Again, by whomever it is done, the guilt is hers and is adequate reason for the authorities to imprison her (Lunde and Ortmann, 1992).

Effects of chronic trauma on subsequent, more specific trauma. There are differing views on how chronic trauma may affect subsequent responses to specific traumatic events. It is likely that the influence does vary with different persons and populations. Manson et al. (1996) cite a study of Native American boarding school students, among whom 37 reported experiencing one or more significantly traumatic events, though only one met the criteria for PTSD. All of these students came from cultural groups and areas in which there is constant and chronic tribal disintegration and demoralization. Manson et al. postulated, "Perhaps the degree of trauma itself is sufficiently greater in many Native communities so that the individual threshold for clinical response has been reset at higher levels as trauma has become more the norm than the exception" (p. 262).

On the other hand, citing studies documenting higher rates of PTSD in blacks than European Americans exposed to the same stresses, Allen (1996) suggests that the greater struggle of African Americans for purpose, meaning, and presence in U.S. society is the reason that

237

traumatic events inflict greater and more long-lasting devastation upon them than upon European Americans.

Spiritual and religious horror of war, of the dead, of killing. Navajo Indians, as part of their religious philosophy stressing beauty and connectedness, believe that being exposed to death or injuries, or having to kill, places them in extreme danger of harm from witchcraft attributed to the spirits of those injured or killed. They are much more traumatized by such experiences than are non-Navajo. Ceremonial rituals such as the Enemy Way and the Beauty Way, supposed to be undergone before and after the experience of war, are protective to traditional believers against much of the psychological damage from such experiences; they help to reintegrate the person's individual and community identity. Manson (1997) found that Navajo veterans for whom such rituals were not available, as in most cases they were not until much later if at all, had much lowered coping ability and greater risk for PTSD.

Indeed, most Native American groups, despite the popular view of them as warlike, regard war as an ultimate evil and form of chaos, though they also often see it as an arena for the warrior to develop as a person and as a means of achievement for the warrior. Therefore, it is seen as a source of extreme spiritual danger; serious spiritual and psychological harm is expected in warriors. Traditionally, in all such groups, warriors are prepared through family- and community-wide rituals. Following exposure, the expected damage must be repaired through rituals that allow and honor the damaged state, that allow for the emergence and expression of the trauma, and (because of the total family and community support and honoring of the warriors) provide for warriors' reintegration into family and community in the posttraumatized state. Traditional Native Americans expect such welcoming reintegration. When they returned from Vietnam, they often suffered greater PTSD than did non–American Indians due to the additional "sanctuary trauma": the disappointment of not finding what they expected and needed in the Anglo settings and hospitals in which they found themselves (Silver, 1994).

Cross-Culturally Different Responses to Traumatized Members

Many of the cross-cultural differences that would logically be discussed under this heading can be understood easily from the previous discussions. Cultures that blame traumatized individuals for what happened obviously do not support them and often even punish them further. There are few, if any, avenues for gaining help, and suffering is increased. Cultures that believe in witchcraft, whether those beliefs exacerbate or ameliorate the traumas associated with witchcraft, generally have developed rituals or ceremonies or shamanistic practices designed to relieve the afflicted individuals. Cultures that place a positive value on certain traumas (such as FC and male circumcision) also embody belief systems that allow for survival of the trauma or solace for family survivors if death ensues (Morris, 1996), and encourage pride in the trauma and its outcome.

In some instances, the cultures that provide ceremonies to relieve the posttraumatic distresses of their members can experience difficulties when those members fail to conform to cultural expectations. Among most Native Americans, warriors are honored, deferred to, and turned to as sources of wisdom. Veterans with PTSD are usually distant, unconnected, and unpredictable; it is often a long time after they return to their cultural communities before they can allow themselves to participate in healing rituals. Their alienation is also very disruptive to their families and communities who, therefore, cannot relate to the warriors in the traditional way (Manson, 1997).

Cultures that accept the normalcy of dissociative and trance states in response to trauma clearly minimize the isolation of such members and facilitate their reintegration as individuals and group members. But the cultures may also be unwittingly doing future members a disservice. In the example of the Balinese trance dance described earlier, the ceremony does allow for externalization and relief from the childhood trauma. But in so doing, it fails to recognize the real-life harmful nature of that particular child-rearing behavior and lessens any need to change the practice (Hegeman, 1995).

The majority of world governments purposefully traumatize and/or torture their own members who openly oppose them. (These are more likely specific governments or organizations within a larger culture than discrete cultural entities.) Those victims can expect no supports built into the institutions that hurt them, other than perhaps reacceptance if they recant. It is likely that these same organizations also have their own ways of helpfully approaching members who are traumatized by other means, but no literature on this split-personality aspect of these groups is known to me.

Individually Different Responses to Equivalent Trauma within Cultures

The concept of resilience.   In a review of 52 major disasters, Rubonis and Bickman (1991) found a 17% increase of psychopathology over baseline in the victims. However, 83% of victims demonstrated no (or no lasting) pathological responses. This clearly raises the issue of resilience. In Harvey's (1996) ecological approach to trauma and recovery, she postulates that individual differences in posttraumatic response and recovery are the result of complex interactions among person(s), event(s), and environmental factors. (She does not expand her discussion into cross-cultural factors.) The interactions may foster or impede individual recovery. The fact that some traumatized individuals recover without clinical intervention calls attention both to individual resilience and to the relevance of community intervention efforts. Her article contains a very good expanded discussion of aspects of recovery.

The concept of temperament.   Strelau (1995) considers that individual temperament is a factor in one's risk for pathological consequences of trauma. Calling upon the Thomas, Chess, and Birch (1968) concept of difficult temperament, Strelau sees this as increasing the risk of pathological emotional or behavioral response to conditions of traumatic stress, because individuals with such a temperament have poorer coping capacity. This would be one aspect of lack of resilience. He also postulates that persons with difficult temperament are more likely to put themselves in situations entailing the risk of stress and trauma.

Greater or lesser acceptance of cultural values.   Movements against FC in the cultures practicing it attest to the fact that some women and men in those cultures strongly reject the procedure (Gruenbaum, 1996; Joseph, 1996; Lane and Rubinstein, 1996). In some instances, this arises from individual inability to tolerate and recover from the trauma. In others, it reflects greater education about the medical hazards and greater appreciation of broader aspects of female and human rights.

Greater or lesser trauma from sexual violence and child–adult sexual interaction.   There is no need to cite studies to show that there is usually significant pathological response to child or adult sexual abuse in Western culture. What is more important for considerations of individual resilience, and perhaps individual differences in the sexual events themselves, are studies that do not find pathological responses to be invariable, even in Western culture, where such harm is expected. Levett (1995) questions the concept of inevitable trauma. Rasmussen (1934) followed up 54 adult women victims of sexual assault between the ages of 9 and 13 years. She found that 46 were functioning normally by community standards. Eight were functioning unsatisfactorily, but there was evidence of emotional instability in those eight prior to the assaults. In Conte and Schurman's (1987) study of 369 sexually abused children, an incidental finding was that 21% had none of the symptoms thought to prove prior sexual abuse, such as behavioral regression, somatic complaints, and fearfulness. The authors caution that undue reliance should not be placed on a child's behavior in determining what experiences a child has had; the same data can be seen as arguing that sexual abuse may not always be damaging. DiPietro (1987) studied 60 adolescents: sexual abuse victims, the sisters of victims, and matched subjects from nonabusive families. She measured neuroticism, adjustment, concept of locus of control, and self-concept. There was no statistical difference between any of the three groups on any of the measures. Although the victims were nonsignificantly poorer functioning in terms of neuroticism, adjustment, and locus of control, they were nonsignificantly higher in self-concept.

It is clear that rape victims in our culture can suffer *very* different degrees of trauma and *very* different successes in outcome, regardless of the severity and violence of the rape. Those whose personal education and philosophy regarding women's rights, and whose family and social networks provide appropriate support in recognizing victimization and encouraging retaking of personal control of one's life, usually suffer far less ongoing damage. Where the family and subculture foster attitudes of "She brought it on herself" and "She'll never be as valuable again," the rape victim will be much more severely traumatized and may never fully recover (Lebowitz and Roth, 1994; Harvey, 1996).

Summary Comments

Severe war stress, whether in childhood or adulthood, transcends cultural and language differences and leads to high levels of diagnosable PTSD. (The only comparative studies found were those involving Cambodian refugees.) There was no significant difference between Cambodian refugees and U.S. trauma survivors in the areas of PTSD, dissociation, anxiety, and depression (Carlson and Rosser-Hogan, 1994). PTSD was found in up to 50% of Cambodian adolescents exposed to Pol Pot atrocities. These findings hold up in both clinical and nonclinical samples (Kinsie et al., 1986; Sack et al., 1996; Sack et al., 1997).

The severity of prerefugee war stress is predictive of PTSD, not depression. Depression is more related to postresettlement stresses (such as whether or not one is reunited with nuclear family members) (Kinzie et al., 1986; Sack et al., 1996). Depression tends to diminish with time, depending on favorable resettlement conditions; PTSD does not (Sack et al., 1994; Sack et al., 1997).

Current information suggests that individuals from cultures that provide family stability, environmental safety, community support, and low rates of drug use might be less vulnerable to PTSD than others. Likewise, we would predict better long-term outcomes for traumatized individuals who are enmeshed in a culture where open discussion of the trauma is encouraged, where survivorship is honored, where victimization is not stigmatized, and where posttraumatic problems are normalized (Friedman and Marsella, 1996, p. 24).

GENDER CONSIDERATIONS

In view of the increase in feminist writings and studies in recent years, it is somewhat surprising that there are relatively few studies that target specifically the differences between males and females in their responses to trauma. In general, available studies can be subdivided into those dealing with sexual abuse and those dealing with other forms of trauma.

Sexual Abuse Studies

A difference of opinion exists as to whether or not there is a gender difference in response to sexual abuse. Finklehor et al. (1989) found no gender differences. Most studies, however, reveal significant differences. Stein et al. (1988) found that female pathology was more likely to consist of affective and anxiety disorders and alcohol abuse, whereas male pathology was more likely to be expressed in other types of substance abuse. Rosen and Martin (1996) studied sexual, physical, and emotional abuse. They found females to be more symptomatic than males on the Global Severity Index and on measures of somatization, interpersonal sensitivity, paranoid ideation, and depression. Heath, Bean, and Feinauer (1996) found that women responded with more internalizing disorders (depressive and anxiety symptoms), whereas men had more externalizing disorders (substance abuse and antisocial behavior). In general, the degree of symptomatology was overwhelmingly related to the severity of abuse. The exception in this study was that males showed a more extreme response to the penetration level of abuse than did females. The authors postulate that this is because for males, when the perpetrator was a male family member, two taboos are violated: incest and homosexuality. Thus, in our society, homosexual violation may be more severe in terms of long-term trauma than is heterosexual violation.

Nonsexual Traumas

Curle and Williams (1996) studied 25 children (mostly adolescents) two years after they were involved in a potentially fatal bus accident. Several children were injured sufficiently to be hospitalized, but there were no fatalities. The girls showed more anxiety, depression, and intrusive phenomena than did the boys. The girls used more coping strategies than the boys (emotional expression, distraction, social withdrawal, and wishful thinking) but found them generally not very effective. The boys used fewer strategies (resignation and cognitive resolution) but found them effective. The authors ascribed the gender differences to different coping strategies.

Dyregrov et al. (1994) studied 63 adolescents one month following the murder of their teacher. They found that the girls talked more openly about it with their friends than the boys did, and this correlated with their feeling more anxiety and depression. The boys were more avoidant and reported fewer symptoms than did girls. Those of both sexes who talked more openly with their parents reported fewer symptoms than those who did not. The authors hypothesized that their findings may correlate with studies that show girls to be more caring about a wider social network; this may predispose them to feel greater distress about others. Their report cites numerous studies demonstrating psychological and physical health benefits resulting from openly talking or writing about painful emotions, but it is not clear how their own work supports that thesis. Are the boys in this study in worse shape than the girls?

Survivors of the Buffalo Creek flood disaster were studied at 2 years and 14 years following the event. At 2 years, women had more social isolation and anxiety than did men; they also had more diagnosable PTSD (52%) than men did (32%). However, at 14 years, women's decrease in PTSD (to 31%) was statistically significant, whereas men's decrease (to 23%) was not (Green, 1995).

In a nonclinical sample of 2180 refugees (all ages) from Laos, Vietnam, and Cambodia (Chi-Ying Chang and Kagawa-Singer, 1993), women from Laos and Vietnam showed more states of anxiety and depression than did men. There was no gender difference in symptomatology among Cambodian refugees. The authors postulated that the enormity of premigration trauma suffered by the Cambodians overrode gender differences.

IMPLICATIONS FOR PSYCHOTHERAPEUTIC INTERVENTION

We know relatively little about how most non-Western cultures deal with trauma within their cultures. I was surprised to find no literature in English regarding the developed Asian cultures. Apparently, as revealed by literature searches, these other cultures have little organized, written research available to Westerners regarding their responses to traumatic events. The knowledge available for this chapter comes chiefly through Western anthropologists' reports; some comes from immigrants and survivors.

Many, if not most, non-Western cultures do not make sharp distinctions among mind, body, and spiritual issues. Indigenous healing for illnesses and emotional distresses (which often have spiritual, magical, or witchcraft explanations as well as perhaps medical and physical explanations) most often involve one or more shamans or healers and group participation with varying composition of the groups. This is also true of most, if not all, Native American groups.

Much of the information that has been developed about different cultural attitudes toward trauma has come from having to deal with victims of large-scale traumas affecting large numbers of people: warfare, torture, and other massive abuses. This, of course, involves mostly Western-culture health professionals working with non-Western persons, not their own indigenous healers working with them. The major exception involves Native American and Alaskan Indians, about whom information is beginning to be developed by researchers from their own cultures.

We can organize this information into implications for interventions with those from different cultures and implications derived from learning what is helpful in other cultures, for interventions with trauma victims in our own culture. Due to the limited information we have from other cultures (more about victims of large-scale trauma rather than about victims of individual traumatic events), the application of this knowledge may have limited value in some of the situations discussed in this chapter.

Implications for Dealing with Trauma Victims from Other Cultures

Westermeyer (1995) has described the training and skills necessary for clinicians to assess and treat PTSD across cultural boundaries, regardless of the culture. He stresses the need to take a pretrauma social and psychiatric history to appreciate fully the impact of the trauma. What life changes have occurred consequent to leaving (or being outside) the original culture? A history of how the decision was made to leave the original culture should also be obtained. Who made the decision? Was it carefully planned or desperately precipitous? Clinicians should ask about the nature and duration of the flight and about traumatic events, losses, and other experiences during flight and in any other countries of refuge. What elements of continuity have there been, pre- and postflight? A history of all areas of experience in the final country of refuge is also needed.

The importance of and availability of indigenous healers should be determined and their participation enlisted, if possible. It may be necessary to work through interpreters; this can cause problems if same-culture interpreters hold similar taboos about what may or may not be inquired or spoken about, and they may not interpret accurately.

Therefore, care must be exercised in choosing interpreters. Counter-transference issues may arise because of the wrenching nature of some victims' experiences or if the victim has had negative experiences of the clinician's culture.

It is meaningful to discuss the problems of some particular non-Western cultures about which we have some knowledge, because they present specific clinical problems for Western health workers. Significant non-Western cultures exist in Western countries, such as those of the Native Americans. And the large numbers of non-Western immigrants and refugees with experiences or customs of trauma present clinical challenges for health care facilities and workers.

Native American trauma victims. It is a generally shared characteristic of the Native American worldview and concept of reality that there is no real distinction between the physical, the psychological, and the spiritual (Silver, 1994). Also, the well-being or distress of an individual affects the family and community as well. Therefore, indigenous healing ceremonies entail much more than healing in the biomedical sense. Because these ceremonies involve family and community, the benefit for the traumatized individual is shared by others, who cannot be whole and untraumatized until the individual is reintegrated. The entire group remains in distress over some members, particularly veterans with PTSD, who have not yet "come home" to their new identities and community roles (Manson et al., 1996).

Because of their view that war is the ultimate chaos and a great spiritual danger, warriors are seen as sacrificing themselves for the good of the group, and thus deserving of the highest respect. They cannot really be honored if they are too numbed and emotionally distant to participate in the ceremonies. There is an explicit expectation that spiritual/psychological damage will occur from the experience of war. The recognition by Native Americans of the numbing and isolation of war veterans predates by millennia our current Western understanding of PTSD. In many traditional postwarfare ceremonies, the numbing and isolation is ritualized and prescribed as part of the healing; the warrior is isolated from everyone except older warriors, specifically forbidden to touch or feed himself, to touch the ground, or to engage in sexual intimacy, for example. The numbing is externalized by such taboos, helping the warrior to get in touch with the psychological phenomena and to resolve them (Silver, 1994).

In response to the overwhelming degree of postwar pathology in Native American Vietnam veterans, many tribes have put aside traditional rivalries and enmities and have shared their rituals or joined together in shared rituals. Intermittent national powwows are held by the Vietnam Era Veterans Intertribal Association; these are specifically designed to offer such veterans the community healing experiences they need (Silver, 1994). The sweat-lodge purification ritual was originally a Northern Plains ceremony but is now practiced by many Native American communities. The nature of healing is described (Silver and Wilson, 1988; Wilson, 1989) as providing physical closeness of the participants in the lodge to promote bonding, individual prayers involving culturally appropriate means of expressing the concerns and needs of the individual and of others, and rituals that promote a sense of continuity of the individual in the community and of the community itself. Such rituals usually employ metaphors of healing, rebirth, and the coming of a new day. These rituals often lead to accepted and normalized altered states of consciousness. Scurfield (1996) describes how a sweat lodge, spiritual leader, and powwows were introduced into the treatment regimen of a Veterans Administration PTSD program. This seems an ideal way to meet the needs of at least some Native American veterans, but it is probably not likely to be widely realized. However, it is possible to help all such veterans avail themselves of what is available to them in their own cultures. Efforts can be made to put them in touch with headquarters and elders of their own tribes. Even if some of the groups are not organized to provide their own healing ceremonies, there are intertribal resources such as that mentioned above.

Southeast Asia trauma victims.   Despite a wide variation in specific religious and cultural beliefs and practices among peoples of this large area, the majority share some philosophies and attitudes. A greater importance is placed on family and community than on the individual. Open expression of emotion is not characteristic, and nonconfrontational interpersonal relationships are favored, with a tendency toward acceptance and passive endurance of life's vicissitudes. And there is widespread belief in reincarnation and karma, which teaches that one's present life conditions are the result of one's behavior in previous lives; one is therefore personally responsible for what happens and has little ability to control life events. There is a further and very severe problem for many women of that region, because their traumas usually include

247

repeated rape, and they are blamed and further punished in the here and now by their families and communities for their loss of purity, if that trauma becomes known (Mollica and Son, 1989; Morris and Silove, 1992; Carlson and Rosser-Hogan, 1994).

Other fears of revealing traumatic events or talking about one's earlier life can affect a wider population of Indonesian refugees. They can fear that questions have a political rather than a scientific purpose, and they can be very suspicious of being questioned, even by a fellow member of their culture, if that questioner or interpreter is not already known and trusted. Questioning can retraumatize them by reminding them of interrogations by hostile forces or governments, when, for example, for those exposed to the Pol Pot regime, a "wrong" answer could lead to summary execution (Sack et al., 1994).

It is important to distinguish the consequences of trauma from other forms of cultural loss and the stress of resettlement, because the different traumas have consequences that follow different clinical pathways, and the modalities of help differ (Sack et al., 1994). Helping victims find and integrate with their own cultural groups is imperative both for their daily lives and in the interests of therapy. This can pose a sticky and perhaps insurmountable dilemma for women who have been raped. Because these peoples do not typically think in terms of individual psychological responses to trauma, they fit more into the medical model of psychopathology. In their indigenous cultures, healers almost always offer medicines of some kind, and they expect medications from Western health workers. They benefit most from medications for their symptoms and from practical help with resettlement issues.

Because of the paramount importance of community, even groups without any specific therapeutic focus can result in major change. Cooke (1991), cited in Hegeman (1995), described a group of refugee Cambodian widows who had developed psychogenic blindness in response to as much as seven years of atrocities and starvation in Khmer Rouge slave labor camps. All had been demonstrated, through electroencephalographic testing, to have intact optical and neurological function. They were formed into a group to learn living skills such as using the phone or the city bus system, yet within a few months, all had recovered sufficient sight to go for a walk or to shop for themselves. There had been no therapeutic focus on their vision; there was only the participation in the community of the group, in contrast with their previous isolation, as a possible explanation.

It is the opinion of several researchers and clinicians (Mollica and Son, 1989; Morris and Silove, 1992), that, despite cultural differences, the rape victim will benefit most if she can openly reveal the rape story in therapy and work toward some degree of reassessment of her role in it and its role in her life. It goes without saying what a delicate therapeutic task this poses. A woman may reveal her rape history only after years in therapy, only to a woman therapist of a totally different culture, and with complete assurance that it will never be revealed to her family or others of her culture. She also requires assurance that her therapy will continue and that she will not be rejected, as she would expect, once her shame is known. This degree of therapeutic intervention is likely possible by only the most highly trained and experienced clinicians in this specific field.

Immigrants from cultures that practice female circumcision. This discussion embraces two groups of women. One involves large groups of immigrants who generally expect and wish to continue the custom of FC in their new Western homes. In France (Winter, 1994), the issue has not been unequivocally dealt with in the law, and some FC continues to be performed under pressure from large African populations, generally by trained physicians so as at least to maintain medical sterility in the procedure.

Another example is the large Somali immigrant group living mostly in San Diego. The vast majority of Somali women have had the most severe (Pharaonic) form of FC and strongly desire it for their daughters. They are frustrated by the fact that the procedure is illegal in California, and it undoubtedly continues through nonmedical practitioners (Morris, 1996). At the time of the cited article, the state legislature was considering introducing a bill making it a felony to perform the procedure or to allow it to be performed on any child under 18 years of age. The problems for health care workers with this population have to do with the medical sequelae and complications arising in those with existing FC, and counseling problems with those who believe their cultural rights are being denied.

A second group consists of students who come to the attention of school health services and other health agencies (Morris, 1996; Wollard and Edwards, 1997). These students may be immigrants or daughters of immigrants, or they intend to return to their home cultures. Circumcised adolescent girls in high schools may be the target of ridicule or ostracism, and they are vulnerable to sexual identity problems. Such a girl who presents to college health services may be uncertain as to what, if any, procedure has been performed due to amnesia covering that time in her life. She may also be concerned about medical and sexual health consequences and about her acceptability in Western culture, if she intends to pursue marriage and family outside her native culture.

Refugees and survivors of torture from South America and other West-ern-culture areas (e.g., Greece, Spain).   Almost all the available litera-ture concerns female torture and sexual abuse victims, most of whom have been raped in addition to suffering other atrocities. The Southern Core (Chile, Argentina, Uruguay, Paraguay, and Bolivia) is a major area of past or present government-sanctioned torture. Victims from that area and those from other Western-culture areas generally share such Western humanistic values as self-assertion, rejection of authori-tarianism, autonomy, and situational ethics. They have grown up ex-posed to Western science and psychology. Given this basic philosophy, they are the victims who most likely would be responsive to Western forms of psychotherapy, which focus on uncovering unconscious mem-ories, analyzing defense mechanisms, actively confronting and reinteg-rating traumatic experiences, and taking personal responsibility for overcoming inappropriate guilt and for control of their lives (Morris and Silove, 1992).

Survivors of torture in general.   Most victims of torture feel very strong guilt, even when they do not come from cultures that blame the traumatized for their own misfortunes. This is because torture is often performed in order to obtain something that the victim does not want to give, most often information that would place others in equally serious danger. And the majority of the tortured will eventually break and betray deeply held allegiances. The guilt over this betrayal of family, friends, or colleagues is intense and destructive to self-esteem. When victims come from areas where the philosophy allows for such concepts as inappropriate personal guilt, they can often be helped by individual and group psychotherapy aimed at helping them realize that the torturers made them face impossible choices. The real guilt for their behavior must be placed on their torturers (Morris and Silove, 1992).

  There are also differences in appropriate therapeutic approach, de-pending on whether or not the victims politicize their torture. This is commonly the case for victims from the Southern Core, South Africa, and other generally Westernized culture areas. For these survivors, one major facet of therapy is to help them turn their pain and rage into realistic political protest movements. Women have been very successful with such actions in many arenas (Chester, 1992). A related aspect of therapy is demonstrated when the victims can be persuaded to give official testimony and can then see it used as a basis for political and social action (Morris and Silove, 1992).

Indochinese torture victims, particularly the women, rarely politicize their torture; essentially, it is seen as their own fault regardless of who inflicted it. Such a goal of therapy would be alien to all but the few who could move beyond ingrained cultural concepts.

Implications for Dealing with Trauma Victims from Our Culture

In our general response to the needs of those who have suffered severe trauma, it might be argued that our culture suffers from a too-narrow focus on the individual and a too-secular view of psychobiological illness. The latter may be considered a complaint without remedy. It may be that cultures such as those of the American Indians can be unusually effective in some of their approaches to healing that are based on their more all-encompassing concept of psychobiospiritual phenomena. If so, there is still no way to change Western culture so that its entire philosophical worldview would be so totally different, even if that were desirable. The religious healing claimed by some religions within Western culture in no way approaches the integration of all aspects of life and the world found in those cultures in which all aspects of existence are one. It is difficult to see what of practical value we might learn from such cultures, even if sometimes we might wish to.

With regard to the former, there probably are ways in which we could implement more and better use of groups to help some trauma victims. Group therapy is already in wide use for treatment of veterans with PTSD. For some in the field, though not all, that is seen as second-best, a modality in part necessitated by funding and manpower shortages that limit the amount of top-quality individual attention that patients receive. Perhaps group approaches could benefit from being elevated to top priority, which would spur serious research, drawing also from other cultures, to ascertain how to achieve the very most out of a, if not the, number-one approach to therapy for such patients.

Outside the Veterans Administration, self-help groups are at least available somewhere for virtually every pathology or disability. Therapy groups run by various types of leaders also exist. But the vast majority of the leaders are not qualified professionals. Many are qualified only by having suffered the same trauma themselves. This can be helpful, but it is in no way equivalent to having the effective training necessary for dealing with the consequences of major trauma. And group therapy has not been openly and scientifically legitimized by the medical, psychiatric, and psychological professions as being the most effective means of dealing with and relieving the consequences of some forms of trauma (Hegeman, 1995). Such legitimization would draw more qualified professionals into the field and spur research that would maximize effectiveness.

Drawing upon insights from other cultures, one can specify some victims of trauma who could benefit especially from group therapy. That would include those whose trauma isolates them, such as incest and sexual abuse victims, whose trauma usually occurs in isolation and leaves them feeling all alone in the experience (and if it occurred in childhood, without the learning experience that there are those who can be turned to and trusted). There are those whose trauma causes symptoms that isolate them, as with some of the symptoms of PTSD and the dissociative symptoms of early chronic sexual trauma. There are those whose trauma causes them to withdraw, as in those who feel some guilt and personal responsibility for the trauma. There are those whose values, derived from their subcultures, lead them to expect that family or community are necessary for them to cope effectively with the trauma, but who live in circumstances such that family members or subculture members do not exist. And there are those whose trauma or the experience causing the trauma is devalued by our culture, such as veterans of unpopular wars.

Most non-Western cultures seem to have much more benign ways, again usually involving groups, of dealing with members who display dissociative states (Hegeman, 1995); they are not stigmatized, and the interventions do not result in the isolation of the individual as they do in our culture. Perhaps it would be helpful for the psychiatric profession to take the lead in destigmatizing dissociative states (such as depersonalization, psychogenic amnesia, and multiple personality disorder) and undertaking a broad public education effort, as is currently the case with depression. Although such symptoms are also present in schizophrenia, it is generally agreed that early severe trauma involving body boundaries being painfully violated is a major cause of dissociative phenomena. In our culture, not only does early sexual abuse cause the victims to feel isolated, but also the dissociative symptoms so often arising from the abuse are further traumatizing and isolating. In addition, the medical, psychiatric, and public responses (hospitalization, medications, ostracism, even electroconvulsive shock therapy) are further traumatizing. If altered states of consciousness follow incest and other early severe traumas as predictably as does pain follow a broken arm, a much more helpfully accepting response to their existence could evolve. We do not regard the pain as something that is wrong with the person with a broken bone. This approach would not depathologize either the trauma or the symptoms but would embody a recognition that there are naturally expectable coping mechanisms in the face of such trauma. Groups such as Survivors of Incest Anonymous (SIA) currently offer some consensual validation for such trauma victims, but a more enlightened psychiatric understanding would lead to more professional involvement with that kind of group therapy (Hegeman, 1995).

General Comments

A theme that runs through many of the studies cited in this chapter supports the general therapeutic benefits of being able to talk about one's emotions and other responses following exposure to trauma. That seems to be an almost unanimous consensus in Western-culture psychiatric and psychological communities. It is puzzling, then, to note the findings in two studies of adolescents exposed to traumatic experiences described earlier. In both of those studies, girls talked more freely about their feelings than boys did, and yet even the girls themselves reported that their ways of coping were less helpful in relieving their distress than the boys found theirs to be. Will the boys pay a higher psychological price later? That is not known. Are adolescents exceptions to a general rule that holds true for other age groups? It is somewhat unlikely that the entire professional mental health community is espousing a false tenet, though that has happened before. It would be useful to devise research to shed further light on such seeming exceptions.

The researcher who described the less-stigmatizing ways that non-Western cultures have of dealing with dissociative states also argues that their practices are not therapeutic, at least in the Western sense (Hegeman, 1995). That raises the question of what constitutes therapy. In our psychiatric philosophy, therapy is grounded in a sense of a closely bounded self, a belief in individual capacity to control how one responds to life events, to recognize the causes of illness and distress, to change traumatogenic conditions, and to recover from trauma; it is a medical concept of illness, trauma, and recovery. In many non-Western cultures, there is no medical model and therefore no concept of cure or stigma or recognition of trauma as the cause of the distress. Hegeman recognizes the culture-bound quality of Western concepts of what is therapeutic but still denies that a practice is therapeutic if it does not lead to recognition of and resolution of the trauma. Helpful and reintegrating rituals in non-Western cultures often exist outside any concept of therapy, but they do enable the victims to tolerate the trauma and do provide relief from debilitating symptoms. It is true that, as in the Balinese example cited earlier, the trance dance does nothing to change the child-rearing practices that continue to cause trauma from generation to generation; in that sense, such ceremonies are not therapeutic for the culture. But it is difficult to deny that they benefit the traumatized individuals. Is that not therapy? There may be some disadvantages in too narrow a concept of what is truly therapeutic, especially to trauma victims whose coping strategies help them to survive, yet leave them stigmatized by falling short of what we define as "recovered."

REFERENCES

Allen, I. M. (1996), PTSD in African Americans. In: *Ethnocultural Aspects of Post Traumatic Stress Disorder,* ed. A. J. Marsella, M. J. Friedman, E. T. Gerrity & R. M. Scurfield. Washington, DC: American Psychological Association, pp. 209–238.

Baker, R. (1992), Psychological consequences for tortured refugees seeking asylum and refugee status in Europe. In: *Torture and Its Consequences,* ed. M. Basoglu. New York: Cambridge University Press, pp. 83–106.

Berkey, J. P. (1996), Circumcision circumscribed: Female excision and cultural accommodation in the medieval Near East. *Int. J. Middle East Stud.,* 28:19–38.

Bourguignon, E. (1971), *Psychol. Anthro.* New York: Holt, Rinehart & Winston.

Carlson, E. B. & Rosser-Hogan, R. (1994), Cross-cultural responses to trauma. *J. Traumatic Stress,* 7:43–58.

Chester, B. (1992), Women and political torture. *Women and Therapy,* 13:209–220.

Chi-Ying Chang, R. & Kagawa-Singer, M. (1993), Predictors of psychological distress among Southeast Asia refugees. *Soc. Sci. & Med.,* 36:631–638.

Conte, J. R. & Schurman, J. R. (1987), Factors associated with increased impact of child sexual abuse. *Child Abuse Negl.,* 11:201–211.

Cooke, P. (1991), They cried till they could not see. *New York Times Magazine,* June 23, 1991, p. 24.

Curle, C. E. & Williams, C. (1996), Post-traumatic stress reactions in children. *Brit. J. Clin. Psychol.,* 35:297–309.

DiPietro, S. B. (1987), The effects of intrafamilial child sex abuse on the adjustment and attitudes of adolescents. *Violence & Victims,* 2:59–78.

Dyregrov, A., Kristoffersen, J. I., Matthiesen, S. B., & Mitchell, J. T. 1994), Gender differences in adolescents' reactions to the murder of their teacher. *J. Adol. Res.,* 9:363–383.

Fabrega, H. Jr. & Nutini, H. (1994), Tlaxcalan constructions of acute grief. *Cult. Med., & Psychiat.,* 18:405–431.

Finklehor, D., Hotaling, G., Lewis, I. A., & Smith, C. (1989), Sexual abuse and its relation to later sexual satisfaction, marital status, religion and attitudes. *J. Interpers. Violence,* 4:379–399.

Friedman, M. J. & Marsella, A. J. (1996), Post-traumatic stress disorder: An overview of the concept. In: *Ethnocultural Aspects of Posttraumatic Stress Disorder,* ed. A. J. Marsella, M. J. Friedman, E. T. Gerrity & R. M. Scurfield. Washington, DC: American Psychological Association, pp. 11–30.

Gordon, D. (1991), Female circumcision and genital operation in Egypt and the Sudan. *Med. Anthrop. Quart.,* 5:3–14.

Green, B. L. (1995), Long-term consequences of disaster. In: *Extreme Stress and Communities,* ed. S. E. Hobfoll & M. W. deVries. Dordrecht/Boston/London: Kluwer Academic Publishers, pp. 307–324.

Gruenbaum, E. (1996), The cultural debate over female circumcision. *Med. Anthrop. Quart.,* 10:455–472.

Harvey, M. R. (1996), An ecological view of psychobiological trauma and trauma recovery. *J. Traumatic Stress,* 9:3–23.

Heath, V., Bean, R. & Feinauer, L. (1996), Severity of childhood sexual abuse. *Amer. J. Family Therapy,* 24:305–314.

Hegeman, E. (1995), Groups and the mediation of dissociative experience. *Group,* 19:31–44.

Joseph, C. (1996), Compassionate accountability. *J. Psychohistory,* 24:2–17.

Kinzie, J. D., Sack, W. H., Angell, R. H., Manson, S. & Rath, B. (1986), The psychiatric effects of massive trauma on Cambodian children: I. The children. *J. Amer. Acad. Child & Adol. Psychiat.,* 25:370–376.

Kirmayer, L. J. (1996), Confusion of the senses. In: *Ethnocultural Aspects of Post-traumatic Stress Disorder,* ed. A. J. Marsella, M. J. Friedman, E. T. Gerrity & R. M. Scurfield. Washington, DC: American Psychological Association, pp. 131–163.

Koskov, F. E. (1991), Primary psychological intervention with families of earthquake survivors in Armenia. *Amer. J. Family Therapy,* 19:54–58.

Lane, S. D. & Rubinstein, R. A. (1996), Judging the other: Responding to traditional female genital surgeries. *Hastings Center Report,* 26:31–40.

Lebowitz, L. & Roth, S. (1994), "I felt like a slut": The cultural context and women's response to being raped. *J. Traumatic Stress,* 7:363–390.

Levett, A. (1995), Discourses of child sex abuse: Regimes of truth? In: *Trends and Issues in Theoretical Psychology,* ed. I. Lubek, R. vanHezewijk, G. Pheterson, C. W. Tolman, pp. 294–300. New York: Springer.

Lunde, I. & Ortmann, J. (1992), Sexual torture and the treatment of its consequences. In: *Torture and Its Consequences,* ed. M. Basoglu. New York: Cambridge University Press, pp. 310–329.

Manson, S. M. (1997), Cross-cultural and multiethnic assessment of trauma. In: *Assessing Psychological Trauma and PTSD,* ed. J. P. Wilson & T. M. Keane. New York: Guilford, pp. 239–266.

———— Beals, J., O'Nell, T. et al. (1996), Wounded spirits, ailing hearts. In: *Ethnocultural Aspects of Post-Traumatic Stress Disorder,* ed. A. J. Marsella, M. J. Friedman, E. T. Gerrity & R. M. Scurfield. Washington, DC: American Psychological Association, pp. 255–283.

Meichenbaum, D. (1995), Disasters, stress and cognition. In: *Extreme Stress and Communities,* ed. S. E. Hobfoll & M. W. deVries. Boston: Kluwer Academic Publishers, pp. 33–61.

Mollica, R. F. & Son, L. (1989), Cultural dimensions in the evaluation and treatment of sexual trauma. *Psych. Clin. N. Amer.,* 12:364–379. Philadelphia: W. B. Saunders.

Morris, P. & Silove, D. (1992), Cultural influences in psychotherapy with refugee survivors of torture and trauma. *Hosp. Comm. Psychiat.,* 43:820–824.

Morris, R. (1996), The culture of female circumcision. *Adv. Nurs. Sci.,* 19:1–53.

Palinkas, L. A., Downs, M., Petterson, J. S. et al. (1993), Social, cultural, and psychological impact of the Exxon Valdez oil spill. *Human Organization,* 52:1–13.

Rasmussen, A. (1934), Die Bedeutung sexualle attentate auf Kinder unter 14 Jahren fur die Entwicklung von Geisteskrankheiten und Characteranomalien. *Acta Psychiatrica et Neurologica,* 9:351–358.

Rosen, L. N. & Martin, L. (1996), Impact of childhood abuse history on psychological symptoms among male and female soldiers in the U.S. Army. *Child Abuse Negl.,* 20:1149–1160.

Rubonis, A. V. & Bickman, L. (1991), Psychological impairment in the wake of disaster. *Psych. Bull.,* 109:384–399.

Sack, W. H., Clarke, G. N. & Seeley, J. R. (1996), Multiple forms of stress in Cambodian adolescent refugees. *Child Devel.,* 67:107–116.

——— McSharry, S., Clarke, G. N., Kinney, R., Seeley, J. & Lewinsohn, P. (1994), The Khmer adolescent project: I. Epidemiologic findings in two generations of Cambodian refugees. *J. Nerv. Ment. Dis.,* 182:387–395.

——— Seeley, J. R. & Clarke, G. N. (1997), Does PTSD transcend cultural barriers? *J. Amer. Acad. Child & Adol. Psychiat.,* 36:49–54.

Scurfield, R. M. (1996), Healing the warrior: Admission of two American Indian war veteran cohort groups to a specialized inpatient PTSD unit. *Amer. Ind. & Alaska Native Ment. Health Res.,* 6:1–22.

Silver, S. (1994), Lessons from Child of Water. *Amer. Ind. & Alaska Native Ment. Health Res.,* 6:4–17.

——— & Wilson, J. (1988), Native American healing and purification rituals for war stress. In: *Human Adaptation to Extreme Stress,* ed. J. Wilson, Z. Harel & B. Kahana. New York: Plenum Press, pp. 337–356.

Stein, J. A., Golding, J. M., Siegel, J. M., et al. (1988), Long-term psychological sequellae of child sexual abuse. In: *The Lasting Effects of Child Sexual Abuse,* ed. G. Wyatt & G. Powell. Newbury Park, CA: Sage, pp. 135–156.

Strelau, J. (1995), Temperament risk factor. In: *Extreme Stress and Communities,* ed. S. E. Hobfoll & M. W. deVries. Boston: Kluwer Academic Publishers, pp. 63–81.

Thomas, A., Chess, S. & Birch, H. G. (1968), *Temperament and Behavior Disorders in Children.* New York: New York University Press.

Toubia, N. (1994), Female genital mutilation and the responsibility of reproductive health professionals. *Int. J. Gyn. Obstet.,* 46:127–135.

Wiesaeth, L. (1995), Preventive psychosocial intervention after disaster. In: *Extreme Stress and Communities,* ed. S. E. Hobfoll & M. W. deVries. Boston: Kluwer Academic Publishers, pp. 401–419.

Westermeyer, J. (1995), Cross-cultural care for PTSD. In: *Psychotraumatology: Key Papers and Core Concepts in Post-traumatic Stress,* ed. G. S. Everly, Jr. & J. M. Lating. New York: Plenum Press, pp. 375–394.

Wilson, J. (1989), *Trauma, Transformation and Healing.* New York: Brunner/Mazel.

Winkel, E. (1995), A Muslim perspective on female circumcision. *Women and Health,* 23:1–7.

Winter, B. (1994), The law and cultural relativism in France. *Signs,* 19:939–974.

Wollard, D. & Edwards, R. M. (1997), Female circumcision: An emerging problem in college health care. *J. Amer. Coll. Health,* 45:230–232.

10   THE NEUROBIOLOGICAL EFFECTS
OF TRAUMA

PATRICIA LESTER, SUSAN W. WONG, AND ROBERT L. HENDREN

Although the precise effects of trauma on the brain are not yet under-stood, there is a consensus that it has significant impact on brain functioning. Studies in animals support the hypothesis that trauma produces long-lasting effects on neurobiological functioning. Intriguing new findings based on neuroimaging suggest that this is also true in humans. To what extent the changes are reversible or permanent is an important unanswered question. Equally important is the question of mitigating versus exacerbating factors.

We know that the developing brain is uniquely vulnerable as well as plastic. The human brain undergoes considerable development during childhood and adolescence (Casey, Giedd, and Thomas, 2000). Current thinking supports the idea that trauma may have particularly devastating effects on immature biological systems (De-Bellis, 2001; Heim and Nemeroff, 2001), but it is less clear what the particular impact of trauma experienced during adolescence may be on the brain. Preliminary mod-els for the neurobiological impact of trauma on development come primarily from research on chronic stress such as child abuse and neglect, and acute stress such as disaster, war, or medical trauma.

An understanding of neurobiological functioning and trauma can inform our selection of treatment. Knowledge about the efficacy of various forms of treatment can likewise suggest possible neurochemical mechanisms underlying the pathogenic actions of trauma. This chapter summarizes research findings and attempts to synthesize them into a state-of-the art discussion of what we know about the neurobiology of trauma and the implications of this knowledge for prevention and treatment. Although some of the literature cited is not specific to adolescence, the discussion and treatment planning are related to the adolescent period.

Models for Stress Response

To determine the effect of trauma exposure on the individual, it is also essential to identify the mediating processes. These include the developmental level of the individual being traumatized, biological factors in the trauma experience, and the social and emotional context (such as the quality of attachment, family involvement, and community and cultural support) in which the effects of trauma are contained (Pynoos, Steinberg, and Piacentini, 1999). The influence of neurobiology in posttraumatic stress disorder (PTSD) involves three interconnected areas:

1. The maturation and reorganization of brain structures and their function and influence
2. Physiological processes such as neuroendocrine and neurotransmitter influences and fluctuations
3. Individual personality resilience and vulnerability expressed in cognition, emotional regulation, and the influence of these on behavior.

These neurobiological components are in a dynamic interplay with the sociocultural context in which the child is or has been located.

Clinical research has described childhood stress responses on the basis of symptom formation. From assessment of children exposed to acute or chronic trauma, Terr (1991) describes two symptom clusters of traumatic reactions. Related primarily to acute reactions, a Type I traumatic response is characterized by full detailed memories, "omens," and misperceptions. Related more to chronic traumatic exposure, a Type II traumatic response includes denial or numbing, self-hypnosis and dissociation, and rage. According to Terr, both Type I and Type II traumatic reactions can coexist in one individual. The symptom of dissociation has important clinical implications.

Dissociative Responses

Dissociative experiences are often an important aspect of response to trauma, both during the traumatic episode and afterward; they may be

260

used as adaptive or maladaptive mechanisms for coping with stressful situations. Retrospective investigations of dissociative symptoms have demonstrated an association with prior childhood abuse, neglect, and other traumatic experiences (Chu and Dill, 1990; Waldinger et al., 1994; Zlotnick et al., 1996). Early predictors of adolescent dissociation include the chronicity and intensity of exposure of earlier childhood trauma (Ogawa et al., 1997).

Several hypotheses have been proposed to explain the relationship between traumatic stress and the development of dissociative symptoms. One is that dissociation is a defense mechanism used during overwhelming trauma, which later develops into an automatic response (Terr, 1991). Another is that dissociation comes from a conflicting model of the self resulting from the irreconcilable behavior of a caretaker who is alternately abusive and protective (Carlson et al., 1989) or who exhibits frightened or frightening behaviors when approached by the child (Hesse and Main, 2000). Dissociation may result from an individual's inability to process traumatic events both cognitively and emotionally. The failure of declarative memory to process trauma may lead to a somatosensory response including symptoms such as visions or physical sensations (van der Kolk, 1994).

Others have found that a dissociative subtype of PTSD occurs in persons who have symptoms of diminished physiological (skin conductance and heart rate) reactivity (Griffin, Resick, and Mechanic, 1997). The startle response is a neuronal response to severe stress that usually normalizes over time. An exaggerated startle response is often found in individuals with PTSD. For instance, women with recent sexual-assault-related PTSD demonstrate a greater startle response than those with long-standing trauma (Morgan et al., 1997). However, the startle response is also influenced by developmental level. Inhibition of startle response occurs at approximately eight years of age, when children are able to construct intervention fantasies that anticipate danger in order to avert or prevent it (Pynoos et al., 1997).

In a longitudinal investigation of developmental risk for later dissociation, findings support theories that dissociative behavior appears more normative in early childhood, whereas it becomes suggestive of psychopathology in adolescence and young adulthood (Ogawa et al., 1997). Ogawa et al. also found that pathological dissociation during adolescence is related to insecure caretaker–infant attachment classification measured during infancy. Others have also identified a relationship between severe psychopathology, insecure attachment classification, and failure to resolve traumatic-stress symptoms (Allen, Hauser, and Borman-Spurrell, 1996).

Thus, the response to trauma is influenced by the individual's developmental level and attachment relationships, prior traumatic exposure, trauma type, and coping strategies surrounding the trauma. Gender also may affect the exposure, processing, and response to trauma, with females reporting more PTSD than males in community samples (see Stein, Walker, and Forde, 2000, for a review). Responses to stress and trauma may also differ depending on the developmental stage of the person involved. For instance, young children in a traumatic situation are likely to react on the basis of their primary caretakers' reactions. Adolescents react on the basis of their previous experiences and the meaning of the trauma to their current life situations. Compared with young children, adolescents may have more control of their responses because they can anticipate or preassign meaning to stressful events. To some extent, the threshold or intensity of reaction is set by previous experience and is then triggered by the later event. This threshold is a biologically and emotionally programmed response.

BIOLOGICAL MARKERS OF STRESS

Stress activates the well-known fight or flight response. The anatomic pathways involve the thalamus, anterior cingulate, amygdala, hippocampus, cerebellum, and, of course, the cortex. Activation of this system involves the autonomic nervous system, the immune system, and the hypothalamic-pituitary-adrenocortical axis, with peripheral release of adrenocorticotropic hormones and cortisol as well as other central nervous system (CNS) neurochemical systems. The nature and extent of this response depends on individual characteristics of the organism such as genetic endowment and previous experience. These, in turn, translate into a neurochemical or signal response in the organism that affects particular brain regions and, ultimately, development. Each of these areas is summarized in the following sections.

Although it may seem a bit far-fetched at first to suggest that genetics can influence the response to stress and trauma, it is easy to appreciate that genetic factors such as temperament (shyness, risk taking), physiological sensitivity (startle response), and neurotransmitter regulation play an important role in the dynamic process between environmental stress and the individual. Genetic factors also may play a role in individual responses to trauma. There is some evidence that a capacity for dissociation is, in part, genetically determined. In addition, early adverse experiences may influence preexisting genetic vulnerability to stress by sensitizing stress-responsive neural circuits, which then manifest a phenotype at risk for further disorder (Heim and Nemeroff, 2001).

BRAIN REGIONS INVOLVED IN STRESS RESPONSE

Maturation of specific brain structures has an important influence on how stress is processed. The amygdala, hippocampus, and prefrontal cortex appear to be most sensitive to the posttraumatic response to danger, but other limbic, midbrain and brain-stem structures are involved as well. Traumatic experiences at periods of neurodevelopmental growth or stabilization can have differential effects on these structures and influence the response to subsequent stress.

The stress response is mediated primarily by the locus coeruleus. The noradrenergic locus coeruleus is located in the pons, a primitive part of the brain that regulates basic bodily functions. It sends noradrenergic projections to the cerebral cortex, the thalamus and hypothalamus, the olfactory bulb, the cerebellum, the midbrain, and the spinal cord. The locus coeruleus is involved in the regulation of attention, arousal, sleep–wake cycles, learning and memory, anxiety, pain, startle response, and behavioral irritability. It increases brain responsiveness and may become more sensitive or sensitized when repeatedly stimulated by stress.

Stress affects a number of brain regions, most particularly the prefrontal cortex, the anterior cingulate, temporal lobe structures, and the cerebellum. The prefrontal cortex subserves executive cognitive functions and modulates limbic information to relate to basal ganglia circuits and to control neurochemical elements of attention and reward. The prefrontal cortex is critical for working memory. It continues to develop throughout adolescence. The anterior cingulate is part of the prefrontal cortex that has been associated with emotional processing, specifically, how a person decides whether a certain behavior, thought, or feeling will be rewarding (Barch, 1999). Diminished response to emotionally relevant stimuli is seen in the anterior cingulate in PTSD and may mediate symptoms such as distress and arousal upon exposure to reminders of trauma (Shin et al., 2001). The number of neurons may actually decrease in the anterior cingulate with repeated stress (De Bellis et al., 1999).

The temporal lobe includes the amygdala, which plays a significant role in the control of emotional behavior and learning, stimulus-reward associations, conditioned emotional responses, and memory for disturbed social interactions. Thus, the amygdala, mediated through stress-related neurochemical events, is involved in the affective response to (and memory for) stress and trauma-related information (LeDoux and Gorman, 2001). This is an evolutionarily adaptive method of creating self-preserving memories. In PTSD, however, these memories can become intrusive or maladaptive.

Patients exposed to scripts of their own traumatic events demonstrate increased activity in the amygdala, median temporal lobe, and the insula, and deactivation in Broca's area on PET-scan measurement (Rauch, 1997). Increased heart rate and subjective reporting of increased anxiety and fear accompany this brain response. It is hypothesized that patients with PTSD have difficulty restructuring recollections of traumatic histories due to the decreased activity of Broca's area, an area responsible for language processing and higher cognitive functioning.

The amygdala receives input from the thalamus and the cortex, with the ultimate emotional reaction reflecting a joint effort of these two inputs. However, the thalamus-amygdala system is several synapses shorter than the cortico-amygdala system, allowing for faster response without cognitive processing. Parallel pathways may become uncoupled, either through experience or genetic endowment. If the thalamus-amygdala pathway is dominant, inappropriate reactions may be common, along with poor insight into the origins of the emotional reactions.

Fear conditioning reactivated by trauma-related stimuli (e.g. hyper-arousal) via explicit and contextual cues encoded in and retrieved from the amygdala may result in intrusive memories. Reactivation by more complex environmental stimuli and aversive events may involve the hippocampus as well. Repeated activation of these memories may produce kindling or increasing activation, resulting in increased intrusive memories with decreased cues (Grillon, Southwick, and Charney, 1996). "Kindling" denotes the phenomenon whereby exposure to stress at a critical time in development becomes encoded in the brain and sensitizes a person to react disproportionally when triggering experiences occur; it is based on assumptions about changes in brain functioning.

The hippocampus is an integral component of neurofunctional pathways involved in learning, memory, attention, processing of polysensory information, and regulation of affect (Zola-Morgan and Squire, 1990). Lesions of the hippocampus result in the loss of the capacity for consolidating short-term memory into long-term memory but retention of memories prior to the lesion. Thus, whereas the amygdala remembers the affect, the hippocampus remembers the circumstances when the amygdala was turned on by the emotional experience.

Studies have shown that patients with PTSD have smaller hippocampal volumes than those without symptoms of PTSD. Gurvitz et al. (1996) found decreased left and right hippocampal volume (26% and 22% respectively) on MRIs of Vietnam veterans with combat exposure compared to those of veterans without combat exposure. They noted, as have others studying women sexually abused in childhood (Stein et al., 1997), that the symptom severity of PTSD was directly proportional to the decreased size of the hippocampus. Bremner et al. (1995) found that Vietnam veterans with PTSD had an 8% reduction in hippocampal volume compared to veterans without symptoms of PTSD. Other studies demonstrate that hippocampal reduction is associated with memory deficits and suggest that trauma at different stages of development may influence the nature of the memory deficits (Bremner and Narayan, 1998).

It is hypothesized that the constant reliving of traumatic events is responsible for cell damage and therefore decreased volume of the hippocampus. It is believed that this may contribute to an individual's difficulty in processing new information, increasing the vulnerability to misinterpretation of even neutral stimuli. One theory is that high levels of glucorticoids secreted in response to stress may contribute to cell death. Although one might be led to assume that the changes in the hippocampus are the result of stress, it is also possible that individuals with preexisting, decreased hippocampal volumes may be predisposed to the development of PTSD (Bremner et al., 1995). This vulnerability may be related to other brain regions as well.

Finally, the cerebellar vermis has also been implicated in the response to stress. Recent studies suggest that the circuitry of the cerebellum is involved in such higher-order behavior as working memory, executive function, visuospatial abilities, linguistic processing, memory, attention, and emotional modulation or coordination (Schmahmann, 1991; Schmahmann and Sherman, 1998). Decreases in functional-MRI-measured blood flow in the cerebellar vermis is associated with repeated childhood abuse in young-adult subjects (Anderson et al., 2002).

Neuromodulators Involved in Stress Response

During a traumatic event, the increase in sympathetic discharge allows maximal mobilization of energy and helps the individual respond to the traumatic situation. Heart rate and blood pressure are increased to increase perfusion of blood to muscles. Skeletal muscles are also supplied with glucose. Pain is suppressed or ignored. The increase in CNS activation is protective, but in many individuals with PTSD, the sympathetic nervous system appears hyperresponsive to stimuli similar to that involved in the trauma (De Bellis et al., 1999).

NEUROTRANSMITTERS

It appears that there are two neurobiological subgroups of patients with PTSD—one with sensitized noradrenergic systems and the other with sensitized serotonergic systems (Southwick et al., 1997). The noradrenergic system is linked to symptoms of fear and anxiety, vigilance, selective attention, consolidation of memory stress response, central and peripheral arousal, affect, irritability, reward dependence, attention, startle response, learning, and consolidation of memory (Southwick et al., 1997). Through these mechanisms, norepinephrine is also linked to subsequent response to stress.

Research with adult combat veterans with PTSD revealed increased excretion of norepinephrine compared with that of control subjects (Yehuda et al., 1992; Southwick et al., 1997). Baseline plasma norepinephrine studies in adults have not found any significant differences between controls and PTSD patients. Receptor studies have found fewer alpha2-adrenergic receptor binding sites in PTSD patients. This is consistent with the theory that down regulation of receptors may take place because of chronically elevated circulating catecholamines. Few studies have been done investigating the pathophysiology of PTSD in children.

Serotonin is linked to the functions of sleep, appetite, perception, hormone secretion, impulse modulation, behavioral inhibition, sexual

266

activity, and mood. Traumatized individuals frequently display changes in impulse control, aggression, mood, and behavior. These factors suggest that serotonin is involved in symptom formation. Decreased serotonin levels have been noted in animals that are shocked and cannot escape and are also related to an inability to modulate arousal, exemplified by an exaggerated startle response and increased arousal (Gerson and Baldessarini, 1980). In addition, serotonin reuptake inhibitors have demonstrated some efficacy in treating PTSD.

Dopamine is involved with modulating movement and cognition, behavioral activation, and novelty seeking. The dopamine mesolimbic system is activated by stressful experiences and plays a role in the responsivity to aversion and pleasure. Postnatal stress experience in mice has been shown to affect mesolimbic dopamine functioning and to increase the adult response to arousing situations but not to aversive uncontrollable situations (Cabib, Puglisi-Allegra, and D'Amato, 1993).

Rodents exposed to stressful experiences show an increase of dopamine release in the nucleus accumbens septi if they are allowed to control the shock experience, while showing a decrease of dopamine release in this brain area if they are not allowed to exert any control. These results indicate that escapable/controllable and inescapable/uncontrollable aversive experiences elicit opposite responses from the mesolimbic dopaminergic system. If environmental conditions allow behavioral control, enhanced mesolimbic dopaminergic release is maintained regardless of the intensity of the aversive stimuli (Cabib and Puglisi-Allegra, 1994).

NEUROENDOCRINE AND OTHER NEUROCHEMICAL SYSTEMS

The hypothalamic-pituitary-adrenal (HPA) axis and glucocorticoids are also involved in modulating the stress response. How this system is affected by acute and chronic stress, what impact dysregulation of glucocorticoid basal levels and stress responses have on the developing brain, and what factors may mediate the glucocorticoid stress response constitute active areas of investigation. In acute stress, cortisol regulates stress hormone release through a negative feedback loop to the pituitary, hypothalamus, and hippocampus resulting in down regulation of glucocorticoid receptors. Organisms exposed to chronic stress will then manage acute stress differently and cope less effectively. The process that is thought to occur is that the HPA axis of a chronically stressed individual becomes sensitized, with decreased resting glucocorticoid levels, decreased secretion of glucocorticoid in response to subsequent stress (Yehuda et al., 1991), and more glucocorticoid receptors in the hypothalamus (Yehuda et al., 1995; Yehuda, 2001). In addition, individuals and children exposed to chronic stress (such as parental neglect) have been found to have disrupted circadian patterns of cortisol release (Cicchetti and Rogosch, 2001; Yehuda, 2001; Gunnar and Gilles, 2002).

Corticotropin releasing factor (CRF) appears to be one of the major regulators in stress response and to have a role in mediating the effects of early-life stress on subsequent psychopathology (Heim et al., 1997b). Although depressed individuals have a pattern of higher cortisol release that is less rhythmic and more chaotic, basal cortisol is generally found to be low in adults with PTSD. This may reflect an exaggerated sensitization of the HPA axis in the PTSD group and dysregulation in the depressed group (Yehuda et al., 1996). Similar results have been found in adolescent earthquake survivors who have low basal cortisol levels (Goenjian et al., 1996). Exposure to parental PTSD has been found to result in decreased 24-hour urinary cortisol excretion in the adult offspring of Holocaust survivors when compared to those whose parents did not have PTSD (Yehuda, Halligan, and Bierer, 2002). Reduced cortisol levels in individuals affected by PTSD may result in impaired stress responses to subsequent trauma (Hart, Gunnar, and Cicchetti, 1995).

Cortisol has a direct effect on a number of physiological systems, including the brain, metabolism, and immune system. Through its effects on specific areas of the brain, cortisol also has an impact on emotional behavior and cognition (McEwen and Sapolsky, 1995; Seeman et al., 1997). Glucocorticoid hormones exert longer lasting responses than do peptide hormones, growth factors, or neurotransmitters. With acute stress, excessive amounts of glucocorticoids may result in a reversible atrophy of dendritic processes, especially in the hippocampus, because it is the most glutamatergic region of the brain (demonstrated by its plasticity during learning). Mediated through the adrenocortical system, exposure to stress may impair hippocampal dependent learning and memory processes (Orchinik et al., 2001). Harmful effects also may result from exposure to excitatory amino acids such as glutamate or kainate acid (Lombroso and Sapolsky, 1998). The consequence of overexposure to glucocorticoids or excitatory amino acids resulting in cell atrophy, cell loss, or decreased neurogenesis is suggested as the cause for this reduced hippocampal volume (Duman and Charney, 1999). Other areas of the brain also have regions with glucocorticoid receptors, including the cingulate gyrus and frontal brain regions, making them vulnerable to high levels of cortisol early in life.

Consequently, the persistence of fear responses may have a long-term negative outcome for developing children. Investigation of the relationship of stress and the HPA axis has also indicated that activity of the adrenocortical system in response to stress is influenced by behavioral and psychological processes. In particular, Gunnar (1998) has proposed that security of attachment with a primary caregiver serves as a buffer of the HPA-axis mediated stress response. In infancy, attachment behaviors are described as the baby's proximity-maintaining activities when sensing discomfort. Closeness to the parent or primary caregiver typically reduces the infant's stress response. For example, for an infant with an inhibited temperament, a secure attachment relationship between infant and caregiver may protect the infant's developing brain by preventing a rise in glucocorticoids (Nachmias et al., 1996). Furthermore, repeated exposure to stress typically results in decreased cortisol responses as behavioral coping strategies are implemented, whereas interference with normal coping strategies, such as seeking a primary caretaker, may lead to marked dysregulation in cortisol. Spangler and Grossmann (1993, 1999) have shown that infants with a disorganized attachment relationship have increased cortisol output when confronted with a stressful situation compared to those infants with an organized attachment relationship, despite similar baseline levels. Mediated in part by attachment relationships, early disruptions in the adrenocortical system secondary to traumatic stress may alter later responses to stress, as well as vulnerability to PTSD, in children and adolescents.

Other neurochemical systems also are implicated in the stress response. Endogenous opioids are secreted in response to stress and serve to decrease pain. Stress-induced analgesia following inescapable stressors has been described in animals. However, opioids can interfere with processing of the traumatic event, therefore contributing to the development of dissociative symptoms and preventing the organism from learning from the experience.

Excitatory amino acids, especially the N-methyl-D-aspartate (NMDA) receptor, have been implicated recently in crucial physiological processes such as synaptogenesis, learning, and memory. NDMA receptor function may thus play an important role in the pathophysiology of PTSD through the creation of permanent emotional memories in the amygdala and its efferents. Blockage of these and other receptors shortly after a traumatic stressor, to mitigate the permanence of the emotional memory, may be a useful strategy in developing new psychopharmacological treatments for the disorder (Heresco-Levy and Javitt, 1998).

EFFECTS OF STRESS ON CNS DEVELOPMENT

In the developing brain, stress-activated neurotransmitters and hormones may alter critical periods of neurogenesis and neurochemical differentiation (Golier and Yehuda, 1998). High levels of maternal prenatal stress and associated CRF hypersecretion appear to be related to later behavioral problems including risk for PTSD in the offspring. Early neglect and abuse, particularly in the presence of genetic susceptibility, permanently alters CRF neurons and increases the risk for PTSD (De Bellis et al., 1999).

Sensitized neurons may organize the brain into new functional networks that provide alternate pathways for integrating experience and memory. Once organized around traumatic experience, these networks can be triggered by reminders and activate trauma-related arousal, cognition, affects, and physical and psychological states that overwhelm ongoing experience. For children exposed to trauma, these networks may organize around experiences of fear, unpredictability, anger, hunger, pain, and helplessness (Schwartz and Perry, 1994).

Sensitized catecholamine receptors in the locus coeruleus and the ventral tegmental region can lead to hypervigilance, increased startle response, affective liability, and autonomic hyperreactivity. Long-term potentiation of traumatic memories also occurs and is thought to be mediated by norepinephrine input to the amygdala. This leads the individual to access memories more readily when aroused, thereby causing repeated experiencing of the trauma (Bremner and Vermetten, 2001; Kaufman and Charney, 2001).

RESILIENCE AND THE ENVIRONMENTAL
CONTAINER AS MEDIATORS OF TRAUMA

The symptomatic outcome of trauma depends on the mediating processes. In terms of neurodevelopment, this includes the sequelae of neurochemical alterations. Chronic alteration in noradrenergic, serotonergic, and glucocorticoid systems are found in many traumatized persons years after the trauma (Southwick et al., 1992). These changes place individuals with PTSD at increased risk for ongoing symptoms of anxiety, depression, and impulsive violence. Physical symptoms such as chronic pelvic pain are also more common in people with PTSD symptoms and may be related to the lack of protective properties of cortisol (Heim et al., 1998).

The sociocultural container may protect against the negative outcome from trauma. It may do this by providing an acceptable way to process the traumatic event so that numbness or dissociation do not need to be used as the primary defensive mechanism. For example, a 12-year-old Navajo girl became psychotic after the trauma of "accidentally" shooting her baby sister when she was repeatedly left alone to baby-sit for her. A cleansing ritual by the tribe's elders (which involved the family and the tribe) resulted in relief of her guilt and the subsequent disappearance of her psychotic symptoms.

CLINICAL IMPLICATIONS OF THE
NEUROBIOLOGY OF STRESS

Assessment of Trauma in an Adolescent

The age of the adolescent at the time of the trauma can affect the presentation of symptoms and the likelihood of the development of PTSD (Perrin, Smith, and Yule, 2000). Unlike younger children, adolescents are more likely to depend on their own and their peers' appraisal of traumatic events. Rather than focusing on escape and protection from the trauma, adolescents are more likely to struggle with their own decision making about what interventions might have altered the event's outcome (Pynoos et al., 1999). Just as at any point in childhood, trauma during adolescence may disrupt the developmental trajectory of the child, and regression to earlier developmental stages may occur.

Previous traumatic experience may increase the individual's likelihood of experiencing subsequent episodes of trauma (Bremner et al., 1993). Depending on the timing, quality, duration, and degree of repetition, traumatic exposure can be associated with lifelong increases in stress-related hormones and peptides, as well as susceptibility to drug and alcohol abuse and learning and memory problems (Post et al., 2001). Trauma also increases the likelihood of anxiety disorders (Heim and Nemeroff, 2001), major depressive disorder (Kaufman and Charney, 2001) and bipolar disorder (Post et al., 2001). Consequently, careful attention to comorbid conditions is warranted.

As noted earlier, dissociative behaviors should be considered within a developmental context. In early childhood, dissociative symptoms following traumatic exposure may represent efforts at resolution through fantasy play (Egeland and Susman-Stillman, 1996), whereas these symptoms in adolescence and young adulthood are more likely to correspond to psychopathology (Ogawa et al., 1997).

A thorough family history is warranted because coexisting parental psychopathology, especially depression and anxiety, may increase the likelihood of the development of PTSD in the child exposed to trauma (Davidson and Smith, 1990). An assessment of parental responsiveness to the adolescent is important, including evaluation of prior trauma and loss in the parent and ongoing parental anxiety and reactivity (Pynoos et al., 1999). It has also been noted that parental reactions to the traumatic event can influence and predict a child's reaction to the trauma. For example, if the child's parents are extremely distressed after a traumatic event, the child may be more likely to develop PTSD (Green, Korol, and Grace, 1991).

The developmental history should include a sociocultural history to assess the extent of support and protection that may be offered. Other factors that should be assessed in order to enhance adaptation and identify increased risk in the adolescent include school history, coping style, problem-solving ability, peer relationships, and the availability of a positive relationship with a competent adult (Masten, Best, and Garmezy, 1990; Pynoos et al., 1999).

Treatment of Trauma Exposure in an Adolescent

Some or many of the neurobiological consequences of early life stress appear to be reversible (Heim and Nemeroff, 2001). In dealing with traumatized adolescents, it is important to consider what part of the brain and what neuromodulator is mediating the affective and behavioral symptoms. The higher-level, thinking cortex may be dissociated from deeper structures in the midbrain and brain stem that regulate the physiological response to stress. Supportive therapy can help the traumatized child tell his or her story through expressive or verbal therapies that lead to an integration of these higher and deeper response centers to build healthier mental images (Perry and Pate, 1996). Categorization at a symbolic level through the use of words and symbols may help extinguish conditioned neurobiological responses. Redirecting memory circuits to alternate pathways through active coping rather than passive fear helps develop successful coping circuits (LeDoux and Gorman, 2001). One example of these therapeutic strategies is successful group psychotherapy for adolescents with PTSD, which incorporates positive coping skills and the integration of traumatic experiences through narrative exposure therapy and cognitive restructuring (Saltzman et al., 2001). Given the important role of early and ongoing caretaker relationships in vulnerability to or exacerbation of traumatic stress symptoms in adolescents, family-based treatment modalities should also be considered, particularly when both parent and adolescent have experienced traumatic exposure and subsequent functional impairment.

Traumatized children and adults may exhibit increased sensitivity to traumatic reminders and may display deficits in their ability to express specific emotions. Cognitive models for understanding stress responses indicate that the highly charged emotional context of traumatic experiences, as well as the relative isolation of these memories from nontraumatic ones, results in the triggering of traumatic memories by reminders. These traumatic memories display stimulus-response associations strong enough to involuntarily disrupt an individual's attention and behavior (Ehlers and Clark, 2000; Fearon and Mansell, 2001). The individual's inability to use cognitive strategies to delay affective reactions to such stimuli has been linked to impulse-control problems, including high-risk behaviors such as substance abuse and risky sexual behaviors, during adolescence (Fish-Murray, Koby, and van der Kolk, 1987). Both psychotherapy and serotonergic medications have been found to decrease the predominance of traumatic perceptions and to enhance cognitive strategies for coping with traumatic reminders (van der Kolk and Fisler, 1994).

Treatment with psychotropic medication can be useful in ameliorating both core and secondary symptoms and may be useful in both primary and secondary prevention (van der Kolk, 2001). It is important to consider the nature of the trauma and the mediators of the expression of its primary effects. It has been suggested that effective treatment may actually help regenerate noradrenergic and serotonergic axons (Duman, 2002). Certain brain areas such as the hippocampus are particularly plastic, and reversal of atrophy is possible (Malberg et al., 2000; McEwen and Magarinos, 2001). The most common psychotropic treatment options include antidepressants, anxiolytics, alpha-adrenergic-receptor partial agonists such as clonidine, and mood stabilizers (Donnelly, Amaya-Jackson, and March, 1999).

Studies that demonstrate that individuals with PTSD have alterations in either norepinephrine or serotonin levels suggest different medication strategies. Patients with increased norepinephrine levels may respond preferentially to medications such as alpha-adrenergic blocking agents like clonidine or propranolol and may respond poorly to antidepressants that increase norepinephrine. Patients with low serotonin levels may be likely to respond preferentially to SSRI medications (Southwick et al., 1997). These intriguing possibilities have yet to be tested clinically in the treatment of PTSD.

High levels of dopamine and norepinephrine are released in the prefrontal cortex during stress exposure and can impair working memory functions. Agents that block catecholamine receptors or prevent catecholamine release such as alpha2-adrenergic agonists (clonidine and guanfacine) or dopamine D1 blockers may improve these prefrontal cortex deficits. Animal research suggests that stress-induced cognitive deficits could be prevented by pretreatment with low doses of neuroleptics or alpha2-adrenergic agonists (Arnsten, 1999). De Bellis (2001) reports that treatment with clonidine of a youth with PTSD resulted in symptom remission and indications of neuronal growth.

Selective serotonin reuptake inhibitors (SSRIs) have shown short- and long-term benefits in treating adults with PTSD. Treatment of PTSD with paroxetine demonstrated significant improvement in primary outcome measures compared to controls (Marshall et al., 2001).

Continued treatment with sertraline lowered PTSD relapse rates over six fold (Davidson et al., 2001).

Anticonvulsant medications have been shown to be efficacious in adults with PTSD (Lipper et al., 1986; Hertzberg et al., 1999). There is some suggestion that they may decrease the kindling response in the limbic system and thus decrease the likelihood of future episodes (Fesler, 1991).

Finally, since disturbance in regulation of the CRF system is impli- cated in both major depression and PTSD, both of which are related to early life stress, selective CRF-receptor antagonists or psychotherapy at the time of the stress may prevent longer-term consequences (Heim et al., 1997a).

IMPLICATIONS FOR A NEUROBIOLOGIC RESEARCH AGENDA

Clearly further understanding of the neurobiology of the effects of trauma holds great promise for early intervention, outcome improve- ment, and prevention. A few of the possible areas for further re- search include:

1. Identification of neurobiological factors related to good and poor outcomes
2. Use of a neurobiological assessment to introduce protective interventions early
3. Determination of neurobiological subtypes and matching of these to treatment interventions
4. Determination of the developmental mediators that suggest risk or provide resiliency in the neurobiological impact of trauma.

REFERENCES

Allen, J. P., Hauser, S. T. & Borman-Spurrell, E. (1996), Attachment theory as a framework for understanding sequelae of severe adoles- cent psychopathology: An 11-year follow-up study. *J. Consult. Clin. Psychol.,* 64:254–263.

Anderson, C. M., Teicher, M. H., Polcari, A. & Renshaw, P. F. (2002), Abnormal T2 relaxation time in the cerebellar vermis of adults sexually abused in childhood: Potential role of the vermis in stress-enhanced risk for drug abuse. *Psychoneuroendocrinology,* 27:231–244.

Arnsten, A. F. T. (1999), Development of the cerebral cortex: XIV. Stress impairs prefrontal cortical function. *J. Amer. Acad. Child & Adol. Psychiat.,* 38:220–222.

Barch, D. M. (1999), Images in neuroscience. Cognition: The anterior cingulate and response conflict. *Amer. J. Psychiat.,* 156:1849.

Bremner, J. D. & Narayan, M. (1998), The effects of stress on memory and the hippocampus throughout the life cycle: Implications for childhood development and aging. *Dev. Psychopathol.,* 10:871–885.

——— Randall, P., Scott, T. M., Capelli, S., Delaney, R., McCarthy, G. & Charney, D. S. (1995), MRI-based measurement of hippocampal volume in patients with combat-related posttraumatic stress disorder. *Amer. J. Psychiat.,* 152:973–981.

——— Southwick, S. M., Johnson, D. R., Yehuda, R. & Charney, D. S. (1993), Childhood physical abuse and combat-related posttraumatic stress disorder in Vietnam veterans. *Amer. J. Psychiat.,* 150:235–239.

——— & Vermetten, E. (2001), Stress and development: Behavioral and biological consequences. *Dev. Psychopathol.,* 13:473–489.

Cabib, S. & Puglisi-Allegra, S. (1994), Opposite responses of mesolimbic dopamine system to controllable and uncontrollable aversive experiences. *J. Neurosci.,* 14: 3333–3340.

——— ——— & D'Amato, F. R. (1993), Effects of postnatal stress on dopamine mesolimbic system responses to aversive experiences in adult life. *Brain Res.,* 604:232–239.

Carlson, V., Cicchetti, D., Barnett, D. & Braunwald, K. (1989), Disorganized/disoriented attachment relationships in maltreated infants. *Dev. Psychology,* 25:525–531.

Casey, B. J., Giedd, J. N. & Thomas, K. M. (2000), Structural and functional brain development and its relation to cognitive development. *Biol. Psychol.,* 54:241–257.

Chu, J. A. & Dill, D. L. (1990), Dissociative symptoms in relation to childhood physical and sexual abuse. *Amer. J. Psychiat.,* 147:887–892.

Cicchetti, D. & Rogosch, F. A. (2001), Diverse patterns of neuroendocrine activity in maltreated children. *Dev. Psychopathol.,* 13:677–693.

276

Davidson, J., Pearlstein, T., Londborg, P., Brady, K. T., Rothbaum, B., Bell, J., Maddock, R., Hegel, M. T. & Farfel, G. (2001), Efficacy of sertraline in preventing relapse of posttraumatic stress disorder: Results of a 28-week double-blind, placebo-controlled study. *Amer. J. Psychiat.,* 158:1974–1981.

———— & Smith, R. (1990), Traumatic experiences in psychiatric outpatients. *J. Traumatic Stress Studies,* 3:459–475.

De Bellis, M. D. (2001), Developmental traumatology: The psychobiological development of maltreated children and its implications for research, treatment, and policy. *Dev. Psychopathol.,* 13:539–564.

———— Baum, A. S., Birmaher, B., Keshavan, M. S., Eccard, C. H., Boring, A. M., Jenkins, F. J. & Ryan, N. D. (1999), A. E. Bennett Research Award. Developmental traumatology part I: Biological stress systems. *Biol. Psychiat.,* 45:1259–1270.

Donnelly, C. L., Amaya-Jackson, L. & March, J. S. (1999), Psychopharmacology of pediatric posttraumatic stress disorder. *J. Child. & Adol. Psychopharm.,* 9:203–220.

Duman, R. S. (2002), Genetics of childhood disorders: XXXIX. Stem cell research, part 3: Regulation of neurogenesis by stress and antidepressant treatment. *J. Amer. Acad. Child & Adol. Psychiat.,* 41:745–748.

———— & Charney, D. S. (1999), Cell atrophy in major depression. *Biol. Psychiat.,* 45:1083–1084.

Egeland, B. & Susman-Stillman, A. (1996), Dissociation as a mediator of child abuse across generations. *Child Abuse Negl.,* 20:1123–1132.

Ehlers, A. & Clark, D. M. (2000), A cognitive model of posttraumatic stress disorder. *Behav. Res. Ther.,* 38:319–345.

Fearon, R. M. P. & Mansell, W. (2001), Cognitive perspectives on unresolved loss: Insights from the study of PTSD. *Bull. Menn. Clin.,* 65:380–397.

Fesler, F. A. (1991), Valproate in combat-related post-traumatic stress disorder. *J. Clin. Psychiat.,* 52:361–364.

Fish-Murray, C. C., Koby, E. V. & van der Kolk, B. A. (1987), Evolving ideas: The effect of abuse on children's thought. In: *Psychological Trauma,* ed. B. A. van der Kolk. Washington, DC: American Psychiatric Press, pp. 89–110.

Gerson, S. C. & Baldessarini, R. J. (1980), Motor effects of serotonin in the central nervous system. *Life Sci.,* 27:1435–1451.

Goenjian, A. K., Yehuda, R., Pynoos, R. S., Steinberg, A. M., Tashjian, M., Yang, R. K., Najarian, L. M. & Fairbanks, L. A. (1996), Basal cortisol, dexamethasone suppression of cortisol, and MHPG in adolescents after the 1988 earthquake in Armenia. *Amer. J. Psychiat.,* 153:929–934.

Golier, J. & Yehuda, R. (1998), Neuroendocrine activity and memory-related impairments in posttraumatic stress disorder. *Dev. Psychopathol.,* 10:857–869.

Green, B., Korol, M. & Grace, M. (1991), Children and disaster: Age, gender, and parental effects on PTSD symptoms. *J. Amer. Acad. Child & Adol. Psychiat.,* 30:945–951.

Griffin, M. G., Resick, P. A. & Mechanic, M. B. (1997), Objective assessment of peritraumatic dissociation: Psychophysiological indicators. *Amer. J. Psychiat.,* 154:1081–1088.

Grillon, C., Southwick, S. M. & Charney, D. S. (1996), The psychobiological basis of posttraumatic stress disorder. *Mol. Psychiat.,* 1:278–297.

Gunnar, M. (1998), Quality of early care and buffering of neuroendocrine stress reactions: Potential effects on the developing human brain. *Prevent. Med.,* 27:208–211.

———— & Gilles, E. (2002), Disturbed daytime cortisol rhythms may reflect adverse factors in the young child's environment. Presented at the International Conference for Infant Studies, Toronto, Canada.

Gurvits, T. V., Shenton, M. E., Hokama, H., Ohta, H., Lasko, N. B., Gilbertson, M. W., Orr, S. P., Kikinis, R., Jolesz, F. A., McCarley, R. W. & Pitman, R. K. (1996), Magnetic resonance imaging study of hippocampal volume in chronic, combat-related posttraumatic stress disorder. *Biol. Psychiat.,* 40:1091–1099.

Hart, J., Gunnar, M. & Cicchetti, D. (1995), Salivary cortisol in maltreated children: Evidence of relations between neuroendocrine activity and social competence. *Dev. Psychopath.,* 7:11–26.

Heim, C., Ehlert, U., Hanaker, J. P. & Hellhammer, D. H. (1998), Abuse-related posttraumatic stress disorder and alterations of the hypothalamic-pituitary-adrenal axis in women with chronic pelvic pain. *Psychosom. Med.,* 60:309–318.

———— & Nemeroff, C. B. (2001), The role of childhood trauma in the neurobiology of mood and anxiety disorders: Preclinical and clinical studies. *Biol. Psychiat.,* 49:1023–1039.

———— Owens, M. J., Plotsky, P. M. & Nemeroff, C. B. (1997a), Persistent changes in corticotropin-releasing factor systems due to early life stress: Relationship to the pathophysiology of major depression and post-traumatic stress disorder. *Psychopharmacol. Bull.*, 33:185–192.

——— ——— ——— ——— (1997b), The role of early adverse life events in the etiology of depression and posttraumatic stress disorder. Focus on corticotropin-releasing factor. *Ann. N.Y. Acad. Sci.*, 821:194–207.

Heresco-Levy, U. & Javitt, D. C. (1998), The role of N-methyl-D-aspartate (NMDA) receptor-mediated neurotransmission in the pathophysiology and therapeutics of psychiatric syndromes. *Eur. Neuropsychopharmacol.*, 8:141–152.

Hertzberg, M. A., Butterfield, M. I., Feldman, M. E., Beckham, J. C., Sutherland, S. M., Connor, K. M. & Davidson, J. R. (1999), A preliminary study of lamotrigine for the treatment of posttraumatic stress disorder. *Biol. Psychiat.*, 45:1226–1229.

Hesse, E. & Main, M. (2000), Disorganized infant, child and adult attachment: Collapse in behavioral and attentional strategies. *J. Amer. Psychoanal. Assn.*, 48:1055–1096.

Kaufman, J. & Charney, D. (2001), Effects of early stress on brain structure and function: Implications for understanding the relationship between child maltreatment and depression. *Dev. Psychopathol.*, 13:451–471.

LeDoux, J. E. & Gorman, J. M. (2001), A call to action: Overcoming anxiety through active coping. *Amer. J. Psychiat.*, 158:1953–1955.

Lipper, S., Davidson, J. R., Grady, T. A., Edinger, J. D., Hammett, E. B., Mahorney, S. L. & Cavenar, J. O. Jr. (1986), Preliminary study of carbamazepine in post-traumatic stress disorder. *Psychosom.*, 27:849–854.

Lombroso, P. J. & Sapolsky, R. (1998), Development of the cerebral cortex: XII. Stress and brain development. *J. Amer. Acad. Child & Adol. Psychiat.*, 37:1337–1339.

Malberg, J. E., Eisch, A. J., Nestler, E. J. & Duman, R. S. (2000), Chronic antidepressant treatment increases in adult rat hippocampus. *J. Neuroscience*, 20:9104–9110.

Marshall, R. D., Beebe, K. L., Oldham, M. & Zaninelli, R. (2001), Efficacy and safety of paroxetine treatment for chronic PTSD: A fixed-dose, placebo-controlled study. *Amer. J. Psychiat.*, 158:1982–1988.

Masten, A., Best, K. & Garmezy, N. (1990), Resilience and development: Contribution from the study of children who overcome adversity. *Dev. Psychopathol.*, 2:425–444.

McEwen, B. S. & Magarinos, A. M. (2001), Stress and hippocampal plasticity: Implications for the pathophysiology of affective disorders. *Hum. Psychopharmacol.,* S1:S7–S19.

——— & Sapolsky, R. M. (1995), Stress and cognitive function. *Curr. Opinions in Neurobio.,* 5:205–216.

Morgan, C. A., Grillon, C., Lubin, H. & Southwick, S. M. (1997), Startle reflex abnormalities in women with sexual assault-related posttraumatic stress disorder. *Amer. J. Psychiat.,* 154:1076–1080.

Nachmias, M., Gunnar, M., Mangelsdorf, S., Parritz, R. & Buss, K. (1996), Behavioral inhibition and stress reactivity: The moderating role of attachment security. *Child Dev.,* 67:508–522.

Ogawa, J. R., Sroufe, L. A., Weinfield, N. S., Carlson, E. & Egeland, B. (1997), Development and the fragmented self: Longitudinal study of dissociative symptomatology in a nonclinical sample. *Dev. Psychopathol.,* 9:855–879.

Orchinik, M., Carroll, S. S., Li, Y. H., McEwen, B. S. & Weiland, N. G. (2001), Heterogeneity of hippocampal GABA(A) receptors: Regulation by corticosterone. *J. Neuroscience,* 21:330–339.

Perrin, S., Smith, P. & Yule, W. (2000), The assessment and treatment of post-traumatic stress disorder in children and adolescents. *J. Child Psychol. Psychiat.,* 41:27–89.

Perry, B. D. & Pate, J. E. (1996), Neurodevelopment and the psychobiological roots of post-traumatic stress disorder. In: *The Neuropsychology of Mental Disorders,* ed. L. F. Koziol & E. S. Chris. Springfield, IL: Charles C. Thomas, pp. 129–146.

Post, R. M., Leverich, G. S., Xing, G. & Weiss, D. B. (2001), Developmental vulnerabilities to the onset and course of bipolar disorder. *Dev. Psychopathol.,* 13:581–598.

Pynoos, R. S., Steinberg, A. M., Ornitz, E. M. & Goenjian, A. K. (1997), Issues in the developmental neurobiology of traumatic stress. *Ann. N.Y. Acad. Sci.,* 821:176–193.

——— ——— & Piacentini, J. C. (1999), A developmental psychopathology model of childhood trauma stress and intersection with anxiety disorders. *Biol. Psychiat.,* 46:1542–1554.

Rauch, S. L. & Shin, L. M. (1997), Functional neuroimaging studies in posttraumatic stress disorder. *Ann. N.Y. Acad. Sci.,* 821:83–98.

Saltzman, W. R., Pynoos, R. S., Layne, C. M., Steinberg, A. M. & Aisenberg, E. (2001), Trauma- and grief-focused intervention for adolescents exposed to community violence: Results of a school-based screening and group treatment protocol. *Group Dynamics: Theory, Res. Prac.,* 5:291–303.

Schmahmann, J. D. (1991), An emerging concept: The cerebellar contribution to higher function. *Arch. Neurol.,* 48:1178–1187.

———— & Sherman, J. C. (1998), The cerebellar cognitive affective syndrome. *Brain,* 121:561–579.

Schwartz, E. D. & Perry, B. D. (1994), The post-traumatic response in children and adolescents. In: *Psychiatric Clinics of North America.* Philadelphia: W. B. Saunders, pp. 311–326.

Seeman, T. E., McEwen, B. S., Singer, B. H., Albert, M. S. & Rowe, J. W. (1997), Increase in urinary cortisol excretion and memory declines: McArthur studies of successful aging. *J. Clin. Endocrin. Metab.,* 82:2458–2465.

Shin, L. M., Whalen, P. J., Pitman, R. K., Bush, G., Macklin, M. L., Lasko, N. B., Orr, S. P., McInerney, S. C. & Rauch, S. L. (2001), An fMRI study of anterior cingulate function in posttraumatic stress disorder. *Biol. Psychiat.,* 50:932–942.

Southwick, S. M., Krystal, J. H., Bremner, J. D., Morgan, C. A. III, Nicolaou, A. L., Nagy, L. M., Johnson, D. R., Heninger, G. R. & Charney, D. S. (1997), Noradrenergic and serotonergic function in posttraumatic stress disorder. *Arch. Gen. Psychiat.,* 54:749–758.

———— ———— Johnson, D. R. & Charney, D. S. (1992), Neurobiology of posttraumatic stress disorder. In: *Review of Psychiatry,* ed. A. Tasman & M. G. Riba. Washington, DC: American Psychiatric Press, pp. 347–370.

Spangler, G. & Grossmann, K. (1993), Biobehavioral organization in securely and insecurely attached infants. *Child Dev.,* 64:1439–1450.

———— & ———— (1999), Individual and physiological correlates of attachment disorganization in infancy. In: *Attachment Disorganization,* ed. J. Solomon & C. George. New York: Guilford Press, pp. 95–124.

Stein, M. B., Koverola, C., Hanna, C., Torchia, M. G. & McClarty, B. (1997), Hippocampal volume in women victimized by childhood sexual abuse. *Psychol. Med.,* 27:951–959.

———— Walker, J. R. & Forde, D. R. (2000), Gender differences in susceptibility to posttraumatic stress disorder. *Behav. Res. Ther.,* 38:619–628.

Terr, L. (1991), Childhood traumas: An outline and overview. *Amer. J. Psychiat.,* 148:10–20.

van der Kolk, B. A. (1994), The body keeps the score: Memory and the evolving psychobiology of posttraumatic stress. *Harv. Rev. Psychiat.*, 1:253–265.

―――― (1997), The psychobiology of posttraumatic stress disorder. *J. Clin. Psychiat.*, 58:16–24.

―――― (2001), The psychobiology and psychopharmacology of PTSD. *Hum. Psychopharmacol. Clin. Experim.*, 16:S49–S64.

―――― & Fisler, R. E. (1994), Childhood abuse and neglect and loss of self-regulation. *Bull. Menn. Clin.*, 58:145–160.

Waldinger, R. J., Swett, C., Frank, A. & Miller, K. (1994), Levels of dissociation and histories of reported abuse among women outpatients. *J. Nerv. Mental Dis.*, 182:625–630.

Yehuda, R. (2001), Biology of posttraumatic stress disorder. *J. Clin. Psychiat.*, 62S:41–46.

―――― Giller, E., Southwick, S., Lowy, M. & Mason, J. (1991), Hypothalamic-pituitary-adrenal dysfunction in post-traumatic stress disorder. *Biolog. Psychiat.*, 30:1031–1048.

―――― Halligan, S. L. & Bierer, L. M. (2002), Cortisol levels in adult offspring of Holocaust survivors: Relation to PTSD symptom severity in the parent and child. *Psychoneuroendocrinology*, 27:171–180.

―――― Kahana, B., Binder-Brynes, K., Southwick S., Mason, J. & Giller, E. (1995), Low urinary cortisol excretion in Holocaust survivors with post-traumatic stress disorder. *Amer. J. Psychiat.*, 152:982–986.

―――― Southwick, S., Giller, E. L., Ma, X. & Mason, J. W. (1992), Urinary catecholamine excretion and severity of PTSD symptoms in Vietnam combat veterans. *J. Nerv. Ment. Dis.*, 180:321–325.

―――― Teicher, M. H., Trestman, R. L., Levengood, R. A. & Siever, L. J. (1996), Cortisol regulation in posttraumatic stress disorder and major depression: A chronobiological analysis. *Biol. Psychiat.*, 40:79–88.

Zlotnick, C., Shea, M. T., Zakriski, A., Costello, E., Begin A., Pearlstein T. & Simpson, E. (1996), Stressors and close relationships during childhood and dissociative experiences in survivors of sexual abuse among inpatient psychiatric women. *Comp. Psychiat.*, 36:207–212.

Zola-Morgan, S. M. & Squire, L. R. (1990), The primate hippocampal formation: Evidence for a time-limited role in memory storage. *Science*, 250:288–290.

11   INTERVENTIONS WITH TRAUMATIZED ADOLESCENTS

MONICA R. GREEN

Other chapters in this special section discuss the nature and prevalence of trauma in adolescence, the cultural and gender aspects of trauma, the neurobiological changes associated with trauma, and the potential pathological sequelae of trauma. This chapter considers the interventions intended to mitigate the effects of trauma. While much work has been done to validate treatments for the sequelae of psychic trauma in adults, to date there are no well-controlled studies that demonstrate completely adequate treatment of the disorder or alleviation of its symptomatology in adolescents. However, given the importance of trauma in the pathogenesis of adolescent psychopathology, a consideration of the available treatments is clinically imperative, because any significant reduction in the extent of pain and suffering is an essential goal.

A related consideration is which forms of sequelae of traumatic stress necessitate intervention. As discussed in the chapter on the impact of trauma (GAP, this volume), most people who experience trauma do not develop PTSD; many experience only transient symptoms, and others develop other kinds of psychopathology. Those whose symptoms are mild or transient obviously do not need treatment, and those who develop other kinds of disorders will need treatment specific to their symptomatology. This chapter will focus specifically on treatment for those who suffer from acute stress reactions and posttraumatic stress disorder (PTSD).

A primary consideration is that of level of intervention. As mentioned previously in the neurobiological section of this work, treatment can occur at the primary, secondary, or tertiary prevention levels. Primary prevention is a method of treatment (such as vaccination in the case

283

of communicable diseases) that involves activities and education to promote health as well as prevent disease. In the case of exposure to trauma, this occurs when we decrease the number of traumatic events. Examples of this is the removal of guns from neighborhoods through buy-back programs, school-based violence-prevention and conflict-resolution programs, public education regarding the adverse effects of physical abuse, and easily accessed mental health services to aid in parenting skills, anger management, and so on. Another example would be the institution of no-tolerance policies in the school systems, which ostensibly prevent violence (at least that involving lethal weapons) in the school setting.

Secondary prevention uses early diagnosis and rapid initiation of appropriate treatment to decrease the severity or progression of a disease after exposure to the disease has occurred. The *DSM-IV-TR* criteria for PTSD include the experience of "intense fear, helplessness, or horror," as well as "clinically significant distress or impairment in social, occupational, or other important areas of functioning" (American Psychiatric Association, 2000, pp. 467–468). As we have seen, not all individuals who live through the same trauma experience it or respond to it in the same way. The responses to trauma Type I and Type II (that is, a single traumatic event vs. a chronic traumatic stressor) may vary significantly. Also, youngsters who fail to meet the full criteria for PTSD may be sufficiently impaired or distressed to warrant intervention. Just as important, some symptoms of trauma may not present as subthreshold PTSD but instead may manifest in entirely different ways, such as aggression or disorganization. This is especially true in adolescents, whose progression through stages of development may change the phenomenology of trauma-related symptoms (i.e., symptoms may appear as regression or lost developmental milestones). Though many individuals may be exposed to the same event, the clinical outcome differs from person to person, depending on resiliency and vulnerability factors such as personal history, biological determinants, and temperament. In time, however, we may discover that specific interventions immediately after the trauma are effective in decreasing the overall rate of development of posttraumatic symptoms and determine that it is appropriate to institute these well before symptoms develop.

In the case of exposure to trauma, secondary prevention involves immediate interventions to mitigate adverse consequences when the exposure to a traumatic event has occurred. An example of this is a program established in the school setting to allow adolescents to discuss a school shooting or the violent death of a peer. Other examples are rape-intervention services such as those established by Foa and colleagues (Foa et al., 1991; Foa, Hearst-Ikeda, and Perry, 1995).

Tertiary prevention is the establishment of rehabilitation and optimization of the patient's functioning after a debilitating disease process has occurred. In the case of exposure to trauma, this involves the optimal treatment (and, therefore, best minimization of symptoms) of well-established clinical sequelae of trauma. Although certainly not the place we as clinicians would like to begin, it is most often this level of prevention at which we find ourselves when the patient presents for treatment.

PSYCHOTHERAPEUTIC INTERVENTIONS

Although challenged by the inroads of managed care, increased patient loads, and the demands for vigorous demonstration of efficacy, the individual therapies have historically been the mainstay of psychotherapeutic intervention. Numerous modalities are encompassed under this category, however, and many discussions of the psychotherapeutic treatment of traumatic sequelae do not distinguish between psychotherapeutic modalities. The main distinction apparent in reviewing the literature is that between cognitive-behavioral treatments and the supportive-psychodynamic psychotherapies. Perhaps this distinction stems from the limited number of rigorous research studies looking at levels of efficacy of the non-cognitive-behavioral individual therapies.

Cognitive-Behavioral Therapies

Evidence for the efficacy of cognitive-behavioral therapies in the treatment of traumatized individuals is fair for adults but less well established for children and adolescents. As early as 1990, positive responses (i.e., decreased symptomatology in all PTSD subcategories) to cognitive-behavioral treatment were observed in sexually abused children (Deblinger, McLeer, and Henry, 1990). Cognitive distortions and misperceptions—the focus of CBT programs—are very common as posttraumatic sequelae (Gillis, 1993). These include inability to realistically assess safety cues (e.g., severe anxiety occurring in a grocery store parking lot in daytime hours, although the assault occurred at night in a deserted lot) and approaching dangerous situations with an apparent abandon suggesting desensitization (e.g., a group of children who continue to play despite a shooting in their playground). The effectiveness of cognitive-behavioral interventions in addressing such cognitive distortions in other psychiatric disorders such as depression is well documented. Perhaps in light of this well-known information, exposure therapy and cognitive therapy were named as two of the three most useful modalities of treatment in the Expert Consensus Guidelines for the treatment of PTSD (Foa, Davidson, and Frances, 1999), with anxiety management listed as the third, as noted in the following section.

Prolonged exposure therapy.   This kind of treatment forces a confrontation with fear-arousing situations and stimuli associated with the trauma. Also known as systematic desensitization, prolonged exposure treatment consists of having the patient tape a narrative of the traumatic experience and listening repetitively to this audiotape at home. (It is analogous to the technique used to treat phobias by forcing a confrontation with feared objects or situations.) The Expert Consensus Guidelines recommend exposure therapy as the first-line technique for treatment of intrusive thoughts, flashbacks, trauma-related fears, panic, and avoidance (Foa et al., 1999). Prolonged exposure treatment, in fact, has been demonstrated to be an effective and durable treatment modality for posttraumatic symptoms (Foa, 1997). Some authors have recommended systematic gradual exposure to upsetting features of the traumatic event in a progressively intensifying fashion (March et al., 1998).

Exposure appears to dissociate the classically conditioned responses from their stimuli (i.e., anxiety and the traumatic experience), as well as disrupting the operant-conditioned avoidance of trauma-related stimuli (Deblinger et al., 1990). This may occur through the repetitive involvement (and therefore, development of more rapid processing time) of corticothalamic tracts that may then supercede the emotive amygdalo-thalamic tracts. In other words, one learns to process the traumatic event in a narrative fashion, developing a context for it, and thereby is better able to consciously manage the emotions that accompany its recovery. Foa et al. (1991) observed that women who received prolonged exposure treatment maintained improvement in symptoms for six months beyond termination of the therapy.

It is important to note, however, that many persons with posttraumatic symptoms are unable to tolerate reliving the experience in exposure therapy, and as many as 50% may be noncompliant, dropping out of treatment (Scott and Stradling, 1997). This statistic is of especial concern when dealing with adolescents, whose compliance with any type of homework will not be easily achieved, much less with an aversive assignment. Certainly, the appropriate use of psychoeducation (see discussion later in this chapter) may increase compliance, as the need for exposure with response prevention may be understood by the adolescent. Parental involvement in cognitive-behavioral treatments for children with anxiety disorders may enhance effects of treatment as well as extend recovery (Mendlowitz et al., 1999). This is not necessarily true for adolescents, who are involved in separating and individuating from their parents.

Anxiety management. Often included under the rubric of cognitive-behavioral therapies is the category of anxiety management (also termed stress inoculation training), which is one of the three most highly recommended psychotherapeutic techniques in the Expert Consensus Guidelines for the treatment of PTSD (Foa et al., 1999). This form of treatment, which encompasses deep breathing techniques and muscle relaxation, was recommended for use specifically with symptoms of sleep disturbance, difficulty concentrating, irritability/anger outbursts, and trauma-related fears, panic, and avoidance. Multiple authors have suggested that anxiety management techniques are effective in the treatment of children and adolescents with posttraumatic sequelae (Terr, 1989; Deblinger et al., 1990; March et al., 1998). The American Academy of Child and Adolescent Psychiatry (AACAP, 1998) Practice Parameters regarding the treatment of PTSD in children and adolescents suggest that "[m]astering these [anxiety management] skills gives the child as sense of control over thoughts and feelings rather than feeling overwhelmed by them" (p. 17S). Foa (1997), writing about adult women who were victims of assault, noted that anxiety management was noted to be effective in the treatment of posttraumatic symptoms. However, although this kind of treatment produced more immediate improvement in victims of rape, prolonged exposure appeared to be the most effective treatment in the long term (Foa et al., 1991). It is unclear to what extent these findings can be applied to adolescents or to other types of trauma.

Supportive-Psychodynamic Therapies

Under the rubric of supportive-psychodynamic psychotherapies are all non-cognitive-behavioral therapies (i.e., interpersonal, psychoanalytic,

287

object relations, self psychology, play therapy, etc.). Although supportive-psychodynamic psychotherapies are mentioned in the literature, the empirical study of this type of technique is plagued by a lack of standardization or specification, unlike cognitive-behavioral therapy, which has a reproducible set of guidelines to be followed by each therapist. Goenjian et al. (1997) demonstrated that the beneficial effects of brief psychotherapy with early adolescents (with decreased symptoms of intrusion, avoidance, and arousal) were sustained up to one and one-half to three years after a natural disaster. Perhaps as a result of the lack of empirical clinical trials, the Expert Consensus Guidelines mention only play therapy as a preferred (yet still secondary) form of therapy in the supportive-psychodynamic psychotherapy category (Foa et al., 1999). In fact, most of the specific guidelines given for the use of these techniques refer to play therapy (Gillis, 1993). Interpretations during play are encouraged by some but considered unnecessary by others (Terr, 1989). Therapeutic interventions that encourage mastery, with movement toward recovery, are encouraged (Pynoos and Nader, 1993). However, play therapy is not a treatment modality suited to the treatment of most adolescents, except perhaps those who are developmentally delayed, regressed, or nonverbal.

Anecdotally, the members of the GAP Committee on Adolescence, in their discussions of trauma and adolescence that led to the production of this special section, cited many successful treatments using both supportive and psychodynamic psychotherapies. Individual therapy is able to more completely and individually address the meaning of trauma in adolescents. In exploratory therapy, the child or adolescent is better able to focus on and process the terrifyingly uncontrollable nature of trauma. This theme is particularly salient during the adolescent period, shattering the defenses of omnipotence and immortality frequently used during these years. This is accomplished by developing a context—a narrative of sorts—into which the inexplicable trauma can be integrated. The theme of reestablishing an internal locus of control figured prominently into these discussions. One cited case was that of a five-year-old girl who was injured in the cross fire of a gang drive-by shooting. In this case, the child's trauma centered largely on blaming herself for not ducking when the situation became violent. Therapy centered largely on processing this blame while reestablishing the internal locus of control by practicing ducking to avoid such dangers. Such cases illustrate the benefits of individual psychotherapy, where the specific characteristics of the patient's trauma can be elucidated, elaborated, and explored in the most complete fashion. Such cases also illustrate that the individual psychotherapies do not use only one type of psychotherapy, incorporating psychodynamic as well as cognitive behavioral and supportive elements.

A related form of nonverbal expression in therapy is found in art therapy, which Terr has used for many years in her treatment of traumatized children (Terr, 1989). This form of therapy can be useful in the treatment of adolescents and adults as well, allowing for expression less hindered by our well-trained verbal defenses. Alternative modes that use similar forms of processing trauma include Lowenstein's resolution scrapbook, akin to the birth history scrapbooks used with adopted children, with the child reconstructing and working through the trauma via development of a pictorial narrative (Lowenstein, 1995). Psychoeducation, another form of psychotherapeutic intervention, may be used in individual treatment. This modality will be discussed subsequently.

Group Psychotherapy

The treatment of posttraumatic symptoms through group therapy is often employed when a large group has been exposed to a common traumatic stressor, such as a natural disaster or school shooting. (This is reminiscent of the tribal interventions discussed in the chapter on cultural issues—see Gadpaille, this volume.) Group therapy allows large numbers of individuals to be reached when such a trauma occurs. The AACAP Practice Parameters (1998) strongly recommend such a group intervention in the case of a shared traumatic event. Much of what occurs in the group setting actually is more properly classified as psychoeducational; this is especially true of school-based interventions (discussed in a later section). Though psychoeducation is certainly invaluable in discussing the etiology and course of posttraumatic symptoms, the group experience has an innate component of healing that extends beyond this. For a child who believes that he or she is the only one who has ever felt this way or had this experience, the group can provide a sense of comfort that, indeed, he or she is not alone (Yule and Williams, 1990). This is especially true of the adolescent period, when the peer group holds such importance for the teen, and deviance from the norm (whether true or imagined) is often devastating. This feeling of being somehow different therefore accentuates the trauma of the event, often leading to greater isolation, denial, or avoidance of reminders of the event; these changes, of course, can prohibit recovery. Group discussion provides an opportunity for the adolescent to view the events and others' reactions from multiple perspectives that may differ from his or her own.

Group therapy also permits the adolescent to see others in the course of recovering, providing hope that recovery is possible as well as models of coping. The inevitable ebb and flow of recovery (with periodic decompensation or even simply discouragement) occurs in the context of observing peers, providing a realistic view that encourages hard work in order to make it through the hard times. The group can find meaning when one member is suffering, because other members take on a helping role. Thus, altruism and helpful interaction with others provides an opportunity to heal one's own wounds and counteracts the tendency for individual members to dwell on their suffering in passive isolation. The group leader must always be aware, however, that reexposure to trauma (while listening to others' stories or telling one's own) may also be potentially harmful if this occurs too early in recovery or is not well managed in the group. Just as sometimes occurs in the PTSD groups of adult male veterans (based upon this author's clinical experience), the group may stalemate, with group members inadvertently retraumatizing one another. Ideally, however, the clinician leading the group will be aware of these potential pitfalls and attempt to discourage them or address them immediately when they occur.

Adolescents today are often under considerable pressure to present themselves as tough or threatening. Similarly, previously traumatized adolescents can develop aggressive behavior in a counterphobic response. (One illustration of this counterphobic response is the Vietnam era T-shirt slogan: "Yea, though I walk through the valley of the shadow of death, I will fear no evil, for I am the meanest m_____ f_____ in the valley.") This can lead to open expression of aggression in the group setting.

Many teens have witnessed multiple episodes of interpersonal violence, such as shootings, stabbings, and beatings in their neighborhoods, including violence against their own families (GAP, this volume). Some come to believe that any demonstration of weakness results in victimization, and it is no surprise that such open aggression becomes part of their repertoire of behaviors (with these same adolescents becoming involved early in the commission of violent crimes). It is worthwhile, then, to consider that such an aggressive stance in the setting of group therapy may be injurious to other recently-traumatized adolescents.

This is not to say that children and adolescents should be discouraged from talking about their anger related to the event (which could possibly erupt at a later point in a very serious fashion). However, guidelines regarding the expression of anger in the group setting should be established, and such volatile aggressiveness should be processed in an individual setting (Gillis, 1993).

School-Based Interventions

The climate of today's world has—all too evidently—invaded our classrooms. The horror of the Columbine High School and other multiple-victim school shootings increased public awareness of this violent reality, but these were, of course, not the first incidents of violence affecting our youth (see Kalogerakis, this volume). But these school-related violent acts made the headlines for weeks, precipitating many copycat crimes throughout the states, and a traumatized public responded with shock. School systems responded by developing crisis management policies and procedures and increasing the emphasis on school-based mental health interventions, combining the modalities of individual and group psychotherapy. Indeed, the suitability of the school as a locus for crisis intervention had already been well demonstrated. For example, a study of Armenian youth after the 1988 earthquake demonstrated the efficacy of brief psychotherapy operating through school-based interventions (Goenjian et al., 1997). In this study (which combined classroom-based group psychotherapy and individual therapy), both intrusion and avoidance symptoms appeared to respond to treatment. The authors explained that the techniques employed decreased physiological and psychological reactivity, which may have directly affected the intrusive symptoms and indirectly led to decreased avoidance of trauma-related stimuli. School-based counseling was the major form of intervention with schoolchildren who received mental health treatment in the aftermath of the Oklahoma City bombing as well as the World Trade Center and Pentagon attacks of September 11, 2001 (Pfefferbaum, Call, and Sconzo, 1999; Stuber et al., 2002).

Trauma that occurs within school walls, however, creates an atmosphere of inadvertent flooding of trauma-related stimuli when the intervention occurs in the classroom. This fact may lead to future research considerations.

The short-term nature of much postdisaster treatment and the lack of sufficiently trained providers raise basic questions about the enduring value of such intervention. "Specialists" from around the country often aggregate at the sight of such tragedies to provide immediate posttraumatic intervention. Unfortunately, these therapists may not be adequately trained and often do not provide ongoing, long-term supportive interventions. As such incidences become more and more common, training of school personnel in the administration of psychotherapy may provide the most immediate, most enduring form of treatment. Pfefferbaum and colleagues (1999) have described the development and implementation of an extensive program for schoolchildren in Oklahoma City following the terrorist bombing there. This program involved collaborations between the university, federal, state and local government, and school districts. Key issues were defining of turf and addressing resistances on the part of some school principals who wanted to put the trauma behind them and opposed talking about it. Nonetheless, it is likely that such interventions will become more generally accepted as knowledge of the impact of trauma on children and adolescents increases. As school-based interventions targeted to all students would be largely psychoeducational in approach (with students in need of more intensive interventions referred to mental health specialists), school staff are natural candidates to be trained to provide such first-line interventions.

Family Interventions

The adolescent's peer group does become crucial in this developmental period, but the context of the trauma often remains that of the family. As has been shown, there is a correlation between the symptoms experienced by the child after an event and those of the parents (McFarlane, 1987). Although adolescents are less likely than younger children to respond in ways that mirror their parents' reactions, they will not respond totally independently either, because coping styles are acquired within the family, and attitudes toward help-seeking will be influenced by parents. The family's ability to work toward resolution, or at least amelioration, of the pain of trauma continues to play a large role in the adolescent's ability to do so. This occurs through modeling by and interventions of the parents. If family members deny any difficulties and refuse treatment, it is much less likely that the adolescent (already receiving covert peer pressure to "get over it") will seek treatment.

Families who have experienced trauma will react based on patterns of interacting established long before the trauma. If these patterns included denial, isolation of affect, and avoidance, then the problematic experience may simply be overlooked. In other words, it is highly improbable that a traumatic stressor will do anything to improve a family's maladaptive patterns. For example, the family that invests much of its energy in meeting the self-interest and emotional needs of one family member at the expense of the others will, in all likelihood, overlook the traumatized child or adolescent to attend to the loudly proclaimed suffering of that member.

The AACAP Practice Parameters (1998) remark that "helping parents resolve their emotional distress related to the trauma, to which the parent usually has had either direct or vicarious exposure, can help the parent be more perceptive of and responsive to the child's emotional needs" (p. 17S). Clearly, family therapy becomes essential when a family already involved in these maladaptive interactions suffers the added stress of a traumatic event. Becker et al. (1999) found a similar result in their investigation of the psychological sequelae of ethnic cleansing, concluding that "family and community context may play a crucial role in determining the course of posttraumatic adaptation during adolescence" (p. 779).

Family intervention may also be mandated in cases of families functioning well until the crisis. Often using psychoeducation as a primary tool, family therapy provides the family with an understanding of what has happened in the family, whether to one member or to all members. It serves to guide the family in coping with a situation that (if they are fortunate) is totally unfamiliar to them, because, although the adolescent is separating and individuating, the traumatic event and subsequent development of posttraumatic symptomatology may lead to regression and a need for unprecedented support from the family.

One necessary consideration is whether the trauma is the result of abuse at the hands of a family member. As children (even adolescent children) have trouble discussing abuse in the presence of the perpetrators of the abuse, family therapy may be contraindicated in such circumstances (Terr, 1989).

Psychoeducation

The Expert Consensus Guidelines (Foa et al., 1999) describe psychoeducation as a technique of choice of many clinicians. The absence of its

293

explicit mention by name in many articles is largely a function of its implicit incorporation into the psychotherapeutic interventions above. Whether the modality of psychotherapeutic intervention be individual, group, or family, the anticipatory explanation of possible expected symptomatology is crucial in the treatment of symptoms. Normalization of this alienating experience allows it to be viewed more clearly, though of course not completely without the use of necessary defenses. Psychoeducation is critical when psychopharmacologic interventions are used, lest the patient and family expect immediate, complete resolution of symptoms on use of the medication. Finally, psychoeducation sets the stage for all interventions that follow, establishing a shared framework and a common language for clinician, patient, and family.

PSYCHOPHARMACOLOGIC INTERVENTIONS

The literature on psychopharmacologic intervention in the treatment of PTSD is growing; however, much of what follows is drawn from the adult literature. The Expert Consensus Guidelines (Foa et al., 1999), in fact, were meant to apply to PTSD in all populations. Most of the experts surveyed in the Guidelines recommended psychopharmacologic interventions to accompany psychotherapeutic interventions from the outset in the treatment of adolescents (as compared with the treatment of children, where psychotherapeutic interventions take precedence). Pharmacotherapy consists of three phases: stabilization (engagement and alliance building), maintenance, and discontinuation (Davidson and Connor, 1999).

Establishment of a therapeutic alliance is crucial in the treatment of adolescents. Adolescents should be treated with respect, and reasons for starting medication should be discussed with them, not simply with their parents. With older adolescents who have obtained a level of abstraction, discussion of theories of the biological changes that can occur as a result of trauma may be in order. With all adolescents (even those younger ones still operating at a concrete level), potential adverse side effects should be openly discussed, with a concurrent discussion that the appearance of such effects does not mean that the drug should be abruptly discontinued. Though such discussions are important in the treatment of adults, they take on an added relevance during this teen period, when body image (potentially adversely affected by the drug, e.g., sexual functioning) is of primary importance. Also, impulse control and frustration tolerance may not be optimal, resulting in the sudden discontinuation of the medication. Perhaps equally important to discuss at the outset is that no medication treats all of the symptoms resulting from exposure to trauma and that accompanying psychotherapy is critical for recovery.

Selective Serotonin Reuptake Inhibitors (SSRIs)

The SSRIs all have anxiolytic effects and all have been reported to have efficacy in reducing symptoms of PTSD. On the basis of double-blind, placebo-controlled studies, sertraline received FDA approval to include PTSD as one of its indications in its labeling in 1999 (Brady et al., 2000; Davidson, Pearlstein, et al., 2001; Davidson, Rothbaum, et al., 2001; Rapaport, Endicott, and Clary, 2002). To a lesser extent, data exist supporting the efficacy of fluoxetine, paroxetine, and fluvoxamine in adult posttraumatic symptomatology. Fluoxetine was found in one double-blind study to improve numbing symptoms, but not avoidance symptoms, after five weeks of treatment (van der Kolk et al., 1994). Other open trials have suggested that the SSRIs can reduce a number of posttraumatic symptoms, including hyperarousal, agitation, anxiety, and insomnia (Marmar et al., 1996; Davidson and Connor, 1999; Tucker et al., 2000; Neylan et al., 2001). Studies of the use of SSRIs in childhood and adolescence are primarily small, open trials rather than controlled studies. However, the low side-effect occurrence and good safety profile of these drugs make them potentially useful components of the armamentarium against the symptoms of trauma exposure. Side effects include agitation, activation, gastrointestinal upset, and sexual dysfunction, as well or malaise and other symptoms following abrupt discontinuation of the shorter-acting agents.

Tricyclic Antidepressants

As with clonidine, the use of tricyclic antidepressants was first advocated for the treatment of PTSD in adults, specifically combat veterans. Studies using amitriptyline (Davidson et al., 1990) and imipramine (Kosten et al., 1991) in these adult populations have demonstrated moderate beneficial effects, with better outcomes obtained in the less severe populations. In an eight-week trial, the amitriptyline study demonstrated significant reduction of avoidant symptoms (but not intrusive symptoms). In contrast, a study of desipramine for the treatment of posttraumatic symptoms demonstrated no significant difference between drug and placebo (Reist et al., 1989). The AACAP Practice Parameters additionally remark that imipramine may be frequently used in children with PTSD and comorbid panic symptoms (AACAP, 1998).

As with clonidine, the use of these medications is associated with certain risks that may be particularly salient for the adolescent population. Among these are frequent somatic side effects: dry mouth, urinary retention, and sexual side effects. Also of concern is the risk of death secondary to overdose, which—in light of teens' foreshortened view of consequences, overvalued belief in immortality, and poor impulse control—is of significant concern in the adolescent population.

Monoamine Oxidase Inhibitors (MAOIs)

Monoamine oxidase inhibitors, specifically phenelzine and the nonreversible MAOIs, have been shown to be effective in the treatment of posttraumatic symptoms in adults—in fact, one study demonstrated greater efficacy of phenelzine when compared with imipramine, primarily in intrusive, but not avoidant, symptoms (Kosten et al., 1991). Another study, however, demonstrated no positive effect of phenelzine on posttraumatic symptoms (Shetatsky, Greenberg, and Lerer, 1988). One possible explanation for this difference in findings may be related to which symptoms were measured, as MAOIs are thought to be less effective for avoidant and numbing symptoms (Southwick et al., 1994). Concern about the potential side effects are especially relevant in considering MAOIs for adolescents. The absolute requirement for a diet free of tyramine (restricting intake of pizza, etc.) is one difficult even for adults to maintain. The risk of hypertensive crisis precipitated by failure to maintain necessary dietary restrictions weighs even more heavily, therefore, against using these drugs in adolescents.

Clonidine

Use of clonidine for the treatment of PTSD in adults, with some encouraging results reported (Friedman, 1988), led to consideration of its use

296

in children and adolescents. Though limited by small sample size, clinical reports in younger children have been positive, with reported decreases in aggression, hyperarousal, and sleep difficulties (Harmon and Riggs, 1996). The risks of hypotension or rebound hypertension, although small, suggest a need for periodic blood pressure monitoring. The most common side effects of clonidine are sedation and/or irritability, especially if given in large doses. Although infrequent, side effects such as arrhythmia underscore the importance of periodic electrocardiograms (EKGs), in addition to an initial EKG on initiation of clonidine. The potential for adverse interactions with other drugs (e.g., stimulants) currently remains under debate. The use of a transdermal clonidine patch results in better compliance but often causes skin irritation, somnolence, or allergic sensitization.

Benzodiazepines

Although widely used to treat acute anxiety, there is no convincing evidence at this time that benzodiazepines are effective for ongoing treatment of posttraumatic symptoms in studies of adults, although there was a slight decrease in the anxiety symptoms noted in one study (Braun et al., 1990) and evidence of decreased stress-induced responses to inescapable shock in another (Drugan et al., 1984). It is generally considered that the undesirable side-effects profile (sedation, potential for behavioral disinhibition, and development of tolerance/dependence) and absence of beneficial effects on the post-traumatic symptoms of reexperiencing, avoidance, or numbing limit the benzodiazepines' usefulness in the long-term treatment of traumatized adults (Friedman, 1998). Similar caveats apply to their use for the long-term treatment of posttraumatic symptoms in adolescents. Though these drugs may be employed temporarily in crisis situations (such as the acute onset of insomnia after a traumatic event), concerns regarding dependence and rebound anxiety paired with the lack of evidence of efficacy advise against long-term use in the treatment of posttraumatic symptoms in this age group.

Antipsychotic Drugs

Although used in the past quite commonly in the treatment of combat-related posttraumatic symptomatology on the basis of its apparent similarity to psychosis (i.e., flashbacks resembled visual and auditory hallucinations), the evolution in the conceptualization of PTSD led to a decline in the use of traditional antipsychotic regimens for the treatment of posttraumatic symptoms. Experts recommend that such medications should only be used for the most severe childhood PTSD (Donnelly, Amaya-Jackson, and March, 1999) due to risks of tardive dyskinesia and other extrapyramidal symptoms.

The newer antipsychotics, however, with their marked anxiolytic properties and relative lack of side effects compared to the older drugs, have become popular among clinicians for a variety of severe anxiety disorders, including PTSD. Fifteen percent of risperidone prescriptions and 20% of olanzapine prescriptions written in a Veterans Administration hospital were for a diagnosis of PTSD (Voris and Glazer, 1999). An open-label study of risperidone used in 18 male children and adolescents with PTSD reportedly showed significant improvement on the Clinical Global Impression Scale in 50% of the boys ("Risperidone Appears Effective for Children, Adolescents with Severe PTDS," *Psychiatric News,* December 18, 1998, p. 8). Details of this study have not been published, however. Even in adults, reports of the efficacy of risperidone have been limited to case reports (Leyba and Wampler, 1998; Krashin and Oates, 1999; Monnelly and Ciraulo, 1999; Eidelman, Seedat, and Stein, 2000), and as of this writing, there are no published studies of the other newer antipsychotic drugs and PTSD.

Propanolol and Other Beta-Blockers

In clinical circles, there is frequent mention of the use of propanolol in the treatment of posttraumatic symptoms in children, but clinical research studies are minimal. Beneficial effects of the use of propanolol have been reported in latency-age children, but the study was not controlled, thereby leaving open the possibility of placebo effect (Famularo, Kinscherff, and Fenton, 1988). Although theoretical consideration suggested that propanolol may be useful for many of the same symptoms that clonidine is thought to ameliorate (hyperarousal, aggression, etc.), more studies are needed to establish it as a proven method of treatment. Propanolol's beta-blocking effects preclude its use in adolescents with the diagnosis of asthma or diabetes, because it may exacerbate asthma or mask the sympathetic signs and symptoms of hypoglycemia. However, one may wish to consider the use of atenolol, with its more peripheral effects and avoidance of the more centrally-mediated side effects, such as sedation.

Anticonvulsants and Lithium

Use of anticonvulsants for the treatment of posttraumatic symptoms was being considered as early as 1986, when Lipper et al. (1986) demonstrated that carbamazepine was effective (in Vietnam veterans) in reducing nightmares of the event, flashbacks, intrusive thoughts, and sleep disturbance. In a 1995 letter to the *Journal of the American Academy of Child and Adolescent Psychiatry,* Looff et al. reported complete remission of posttraumatic symptoms in 22 of 28 children receiving carbamazepine. Valproic acid has been demonstrated in an open-label study (also with Vietnam veterans) to aid in reduction of avoidant and hyperarousal symptoms (Fesler, 1991).

Although lithium has demonstrated beneficial effects in the treatment of adult PTSD in open trials (Donnelly et al., 1999), there are currently no published trials in children or adolescents.

As in the treatment of adults, one must consider the potential side effects of each of these medications: bone marrow suppression with carbamazepine, diabetes insipidus and weight gain with lithium, and weight gain and growth-hormone dysregulation with valproic acid. Of great importance in the treatment of adolescents with valproic acid is the recent evidence of increased incidence of polycystic ovary disease in postpubertal females.

POTENTIAL FUTURE INTERVENTIONS

The preceding discussion of interventions for use in adolescent posttraumatic symptoms was largely drawn from the adult—and some limited child and adolescent psychiatric—literature. References to adolescents (as distinct from either children or adults) are few and far between. In a society in which traumas of all types (accidents, suicide, and homicide) are the primary causes of death of adolescents, this paucity of research directed at adolescents is shocking. Perhaps the most important future intervention, therefore, will be the differential clarification of the efficacy of specific interventions in the treatment of adolescent posttraumatic symptoms. Once these issues are addressed, considerations of optimal dosing and responses at different intervals of treatment (because the treatment duration may be longer than that needed for depressive or anxiety disorders) should be examined (Davidson et al., 1990).

Universally, in the treatment of the posttraumatic symptoms, we must continue to explore new pharmacological possibilities. Although there have been limited reports of success with carbamazepine, valproic acid, neuroleptics, and lithium, there is a great need for controlled studies. Some success was demonstrated in both the United States and Europe with the drug brofaromine, a reversible inhibitor of MAO type A and the uptake of serotonin, suggesting that there may be new, safer drugs that could be developed (Katz et al., 1994). Based on the hypothesized role of cortisol-releasing factor (CRF) in posttraumatic stress and resulting depression (Yehuda, 1998), development of CRF-receptor antagonists could provide a radically different approach to the treatment of PTSD.

Finally, it is worthwhile to note that assault victims have been found to use medical services at twice the rate of those who have never experienced such trauma. This suggests that involvement of primary care physicians and nurses in the treatment should be great, with training developed to assist these caregivers in providing appropriate interventions and, when necessary, referrals to mental health specialists (Koss, Woodruff, and Koss, 1991). As we well know, the stigma associated with many other illnesses in psychiatry has not forgotten PTSD, and our patients may find identification of a somatic symptom a much more socially acceptable expression of distress. We, as professionals, must work to provide public outreach education to facilitate our patients' revealing their symptoms without fear of stigmatization, to provide them with appropriate treatment.

REFERENCES

American Academy of Child & Adolescent Psychiatry (1998), Practice parameters for the assessment and treatment of children and adolescents with posttraumatic stress disorder. *J. Amer. Acad. Child & Adol. Psychiat.*, 37(10S):4S–26S.

American Psychiatric Association (2000), *Diagnostic and Statistical Manual of Mental Disorders*, 4th ed. (*DSM-IV-TR*). Washington, DC: American Psychiatric Association.

Becker, D. F., Weine, S. M., Vojvoda, D. & McGlashan, T. H. (1999), Case series: PTSD in adolescent survivors of "ethnic cleansing." Results from a 1-year follow-up study. *J. Amer. Acad. Child & Adol. Psychiat.*, 38(6):775–781.

Brady, K., Pearlstein, T., Asnis, G. M., Baker, D., Rothbaum, B., Sikes, C. R. & Farfel, G. M. (2000), Efficacy and safety of sertraline treatment of posttraumatic stress disorder: A randomized controlled trial. *J. Amer. Med. Assn.*, 283:1837–1844.

Braun, P., Greenberg, D., Dasberg, H. & Lerer, B. (1990), Core symptoms of posttraumatic stress disorder unimproved by alprazolam treatment. *J. Clin. Psychiat.*, 51(6):236–238.

Davidson, J. R. T. (1997), Biological therapies for posttraumatic stress disorder: An overview. *J. Clin. Psychiat.*, 58(suppl.) 9:29–32.

———— & Connor, K. M. (1999), Management of posttraumatic stress disorder: Diagnostic and therapeutic issues. *J. Clin. Psychiat.*, 60(suppl.) 18:33–38.

———— Kudler, H., Smith, R., Mahorney, S. L., Lipper, S., Hammett, E., Saunders, W. B. & Cavenar, J. O., Jr. (1990), Treatment of posttraumatic stress disorder with amitriptyline and placebo. *Arch. Gen. Psychiat.*, 47:259–266.

———— Pearlstein, T., Londborg, P., Brady, K. T., Rothbaum, B., Bell, J., Maddock, R., Hegel, M. T. & Farfel, G. (2001), Efficacy of sertraline in preventing relapse of posttraumatic stress disorder: Results of a 28-week double-blind, placebo-controlled study. *Amer. J. Psychiat.*, 158:1974–1981.

———— Rothbaum, B. O., van der Kolk, B. A., Sikes, C. R. & Farfel, G. M. (2001), Multicenter, double-blind comparison of sertraline and placebo in the treatment of posttraumatic stress disorder. *Arch. Gen. Psychiat.*, 58:485–492.

Deblinger, E., McLeer, S. V. & Henry, D. (1990), Cognitive behavioral treatment for sexually abused children suffering post-traumatic stress: Preliminary findings. *J. Amer. Acad. Child & Adol. Psychiat.*, 29:747–752.

Donnelly, C. L., Amaya-Jackson, L. & March, J. S. (1999), Psychopharmacology of pediatric posttraumatic stress disorder. *J. Child & Adol. Psychopharmacol.*, 9:203–220.

Drugan, R. C., Ryan, S. M., Minor, T. R. & Maier, S. F. (1984), Librium prevents the analgesia and shuttlebox escape deficit typically observed following inescapable shock. *Pharmacol. Biochem. Behav.*, 21:749–754.

Eidelman, I., Seedat, S. & Stein, D. J. (2000), Risperidone in the treatment of acute stress disorder in physically traumatized in-patients. *Depress. Anxiety,* 11:187–188.

Famularo, R., Kinscherff, R. & Fenton, T. (1988), Propanolol treatment for childhood posttraumatic stress disorder, acute type. *Amer. J. Dis. Child.,* 142:1244–1247.

Fesler, F. A. (1991), Valproate in combat-related post-traumatic stress disorder patients. *J. Clin. Psychiat.,* 52:361–364.

Foa, E. B. (1997), Trauma and women: Course, predictors, and treatment. *J. Clin. Psychiat.,* 58(suppl.) 9:25–28.

———— Davidson, J. R. T. & Frances, A. (1999), The expert consensus guideline series: Treatment of posttraumatic stress disorder. *J. Clin. Psychiat.,* 60(suppl.) 16:10–33.

———— Hearst-Ikeda, D. & Perry, K. I. (1995), Evaluation of a brief cognitive-behavioral program for prevention of PTSD in recent assault victims. *J. Consult. Clin. Psychol.,* 63:948–955.

———— Olasov-Rothbaum, B., Riggs, D. S. & Murdock, T. B. (1991), Treatment of posttraumatic stress disorder in rape victims: Comparison between cognitive behavioral procedures and counseling. *J. Consult. Clin. Psychol.,* 59:715–723.

Friedman, M. J. (1988), Toward rational pharmacotherapy for posttraumatic stress disorder: An interim report. *Amer. J. Psychiat.,* 145:281–285.

———— (1998), Current and future drug treatment for post-traumatic stress disorder patients. *Psychiat. Annals,* 28:461–468.

Gillis, H. M. (1993), Individual and small-group psychotherapy for children involved in trauma and disaster. In: *Children and Disasters,* ed. C. F. Saylor. New York: Plenum Press, pp. 165–186.

Goenjian, A. K., Karayan, I., Pynoos, R. S., Minassian, D., Najarian, L. M., Steinberg, A. M. & Fairbanks, L. A. (1997), Outcome of psychotherapy among early adolescents after trauma. *Amer. J. Psychiat.,* 154:536–542.

Harmon, R. J. & Riggs, P. D. (1996), Clonidine for posttraumatic stress disorder in preschool children. *J. Amer. Acad. Child & Adol. Psychiat.,* 35:1247–1249.

Katz, R. J., Lott, M. H., Arbus, P., Crocq, L., Herlobsen, P., Lingjaerde, O., Lopez, G., Loughrey, G. C., MacFarlane, D. J. & McIvor, R. (1994), Pharmacotherapy of post-traumatic stress disorder with a novel psychotropic. *Anxiety,* 1:169–174.

Koss, M. D., Woodruff, W. J. & Koss, P. G. (1991), Criminal victimization among primary care medical patients: Prevalence, incidence, and physician usage. *Behav. Sci. Law,* 9:85–96.

Kosten, T. R., Frank, J. B., Dan, E., McDougle, C. J. & Giller, E. L. Jr. (1991), Pharmacotherapy for posttraumatic stress disorder using phenelzine or imipramine. *J. Nerv. Ment. Dis.,* 179:366–370.

Krashin, D. & Oates, E. W. (1999), Risperidone as an adjunct therapy for post-traumatic stress disorder. *Mil. Med.,* 164:605–606.

Leyba, C. M. & Wampler, T. P. (1998), Risperidone in PTSD. *Psychiatr. Serv.,* 49:245–246.

Lipper, S., Hammett, E. B., Davidson, J. R. T., Edinger, J. D., Hammett, E. B., Mahorney, S. L. & Cavenar, J. O. Jr. (1986), Preliminary study of carbamazepine in posttraumatic stress disorder. *Psychosomatics,* 27:849–854.

Looff, D., Grimley, P., Kuller, F., Martin, A. & Shonfield, L. (1995), Carbamazepine for posttraumatic stress disorder (letter). *J. Amer. Acad. Child & Adol. Psychiat.,* 34:703–704.

Lowenstein, L. B. (1995), The resolutions scrapbook as an aid in the treatment of traumatized children. *Child Welfare,* 74:899–904.

March, J. S., Amaya-Jackson, L., Murray, M. C. & Schulte, A. (1998), Cognitive-behavioral psychotherapy for children and adolescents with posttraumatic stress disorder after a single incident stressor. *J. Amer. Acad. Child & Adol. Psychiat.,* 37:585–593.

Marmar, C. R., Schoenfeld, F., Weiss, D. S., Metzler, T., Zatzick, D., Wu, R., Smiga, S., Tecott, L. & Neylan, T. (1996), Open trial of fluvoxamine treatment for combat-related posttraumatic stress disorder. *J. Clin. Psychiat.,* 57(suppl.) 8:66–70; discussion pp. 71–72.

McFarlane, A. C. (1987), Posttraumatic phenomena in a longitudinal study of children following a natural disaster. *J. Amer. Acad. Child & Adol. Psychiat.,* 26:764–769.

Mendlowitz, S. L., Manassis, K., Bradley, S., Scapillato, D., Miezitis, S. & Shaw, B. F. (1999), Cognitive-behavioral group treatments in childhood anxiety disorders: The role of parental involvement. *J. Amer. Acad. Child & Adol. Psychiat.,* 38:1223–1229.

Monnelly, E. P. & Ciraulo, D. A. (1999), Risperidone effects on irritable aggression in posttraumatic stress disorder. *J. Clin. Psychopharmacol.,* 19:377–378.

Neylan, T. C., Metzler, T. J., Schoenfeld, F. B., Weiss, D. S., Lenoci, M., Best, S. R., Lipsey, T. L. & Marmar, C. R. (2001), Fluvoxamine and sleep disturbances in posttraumatic stress disorder. *J. Traum. Stress,* 14:461–467.

Pfefferbaum, B., Call, J. A. & Sconzo, G. M. (1999), Mental health services for children in the first two years after the 1995 Oklahoma City terrorist bombing. *Psychiatr. Serv.,* 50:956–958.

Pynoos, R. S. & Nader, K. (1993), Issues in the treatment of posttraumatic stress in children and adolescents. In: *International Handbook of Traumatic Stress Syndromes,* ed. J. P. Wilson & B. Raphael. New York: Plenum Press, pp. 535–549.

Rapaport, M. H., Endicott, J. & Clary, C. M. (2002), Posttraumatic stress disorder and quality of life: Results across 64 weeks of sertraline treatment. *J. Clin. Psychiat.,* 63:59–65.

Reist, C., Kauffmann, C. D., Haier, R. J., Sangdahl, C., DeMet, E. M., Chicz-DeMet, A. & Nelson, J. N. (1989), A controlled trial of desipramine in 18 men with posttraumatic stress disorder. *Amer. J. Psychiat.,* 146:513–516.

Scott, M. J. & Stradling, S. G. (1997), Client compliance with exposure treatments for posttraumatic stress disorder. *J. Traum. Stress,* 10:523–526.

Shetatsky, M., Greenberg, D. & Lerer, B. (1988), A controlled trial of phenelzine in posttraumatic stress disorder. *Psychiat. Res.,* 24:149–155.

Southwick, S. M., Yehuda, R., Giller, E. L. & Charney, E. S. (1994), Use of tricyclics and monoamine oxidase inhibitors in the treatment of PTSD: A quantitative review. In: *Catecholamine Function in Posttraumatic Stress Disorder: Emerging Concepts,* ed. M. M. Marburg. Washington, DC: American Psychiatric Press, 2:293–305.

Stuber, J., Fairbrother, G., Galea, S., Pfefferbaum, B., Wilson-Genderson, M. & Vlahov, D. (2002), Determinants of counseling for children in Manhattan after the September 11 attacks. *Psychiatr. Serv.,* 53:815–822.

Terr, L. C. (1989), Treating psychic trauma in children: A preliminary discussion. *J. Traum. Stress,* 2:3–20.

Tucker, P., Smith, K. L., Marx, B., Jones, D., Miranda, R. & Lensgraf, J. (2000), Fluvoxamine reduces physiologic reactivity to trauma scripts in posttraumatic stress disorder. *J. Clin. Psychopharmacol.,* 20:367–372.

van der Kolk, B., Dreyfuss, D., Michaels, M., Shera, D., Berkowitz, R., Fisler, R. & Saxe, G. (1994), Fluoxetine in posttraumatic stress disorder. *J. Clin. Psychiat.,* 55:517–522.

Voris, J. C. & Glazer, W. M. (1999), Use of risperidone and olanzapine in outpatient clinics at six Veterans Affairs hospitals. *Psychiat. Serv.,* 50:163–164, 168.

Yehuda, R. (1998), Psychoneuroendocrinology of post-traumatic stress disorder. *Psychiat. Clin. N. Amer.,* 21:359–379.

Yule, W. & Williams, R. M. (1990), Post-traumatic stress reactions in children. *J. Traum. Stress,* 3:279–295.

12 LATE ADOLESCENCE AND COMBAT PTSD

MAX SUGAR

Studies of combat veterans from the wars of the 20th century have raised many questions. Are those who develop combat PTSD vulnerable due to having a preexisting condition, less resilience to stress, or a problem in their emotional stability or character? Alternatively, is it possible that combat PTSD occurs regardless of premilitary status? There are many proponents with persuasive notions for each of these views (Boman, 1982). Because most combatants are older adolescents or young adults, these questions are of particular interest to adolescent psychiatrists. An examination of the ways in which the adolescent developmental process itself might contribute to vulnerability to combat trauma may suggest answers to some of these questions.

Two hypotheses are presented as follows: 1) although company grade combat military officers are exposed to similar combat trauma as combatants of lower ranks (OR), they have a much lower incidence of PTSD compared to OR; and 2) since the officers are about five years older than OR, they have completed the developmental tasks of adolescence and have a stable adult identity. In addition, due to the selection process, officers have a higher IQ, a better education, and leadership abilities, all of which the modal OR do not have. These differences appear to account for the differences in the incidence of PTSD between officers and OR.

The methods used are a review of the available literature on combat stress-related syndromes in veterans of U.S. wars, and my clinical experience with combat veteran patients. The hypotheses advanced here are based on the limited data in the literature, which support my clinical experiences in private practice, the military, and the Veterans Administration (VA). For both OR and officers, veterans of combat from all branches of the military are considered. The term military officers is limited here to U.S.-commissioned officers at the company-grade level, that is, lieutenant or captain (equivalent ranks in the Navy and Coast Guard are included), because they are the officers most often engaged in combat alongside the OR. Higher-ranking officers are less likely to be exposed to direct combat.

EVOLUTION OF DIAGNOSTIC TERMS

Previous diagnoses for reactions to combat were shell shock in World War I, and combat fatigue and operational fatigue in World War II, the Korean War, and the Vietnam War. The diagnosis of PTSD replaced them in 1980 (American Psychiatric Association [APA]). The accepted, and usual, psychiatric casualty rate of 25% in military combat (Glass, 1958) is composed of diverse diagnoses. The current *DSM-IV* (APA, 1994) listings of acute distress reaction, anxiety disorder, depressive disorder, and schizophreniform reaction would probably be applicable to a large percentage of the acute diagnoses. PTSD, which requires a month's duration of symptoms for the diagnosis (APA, 1994), would probably constitute a much smaller percent of the initial total casualties.

BIOLOGICAL CONSIDERATIONS

Van der Kolk and colleagues (1985) noted that inescapable shock leads to catecholamine depletion and subsequent stress-induced analgesia due to endogenous opioids. After the stress ends, opioid withdrawal symptoms and hyperactivity develop due to noradrenergic hypersensitivity. They suggested that this could account for the voluntary reexposure to trauma that many with combat PTSD seek.

Bremner and colleagues (1995) found right hippocampal atrophy in combat veterans with PTSD. The study cohort and the control group were alcohol abusers, and the authors noted that alcohol abuse has been implicated as a possible cause of lower hippocampal volume. This raises the question of the validity of the relationship of PTSD to lower hippocampal volume. Could a smaller hippocampus lead to a combat assignment instead of a skilled job in headquarters due to the relation of cognitive ability to the size of the hippocampus? Since those with combat PTSD had high rates of learning disorders and developmental delay, Sapolsky (1996) asked if a small hippocampus could be the cause, instead of the result, of trauma. It is puzzling to see postcombat findings extrapolated retrospectively to infer a preexisting low-volume hippocampus. A detailed past history of combat PTSD patients would be needed, along with MRIs of their hippocampi, in order to make any comparison between premilitary and postmilitary conditions. Even then, no differentiation could be made between officers and OR without clarification of age and rank at the time of combat.

The observation by Bremner and colleagues (1997), that low volume in the right hippocampus in combat PTSD is related to childhood physical and sexual abuse, raises further questions about a linear relationship between hippocampal volume and combat. Both of these studies by Bremner and others (1995; 1997) lacked classifications of the veterans by rank or age and listing of the age of the combatants at the time of combat; furthermore, each cohort had small numbers.

Shay (1994) stated that combat soldiers have a limited temporal, moral, and social view, with only one meaningful goal—that of "getting through now" (p. 176). He added that there is a loss of a significant personal narrative, which leads to a decrease in exercise of will and future planning. These adaptations often remain after combat when they are no longer needed for survival. The concepts from biological and psychiatric studies should apply uniformly to all ranks with combat PTSD, and all ranks would then have a similar rate of PTSD from exposure to equivalent combat stress. However, this does not appear to be the case.

COMBAT EXPOSURE OF OFFICERS AND OR

The tour of combat duty for infantry officers in the Vietnam War consisted of three months in combat, then rotation to a position behind the lines, followed by combat in another unit for three months, after which they were rotated to another unit behind the lines for three months. This gave them six months of actual combat duty during their 12 months in Vietnam, compared with the 12 months of combat that the OR had. When the very high rate of fragging (assaults with fragmentation grenades) and murders of junior officers in their tents by OR (Bond, 1976) is added to the officers' trauma-duration-exposure dose, then it probably comes close to that of OR. Company-grade officers in the other branches of the military had tours of combat duty equivalent to that of the infantry officers.

RETURNING FROM COMBAT

Grinker and colleagues (1946) and Grinker and Spiegel (1945) observed an anxious reaction to leaving one's unit for stateside hospitalization or another assignment. This was a reaction to separation from the group and the loss of support from it. During combat, the group was a very important positive. The loss of a buddy was often the precipitating factor that led to psychiatric hospitalization (Grinker and Spiegel, 1945).

The presence of a strong friend with a sympathetic and supportive attitude on a combat team "may see a man through a most difficult combat tour in spite of a weakened ego and much anxiety" (Grinker and Spiegel, 1945, p. 164). Similarly, Steiner and Neumann (1978) noted that the positive social support offered by the soldiers' group played a large part in protecting the Israeli soldiers against combat neurosis.

Returning from combat in Vietnam was different for the U.S. military than for soldiers returning from other wars, because the soldier returned by air in 24 hours without his unit. There was also a negative reaction instead of welcoming parades from those at home. In contrast, Australian combat troops in the Vietnam War came home with their units, and there was some public support and greeting for them on returning home (Boman, 1982).

Bourne (1972) felt that, although the policy for the U.S. troops of rotation out of Vietnam after 12 months of combat probably reduced psychiatric casualties, it also affected the cohesiveness of the small unit negatively and made the task of returning home more difficult. With a rate of 38% just for PTSD in Vietnam combat veterans six years after the war ended (Kulka et al., 1990), perhaps this policy of isolation on separation from combat contributed to an increased rate of psychiatric disorders in Vietnam combat veterans compared with veterans of other wars.

Borus (1976) suggests that factors facilitating the reentry of a soldier to civilian life on return from Vietnam were related to protection against loss of his support system. If reentry had been done properly for U.S. combat veterans of Vietnam, the soldiers would have been given a gradual rather than a precipitous transition from combatant to noncombatant status, a reorientation to civilian roles and routines, a formal and ceremonious acknowledgment noting the significance of their performance, some focus on the helpfulness of the immediate unit group by sharing experiences to facilitate readjustment, preparation and forewarning to the veterans about the new stresses accompanying the transition, and a meaningful view of the noncombat role.

RATES OF COMBAT REACTIONS IN OR AND OFFICERS

Most of the literature on combat PTSD does not give data about rank or age of the combatants at the time of combat. Solomon, Mikulincer, and Hobfoll (1986); Lee et al. (1995); Mellsop, Duraiappah, and Priest (1995); and Bower and Sivers (1998) mention combat PTSD in officers and OR but provide no rates for either group. The extensive study by Egendorf and colleagues (1981) of Vietnam veterans has no data for combat PTSD by rank or age.

Although company grade officers and OR served together in the trenches in World War I, officers seem to have been affected psychiatrically less often than OR. Nevertheless, some shell-shocked officers were treated in a special psychotherapy unit (Rivers, 1923). Yealland (1918) described treatment of a few shell-shocked officers but many OR in WWI. Neither he nor Rivers (1923) gave the prevalence of shell shock in officers or OR.

Grinker and Spiegel (1945) noted that operational fatigue among air crew in World War II was three times more frequent in OR than in officers, but rates for officers and OR were not provided. They observed that the prognosis for officers who had aspirations for postmilitary life was better than for OR. This seems to indicate that the officers had a future orientation and, perhaps, formal operational thinking.

McDuff and Johnson (1992) observed that there were only three officers in a cohort of 158 casualties with combat stress in the U.S. Army Seventh Corps in Operation Desert Storm in the Gulf War. They gave no details about the officers or rates or prevalence of psychiatric casualties in either group. Similarly, Brailey and colleagues (1997) did not mention any officers in noting that higher IQ and verbal skills seemed to protect veterans of the Gulf War against the development of stress-related psychopathology following combat trauma.

Levav, Greenfield, and Baruch (1979), who studied the 1967 Yom Kippur War in Israel, found that OR were five times more vulnerable to war stress than officers, and that the younger soldiers were especially at risk for war stress regardless of their rank. In addition, those with lower sociopsychological ratings were also at higher risk for war stress. They did not record prevalence of stress-related psychopathology for the various groups, nor did they specify an age range for the younger soldiers.

CONFOUNDING RATES OF COMBAT REACTIONS IN THE VW

Glass (1969) noted the following:

1. Anyone may develop combat fatigue with a severe enough stressor of sufficient duration.
2. After 80 to 100 days of combat, there is an increased risk of becoming a psychiatric casualty.
3. The number of psychiatric casualties is related to the severity of the danger.
4. The support and cohesion of the soldier's primary unit is the major protective influence against combat stress.

Rates of reported psychopathology changed during the course of the Vietnam War, owing to changing political views as the war progressed. Initially, low rates of psychiatric diagnoses and reports of psychiatric casualties were reported, with only 6% diagnosed with combat fatigue, but 40% given diagnoses of character and behavior disorders. Despite somnambulism, anxiety dreams, amnesia after exposure to explosions, and conversion or dissociative reactions, the latter two groups were managed administratively, not psychiatrically. Concomitantly, military psychiatrists felt that combat fatigue occurred only in healthy "normal" personalities, whereas those with preexisting adjustment or personality problems had pseudocombat fatigue, which was unrelated to the stress of combat (Boman, 1982). Early in the Vietnam War, there was a warning that combat fatigue was often expressed via antisocial behavior (Copen, 1964), but it was ignored (Boman, 1982). It seems that individual vulnerability factors were emphasized to minimize the role of war trauma in psychiatric diagnoses. A broken home was frequently used as a predisposition to combat stress, anxiety reaction, or depression.

Glass (1958) was skeptical of low reported psychiatric military casualty rates in war. Egendorf et al. (1981) reconfirmed the opinion of Glass (1969) in their five-volume study of the Vietnam War when they stated: "While predisposition may play some role, problems among Vietnam veterans cannot, on the average, be ascribed solely to conditions that pre-date military service" (p. xxviii). Kulka et al. (1990) found that male veterans of the Vietnam War had a 53% lifetime rate of clinical stress-reaction symptoms, that is, full or partial PTSD, and that by 1981, 38% of Vietnam combatants had been diagnosed with PTSD.

LONG-TERM EFFECTS OF COMBAT STRESS

The long-term effects of PTSD on adolescents include problems in learning, vocational choice, interpersonal relations, major depression, substance abuse, hypertension, group delinquent behavior, unwed pregnancy, and continued PTSD symptoms (Sugar, 1999). At their 20-year follow-up of the adolescents in the Buffalo Creek disaster, Honig et al. (1999) found previously overlooked PTSD symptoms in videotaped clinical interviews, as well as trauma-induced character change, displacements, and survivor guilt.

Koenig (1964); Carmil and Carel (1986); Nadler and Ben-Shushan (1989); Krell (1990); Ryn (1990); Southwick, Yehuda, and Giller (1993); Robins, Rapport-Bar-Sever, and Rapport (1994); Shay (1994); and Honig et al. (1999) also indicated that alteration in character structure occurs in adolescents with PTSD. Whether a biological substrate or psychiatric issues are causative for all these changes remains for further research.

Some caveats are necessary. The subject of the long-term impact of combat trauma on soldiers is difficult to study. Because many veterans of combat with PTSD symptoms may not present for evaluation until years or decades after combat, it is difficult to obtain an accurate percentage of the total psychiatric casualties of military combat, much less of combat PTSD. For officer veterans with such symptoms, this is even more difficult to obtain, because very few attend VA clinics;

313

they probably seek private therapy. Over a 20-year period, only three or four officers have been in the PTSD program at the New Orleans VA Medical Center (H. Woodside, 1999, personal communication).

LATE-ADOLESCENT DEVELOPMENT

Most military combatants are late adolescents, and, thus, attention to the psychological aspects of this developmental period may offer some understanding of vulnerability and resistance to combat-related PTSD. Reaching the developmental stage of formal operations allows adolescents to think and plan in a new, trial-action, less limited fashion than in the preceding stage of concrete operations, but formal operational thinking is present in only 20% to 35% of late adolescents (Dulit, 1972). This advanced form of cognitive functioning is more likely to be present in officers than OR, because formal operational thinking is correlated with higher IQ, education, socioeconomic status, intellectual stimulation from adults, and culture (Piaget, 1972).

During adolescent development, a second individuation occurs, with the result that, if it is successful, individuals assume responsibility for their actions and cease to attribute their difficulties to parents or others (Blos, 1968). During this second individuation process, a concomitant normal adolescent mourning process occurs as the young person adjusts to infantile object loss, that is, lesser emotional dependence on the parents. This adolescent mourning is a process with three stages— protest, disorganization, and reorganization. The latter occurs in late adolescence as the acceptance and adjustment to the object loss continues. The reorganization stage involves wishes to be free of parental and other authorities' restrictions, testing one's omnipotentiality, achieving a sense of fidelity and commitment to self and object choice, and the need to explore and manage reactions in relation to same- and opposite-sex individuals. All the while, the adolescent is still adjusting to object loss, with a less fluid superego (Sugar, 1968).

The late adolescent has many developmental tasks to complete before adulthood begins. These are identity consolidation, the attainment of some emotional separation from parents, dealing with residual trauma from childhood, ego continuity, achieving genital primacy, and developing a sexual identity (Blos, 1968). Additional important tasks of late adolescence include developing a time perspective (Buhler, 1968;

314

Neugarten, 1969), identity formation, having a commitment to a life goal, development of intimacy and friendships (Erikson, 1959), and the further development and harmonizing of the ego, superego, and ego ideal. Issues from previous developmental stages need to be reworked, refined, and harmonized. Identity formation in late adolescence involves a sense of self, as well as competence that harmonizes, and has continuity, with the community, culture, and region.

SELECTION CRITERIA FOR OFFICERS AND OR

Acceptance in officers' candidate school (OCS) requires that an applicant be at least age 21, with an above-average IQ (minimum of 120 on the Armed Forces Qualifying Test) and a college diploma. Graduation from OCS involves further training, testing, and achievements, as well as demonstrated leadership skills. Not all OCS candidates graduate to become officers. Company combat officers are usually about age 24. The selection criteria ensure that they have relatively high IQs, coping skills, and educational attainment. With these characteristics, which are signs of good functioning, they are likely to have a view of the future possibilities for themselves (beyond being combatants) and to have attained the formal operations stage and stable identities. Their late-adolescent development has been completed, and they are now young adults.

To be a private in the U.S. army or its equivalent in other branches of the military in wartime, an individual must be age 18, with at least a low-average IQ and a third-grade reading ability. In peacetime, a high-school diploma or its equivalent is the educational standard for acceptance as a private. During war, the requirements for enlistment may be reduced; for example, remedial reading may be offered, if needed.

Due to the differences in selection criteria, the average OR in combat is about age 18 or 19, that is, at the beginning stage of late adolescent development. As a result of their younger age and the less stringent requirements for them compared to officers, they are more likely to have lower IQs (on average), concrete thinking, fewer coping skills, less education, fewer (or no) goals for the future, less ability to translate their potential into a meaningful future orientation vocationally, and foreclosed identities.

Thus, officers and enlistees are distinctively different. Officers have decreased dependency, increased learning opportunities, the capacity for self-observation, consolidation of character, a sense of independence and autonomy. Officers have had the opportunity to try out different ego ideals and have a completed sense of identity. In contrast, very few OR have attained these developmental milestones. Table 1 presents an hypothesized comparison of factors involved in consolidation of personality by company-grade military officers and by OR.

Table 2 is a speculative comparison of the completion of the tasks of adolescence by company-grade military officers and by OR. The officers are considered to have consolidated the personality, attained the development of intimacy, acquired a time perspective, and harmonized the ego, superego, and ego ideal. In contrast, few of the OR have achieved these milestones.

CASE ILLUSTRATION

Despite good grades, this 17-year-old left high school in his senior year to join the Navy early in World War II. He served as a machine gunner in landing craft to clear the beaches of the enemy before the

TABLE 1

THEORETICAL COMPARISON OF FACTORS INVOLVED IN CONSOLIDATION
OF PERSONALITY, BY MILITARY RANK

Factors	Officers	Other Ranks (OR)
Dependency	No	Yes
Learning opportunity	Yes	No
Capacity for self-observation	Yes	No
Consolidation of character	Yes	No
Sense of independence	Yes	No
Autonomy	Yes	No
Opportunity for identification with mentors	Yes	Yes
Trying out different ego ideals	Yes	No
Completion of sense of identity	Yes	Yes

316

TABLE 2

THEORETICAL COMPARISON OF COMPLETION OF TASKS
OF LATE ADOLESCENCE BY MILITARY RANK

Tasks	Officers	Other Ranks (OR)
Consolidation of identity	Yes	No
Separation from parents	Yes	No
Achievement of genital primacy	Yes	No
Attainment of sexual identity	Yes	Yes
Development of a time perspective	Yes	No
Capacity for intimacy	Yes	No
Development of friendships	Yes	Yes
Harmony of ego, superego, and ego ideal	Yes	No

assault on islands in the South Pacific, then he was helpless in the landing craft while the Marines disembarked. During and after five such assaults, he experienced a great deal of fear and anxiety, because he was a sitting target who witnessed a great deal of death and mutilation. After the fifth landing, his agitation led to a diagnosis of combat fatigue, a stay in the sick bay, and hospitalization for several years in naval and Veterans Administration hospitals.

After wandering about unemployed for several more years, he obtained an undemanding low-skill job. Then he married and had a stable family life. He was withdrawn and eschewed alcohol and socialization. His main involvements were work, the VA clinic for combat PTSD, and occasionally going fishing. In his sessions he often spoke of being "too young, immature, and unprepared at 17" for military service. He felt that he had done his duty but wished it had never happened, because it "messed up" his life, and he still suffered from the symptoms of PTSD 55 years later.

This case highlights incomplete late adolescent development with foreclosure of identity during military service. His sense of identity was incomplete, and he had no ideas about a future vocation during or after military service.

It seems that these features, combined with his PTSD, led to character problems. He had not achieved identity consolidation, genital primacy, a time perspective, the capacity for intimacy, or harmonized his psychic

317

apparatus while in, or for many years after, military service. While on active military duty and in psychiatric hospitals, his dependency increased.

CONCLUSIONS

The literature and clinical observation support the first hypothesis that company grade military officers have a much lower incidence of combat PTSD compared to other ranks. Enlisted men appear to be more vulnerable to combat stress. The data confirm the hypothesis that due to about five years difference in age between company grade officers and enlisted personnel, the former have completed late adolescent development. Alongside this is the fact of the stringent selection process for military officers, which requires them to have high IQ, a college degree, and demonstrated leadership skills. These features are not found frequently in enlisted personnel.

These developmental and psychosocial differences appear to be positive factors for company-grade commissioned officers to have a lower incidence of combat-related PTSD than enlisted personnel. Further research is indicated on officers and enlistees by age and rank, pre- and postcombat, to confirm these hypotheses. Given the preponderance of older adolescents and young adults among soldiers in combat, the effects of combat trauma on this age group are of particular interest to adolescent psychiatrists.

REFERENCES

American Psychiatric Association. (1980), *Diagnostic and Statistical Manual,* 3rd ed. (*DSM-III*). Washington, DC: American Psychiatric Association.

———— (1994), *Diagnostic and Statistical Manual,* 4th ed. (*DSM-IV*). Washington, DC: American Psychiatric Association.

Blos, P. (1968), Character formation in adolescence. *The Psychoanalytic Study of the Child,* 23:245–268. New Haven, CT: Yale University Press.

Boman, B. (1982), The Vietnam veteran ten years on. *Austral. New Zealand J. Psychiat.,* 16:107–127.

Bond, T. C. (1976), The why of fragging. *Am. J. Psychiat.,* 133:1328–1331.

Borus, J. F. (1976), The re-entry transition of Vietnam veterans. In: *Social Psychiatry in Military Service,* ed. A. L. Goldman & D. R. Siegel. Beverly Hills, CA: Sage.

Bourne, P. G. (1972), The Vietnam veteran: Psychological casualties. *Psychiat. Med.,* 3:23–27.

Bower, B. H. & Sivers, H. (1998), Cognitive impact of traumatic events. *Develop. & Psychopath,* 10:625–653.

Brailey, K., Constans, J. I., Vasterling, J. J., Borges, A. & Sutker, P. E. (1997), Assessment of intellectual resources in the Gulf War. *Assessment,* 4:51–59.

Bremner, J. D., Randall, P., Scott, T. M., Bronen, R. A., Seibyl, J. P., Southwick, S. M., Delaney, R. C., McCarthy, G., Charney, D. S. & Innis, R. B. (1995), MRI-based measurement of hippocampal volume in patients with combat-related posttraumatic stress disorder. *Amer. J. Psychiat.,* 152:973–981.

————— ————— Vermetten, E., Staib, L., Bronen, R. A., Mazuro, C., Capelli, S., McCarthy, G., Innis, R. B. & Charney, D. S. (1997), Magnetic resonance imaging-based measurement of hippocampal volume in posttraumatic stress disorder related to childhood physical and sexual abuse—A preliminary report. *Biol. Psychiat.,* 41:23–32.

Buhler, C. (1968), The course of human life as a psychological problem. *Human Develop.,* 11:184–200.

Carmil, D. & Carel, R. S. (1986), Emotional distress and satisfaction in life among Holocaust survivors—A community of survivors and controls. *Psychol. Med.,* 16:141–149.

Copen, E. G. (1964), Psychiatric service to military personnel in Vietnam. In: *Proceedings of Social and Preventitive Psychiatry Short Course.* Washington, DC: Walter Reed Army Institute of Research.

Dulit, E. (1972), Adolescent thinking à la Piaget: The formal stage. *J. Youth & Adol.,* 1:281–301.

Egendorf, A., Kadushin, C., Laufer, R. S., Rothbart, G. & Sloan, L. (1981), *Legacies of Vietnam.* Vol. 1. Springfield, VA: U.S. Department of Commerce, National Technical Information Service.

Erikson, E. H. (1959), *Identity and the Life Cycle.* New York: International Universities Press.

Glass, A. J. (1958), Observations upon the epidemiology of mental illness in troops during warfare. In: *Symposium on Preventative and*

Social Psychiatry. Washington, DC: Walter Reed Army Institute of Research.

———— (1969), Introduction. In: *The Psychology and Physiology of Stress,* ed. P. G. Bourne. New York: Academic Press.

Grinker, R. R. & Spiegel, J. P. (1945), *Men Under Stress.* Philadelphia: Blakiston.

———— Willerman, B., Bradley, A. D. & Fastovsky, A. (1946), A study of psychological predisposition to the development of operational fatigue: I. In officer personnel. II. In enlisted flying personnel. *Amer. J. Orthopsychiat.,* 16:191–274.

Honig, R. G., Grace, M. C., Lindy, J. D., Newman, C. J. & Titchener, J. L. (1999), Assessing the long-term effects of disaster occurring during childhood and adolescence. In: *Trauma and Adolescence,* ed. M. Sugar. Madison, CT: International Universities Press, pp. 203–224.

Koenig, N. (1964), Chronic or persisting identity diffusion. *Amer. J. Psychiat.,* 120:1081–1084.

Krell, R. (1990), Holocaust survivors: A clinical perspective. *Psychiat. J. Univ. Ottawa,* 15:18–21.

Kulka, R. A., Schlenger, W. E., Fairbank, J. A., Hough, R. L., Jordan, E. K., Marmar, C. P. & Grady, D. S. (1990), *Trauma and the War Generation.* New York: Brunner/Mazel.

Lee, K. A., Vaillant, G. E., Torrey, W. D. & Elder, G. (1995), A 50-year prospective study of the psychological sequelae of World War II combat. *Amer. J. Psychiat.,* 152:516–522.

Levav, I., Greenfield, H. & Baruch, E. (1979), Psychiatric combat reactions during the Yom Kippur War. *Amer. J. Psychiat.,* 136:637–641.

McDuff, D. R. & Johnson, J. L. (1992), Classification and characteristics of army stress casualties during Operation Desert Storm. *Hosp. Commun. Psychiat.,* 43:812–815.

Mellsop, G. W., Duraiappah, V. & Priest, A. J. (1995), Psychiatric casualties in the Pacific during WWII: Servicemen hospitalized in a Brisbane mental hospital. *M. J. Australia,* 163:619–621.

Nadler, A. & Ben-Shushan, D. (1989), Forty years later: Long-term consequences of massive traumatization as manifested by Holocaust survivors from the city and the kibbutz. *J. Consult. Clin. Psychol.,* 57:287–293.

Neugarten, B. L. (1969), Continuities and discontinuities of psychological issues in adult life. *Human Dev.,* 12:121–130.

Piaget, J. (1972), Intellectual evolution from adolescence to adulthood. *Human Dev.,* 15:1–12.

Rivers, W. H. R. (1923), *Conflicts and Dreams.* London: Kegan Paul.

Robins, S., Rapport-Bar-Sever, M. & Rapport, J. (1994), The present state of people who survived the Holocaust as children. *Acta Psychiat. Scand.,* 89:242–245.

Ryn, Z. (1990), The evolution of mental disturbances in the concentration camp syndrome (K–Z syndrome). *Genet. Soc. Gen. Psychol. Monog.,* 116:21–36.

Sapolsky, R. (1996), Why stress is bad for your brain. *Science,* 273:749–750.

Shay, J. (1994), *Achilles' Heel in Vietnam.* New York: Touchstone.

Solomon, Z., Mikulincer, M. & Hobfoll, S. F. (1986), Effects of social support and battle intensity on loneliness and breakdown during combat. *J. Pers. & Soc. Psychol.,* 51:1269–1276.

Southwick, S. M., Yehuda, R. & Giller, E. L. (1993), Personality disorders in treatment-seeking combat veterans with post-traumatic stress disorder. *Amer. J. Psychiat.,* 150:1020–1023.

Steiner, M. & Neumann, M. (1978), Traumatic neurosis and social support in the Yom Kippur War returnees. *Milit. Med.,* 143:866–868.

Sugar, M. (1968), Normal adolescent mourning. *Amer. J. Psychother.,* 22:258–269.

———— (1999), Severe physical trauma in adolescence. In: *Trauma and Adolescence,* ed. M. Sugar. Madison, CT: International Universities Press, pp. 183–201.

van der Kolk, B., Greenberg, M., Boyd, H. & Krystal, J. (1985), Inescapable shock, neurotransmitters, and addiction to trauma: Toward a psychobiology of posttraumatic stress. *Biol. Psychiat.,* 20:314–325.

Yealland, L. R. (1918), *Hysterical Disorders of Warfare.* London: Macmillan.

PART IV

CLINICAL
CONSIDERATIONS

13 THE SELF-DECEPTIONS AND MISCONCEPTIONS OF PSYCHIATRISTS, PSYCHOLOGISTS, AND OTHER MENTAL HEALTH PROFESSIONALS

SAUL LEVINE

In this scientific and managed-care era, one could expect that the current clinical practices of mental health professionals would be entirely data based and outcome substantiated. Of course, this is still far from reality, for many reasons, not the least of which are the inherent difficulties in rigorously, reliably, and validly evaluating those practices. But numerous practitioners nonetheless feel that their own unique techniques are unequivocally efficacious, and they act as if they have achieved the psychotherapeutic Holy Grail. Are they deceiving themselves, or others?

The word deception connotes or implies the active and conscious misrepresentation of reality with the express purpose of manipulating or deceiving others. Self-deception, on the other hand, like myths or misconceptions, has a less malevolent connotation (Mele, 1997; Trivers, 2000). Instead of duplicity, we are witnessing lack of knowledge, cognitive dissonance (Festinger and Carlsmith, 1959), or even denial and defenses, and entrenched beliefs, that enable individuals to unconsciously act in a manner that protects and enhances their own senses of self. Although usually not volitionally deceitful, the self-deceptions of some psychiatrists, psychologists, and other mental health professionals might well enable these "providers" (a decided minority of all mental health professionals) to espouse attitudes, behave therapeutically, or promulgate expert opinions in ways that are less than justified or not substantiated by empirical research.

MYTHS ABOUT PSYCHOPATHOLOGY

Let us review some of the myths and misconceptions that may have crept into some of our professional beliefs and actions, or into the way we are perceived.

Sturm und Drang in Adolescence Is Inevitable

There are still some mental health professionals (and certainly, many parents) who cling to this long-discredited notion. First postulated by Anna Freud (1966) a half century ago, it became a sacred belief and part of the professional teaching of many psychotherapists. But its roots lay in ancient cultural anlages. Hesiod complained:

> Our adolescents now seem to love luxury. They have bad manners and contempt for authority. They show disrespect for adults and spend their time hanging around places gossiping with one another. . . . They are ready to contradict their parents, monopolize the conversation in company, eat gluttonously, and tyrannize their teachers.

Even Shakespeare (1610) is often quoted: "I would there were no age between ten and three and twenty, or that youth would sleep out the rest for there is nothing in the between but getting wenches with child, wronging the ancientry, stealing and fighting" (*A Winter's Tale,* Act 2, Scene 2).

Thus, adolescents have long been seen as inevitably tormented, wanton, selfish, and irresponsible. Nevertheless, longitudinal studies in different cultures have confirmed that most adolescents go through those years with fairly smooth and stable trajectories. It is an unfortunate myth that is disrespectful to that entire age group, the vast majority of whom progress relatively seamlessly and remarkably productively (Offer and Sabshin, 1984; Levine, 2000). It is also a dangerous belief: it is a self-fulfilling prophecy, an example of how expectations can and do shape behavior. Adolescents, expected to get into trouble, are more likely to use drugs, explode, act out, get pregnant, and so on by way of fulfilling their parents' and society's expectations. In addition,

326

not only does this purview enable some behaviors to be ignored or excused as merely stage-related, but it can minimize pathological symptomatology. If it is expected that adolescents are by definition troubled beings, how is one to discern serious symptomatology and disorders?

Early Destitution Inevitably Leads to Later and Permanent Emotional Scarring and Disability

Prevailing conventional wisdom has been that early life deprivation can predict later adult suffering and scarring with absolute certainty. That this is not, in fact, the case has become abundantly clear via a variety of new research studies (Skeels, 1966; Garmezy, 1991; Richters and Martinez, 1993). Although early trauma can be a severe impediment, there are myriad accounts of people who have been born into lives of abject destitution, yet who have grown into mature, stable, productive, and generative adults (Brown, 1965).

Even children who were born into circumstances of tragic loss, war, brutality, forces majeurs, abuse, disease, disfigurement, and severe deprivation have developed and evolved into productive, generative, fulfilled and optimistic adults (Werner and Smith, 1992; Levine and Ion, 2001). There are known personal and social risk factors, to be sure, which can contribute to the more likely occurrence of psychological problems and obstacles, potentially leading to frailty and failure. But the obverse is equally valid, and, in fact, has much more valence in eventual maturation: human beings are remarkably resilient. Personal and social resources (both internal and external) are extremely influential in enhancing one's life and overcoming adversity (Rutter, 1990).

The Certitude and Absolutism of Diagnoses: DSM-IV as a Sacred Text

The authors of the series of *Diagnostic and Statistical Manuals* (*DSMs*) have done our professions a major service, bringing organizational coherence, uniform standards, and elucidated criteria to the heretofore confusing state of psychiatric nosology and diagnosis (American Psychiatric Association, 1994). *DSM* was the first significant attempt to impose uniformity, reliability, and validity on defined aberrant behaviors. It moved us away from unsubstantiated etiologies and toward

327

rigorous description and documentation. It has furthered the cause of consensual validation of diagnosis and the study and evaluation of the efficacy of various interventions.

As salutary as the *DSM* has been in its accomplishments and aspirations, and however historically and scientifically based the motivation behind it, the exclusive or undue reliance on *DSM-IV* definitions as our sole guide to disease entities has made us prisoners of our human need to label and categorize. Most of the diagnoses have been based on consensual perceptions of clinical psychiatrists and psychologists and not on known causations. Furthermore, many of the diagnoses are representative of spectrum or continuum disorders, in which symptoms, signs, feelings, and behaviors deemed normative in some situations take on a pathological cast when they exceed a certain arbitrary number, intensity, and longevity, based on subjective professional consensual validation.

Arbitrary designation (as pathological) differs markedly from country to country, and even from jurisdiction to jurisdiction in the same country. What is deemed pathological by one group of mental health professionals harboring certain cultural norms and expectations may be viewed in a markedly different way by another group of colleagues elsewhere. Hence the remarkable geographic differences in prevalence and incidence of ADHD, for example (Mann et al., 1992; Bird, 2001). Is identity-related disorder really a certified, diagnosable psychiatric condition? The number of young children currently being diagnosed with bipolar disorder is astounding, given that, 10 years ago, it was rarely used as a diagnosis for anyone other than adults (Taylor et al., 1991). Is a repetitively misbehaving youth oppositionally defiant, conduct disordered, behaviorally disruptive, antisocial, merely misbehaving ("Boys will be boys"), or a bad kid? (See "He's not bad, he's mad.") Are the characterological and personality disorders epidemiologically substantiated as discrete entities? The specific diagnoses of personality disorders are rife with personal subjectivity and controversy, not only as to their reliability and validity as distinct medical pathological entities, but also in the realm of personal responsibility and accountability for untoward behavior. Hence, we unfortunately see use of these terms as epithets at times, rather than as clinical diagnostic phenomena.

Pathologizing of Behaviors in America

We seemed to have reached the stage where many feelings and thoughts that are unusual or problematic to individuals, and many other behaviors that are somehow troublesome to others, are described, categorized, and classified to fit into a *DSM-IV* diagnostic category. If fully 20% of our population have diagnosable mental illnesses in a single year (Robins and Regier, 1996), we have what is tantamount to an epidemic; even the Great Flu of 1917 did not permeate the population to this extent.

When so many of our male children are on medication to control their distractibility and lack of *zitzflaish* (ability to sit still), what exactly are we saying about our expectations of youngsters, or about our inability to command their respect and attention? As mentioned above, the prevalence rates of ADHD (and its drug treatment), bipolar disorders, and borderline personality disorders are widely disparate (see the section on *DSM* as sacred text). When so many millions around the world are labeled as having some form of depressive disorder and treated with serotonin reuptake inhibitors, what are we saying about the validity of that diagnosis? Individuals who have suffered abuse or serious loss in their early years and have committed heinous acts too often have their legal culpability or responsibility rationalized on the basis of early suffering and the inevitably inferred and ascribed diagnosis of posttraumatic stress disorder (PTSD). Merely being the child of an alcoholic, or having witnessed or experienced early abuse, is too often used not only in courts of law, but even as a way of defining the totality of individual identities ("I am a child of . . . "). We should not be complicit in encouraging the sum total of an individual's self-image to be defined by what we have labeled, either developmentally or diagnostically, a psychiatric disorder.

The repetitive and compulsive use of drugs or alcohol and now, by extension, other so-called addictive behaviors (eating, sex, gambling, and so on) are also removed from personal volition and the realm of individual responsibility, and pathologized. Then credence is given for explaining, rationalizing, or even excusing untoward, uncivil, or destructive actions. In the guise of compassion, understanding, and treating, we too often infantilize, tolerate, indulge, and obfuscate.

"He's Not Bad, He's Mad"

Bernstein and Sondheim caught the essence of this dilemma accurately (and brilliantly) in the insightful lyrics of Officer Krupke's song in *West Side Story*—"We're not depraved, we're deprived!"

When is a youth's destructive behavior seen as pathological, when is she just misbehaving, and when is she being bad? The designation of some identical behaviors, even in the same city, as merely trouble-some or as normative; as conduct disorder, or oppositional defiant disorder; or as just plain bad—or even evil—is seen repetitively. Al-though *DSM-IV* carefully delineates a number of diagnostic states that could account for misdemeanors, even we too often use personal, societal, and cultural factors in our own lives as the basis for characteriz-ing misbehavior.

It is clear that our beliefs cloud or determine our perceptions. To what extent do we excuse wanton behavior by labeling, diagnosing, and pathologizing it (Levine, 1997)? When we say, "not guilty by reason of insanity," what is the message we are giving to the victim's family and to society? Guilt (not as in feeling remorseful, but rather as being responsible and accountable) can and should be determined before we interject our imperfect rationales, postulations, and diagnoses. McNaughton and Durham Rules notwithstanding, even a clear lack of competence should not imply that a perpetrator, even a juvenile, is not to be held responsible for a heinous act.

"Expert" Forensic Opinions

It is especially in the courtroom or in the realms of adversarial litigation that the depiction of mental health professionals as hired guns is most frequent and salient. This is a consequence of a frequent and unseemly scenario: equally reputable mental health professionals hired by con-testing parties as experts in civil suits, or by prosecutors and defense in courts of law or in depositions, offering equally erudite and rational opinions that are diametrically opposed.

This is certainly seen in the validly debated mad versus bad disputes (see "He's Not Bad, He's Mad"), but it has now become ubiquitous in injury suits, posttraumatic stress disorder evaluations, criminal cases, divorce and custody disputes, diagnostic and clinical management con-flicts, medical and labor compensation conflicts and deliberations, com-petitive medical negligence suits, and any other potentially disputatious areas of human endeavor that easily lend themselves to involvement of psychological influences. Aside from the egregious conclusion that experts can be bought, this myth points to the lack of rigor in diagnoses. There is little room for absolutism in our clinical deliberations concern-ing etiology, diagnosis, and treatment. The conceit of our infallibility is not only pernicious to the credibility of our work; it also raises legitimate concerns among the public about the validity and worthiness of even some of our most cogent opinions (Levine, 1983; Faust and Ziskin, 1988).

MYTHS ABOUT INTERVENTION

Psychopharmacology über Alles

The myth referred to here, as practiced and promulgated by some practitioners, is that there is no better mood, cognition, and behavior modifier than some form or other of psychotropic medication. These clinicians see all aberrant or troublesome behaviors as organically based symptoms and syndromes that can be ameliorated or eradicated by highly specific pharmacological agents. In the extreme form of this perspective, they indeed see no need for any type of psychosocial intervention. Prescription drugs are considered to be the universal panacea for psychiatric and psychological ills, and clinical trial data are used to substantiate this bias. The problem is, of course, that very little of the latter empirical evidence is clear and unequivocal, especially when the validity of many of our current diagnoses have recently been under scrutiny and debate. There is no doubt that medication can be of remarkable utility in many instances, but very seldom is it maximally efficacious without psychosocial intervention, support, counseling, psychotherapy, and so on (Thase et al., 1997; Van Balkom et al., 1997; Walsh et al., 1997; De Oliveira, 1998; Fava et al., 1998; Peterson and Mitchell, 1999).

There are even some psychiatric practitioners who have portable functional neuroimaging equipment in their offices and claim to be able to prescribe (based on their cogent study of the resultant scans and their expert knowledge of the current literature) esoteric medication with exactitude, certainty, and confidence. (Is this a scan or a scam?) They claim to be able to correlate observed discrete and pathognomonic neuroanatomical changes with behavioral or affective symptoms and signs, and to prescribe accordingly. (Would that the current state of our craft were so.) And, most recently, there have been similarly premature and grandiose (if not dishonest) claims of pathognomonic genetic markers for common psychiatric disorders and their medical treatment—at considerable cost to patients and families, I might add.

Psychoanalytic Therapies über Alles

Although their numbers are considerably fewer than in decades past, there are still some doctrinaire true believers who look with disdain and derision at other forms of psychotherapy, considering them to be ersatz or inferior (for example, cognitive-behavioral, family, group, transactional, short-term therapy, and so on). Aside from the fact that there are precious few studies supporting grandiose claims of the efficacy of pristine psychoanalysis, these practitioners still hold to a blind and abiding belief in the supremacy of their theory and practice. Even more so, their condescending view of medication is that it serves as a potential adulteration of the therapeutic process. They see the advent of other modalities, and certainly any constraint on unlimited psychoanalysis, as unwarranted interference in their professional autonomy and function. They feel that theirs is the only real way to genuinely transform troubled personalities and individuals. The paradox is that it is the most affluent, educated, sophisticated, urbane—and healthy—individuals who gravitate to these therapies. Yet, there have been far too many depressed individuals, for example, in long-term psychoanalytic therapies, who have not had the option of getting appropriate medication, and who have languished on the couches of some of these practitioners for unconscionable lengths of time (Dawes, 1994). There is now ample evidence that psychotherapies of various kinds can be extremely effective and can augment pharmacological treatment (see section on psychopharmacology). Aside from substantiated and specific techniques (of cognitive–behavioral therapy, for example), there are nonspecific factors that contribute to patient and client improvement (Strupp, 1989; Frank, 1993).

Wraparound Services for Troubled Youth and Their Families Are Unequivocally Clinically Effective, Save Money, and Should Be Immediately Implemented Universally

The latest mental health services campaign in child and adolescent psychiatry taken on with the zeal of proselytization is the so-called wraparound movement. This refers to simultaneous and multidimensional intervention with a severely emotionally disturbed child and his or her family, by all the key stakeholders in the child's development and improvement. This team would always include, literally (or figuratively) around the table the parents, school personnel, case coordinator or manager, mental health professionals, and anyone else involved with that child's specific areas of concern (e.g., recreation, fiscal support, child welfare, pediatrics, counseling, juvenile justice, and so on).

Theoretically, such a comprehensive approach makes a great deal of sense. We have too often seen children trapped in separate silos of intervention by virtue of their portal of entry to the system of care (e.g., juvenile justice, mental health, education, social services), with no integration or cooperation among different caretakers or professionals. And parents are often left out of the planning and discourse or are totally unsupported with their overwhelming and related problems.

The truth is not that wraparound is a useless endeavor; there are some early promising results, especially with antisocial youth and seriously troubled families (Henggeler et al., 1996; Kazdin and Wassell, 2000). Rather, it is the grandiose claim made by fervent proponents of this movement that causes difficulties for providers, policymakers, and social scientists. The fact is that current empirical research data are equivocal concerning any long-term clinical difference in amelioration, efficacy, or outcomes with wraparound (Bickman, 1996; Levine, 1999). Furthermore, the oft-repeated mantra of saving money is self-defeating. If not enough money is invested at the front end, or if the major rationale for implementation of wraparound programs is to save public mental health expenditures (on hospitalization, for example), these programs cannot succeed. It may well be that a properly and carefully organized and instituted program will have its most decided and beneficial effects well down the road in the child's development. Furthermore, these programs, if they are to be done well, are expensive, but they may be more than worth it, if they are not set up with severe cost and resource constraints a priori.

Unequivocal, Absolute Data-Based Outcomes

The managed care industry, as well as most levels of government (federal, state, county) have mandated voluminous prospective and follow-up outcome measures to evaluate and measure the effectiveness of various modalities and interventions (California Mental Health Planning Council, 1997). There are those who believe that the mandated outcome measures are, in themselves, highly standardized, reliable,

333

valid and foolproof, particularly in the realm of child and adolescent behavioral health services. Outcome measures are too often used as mantras and cudgels, so much so that there is a perception that a therapeutic Holy Grail has been achieved. A plethora of tests and measures is then instituted, and the collected results become the crucial determinants of utilization, performance, and efficacy. Although the theory behind this impetus is laudatory, the validity of the measures in particular and their real life applicability and utility still leave much to be desired (Breda, 1996; Bickman et al., 1998; Kessler and Mroczek, 2000; Garland, Kruse, and Aarons, in press). We used to criticize the automatic imposition of a clinical approach solely on the basis of the practitioner's beliefs, biases, and anecdotal reports; now we institute so-called best practices, too often based on inadequate data gleaned in doctrinaire fashion from a battery of mandated written evaluative scores.

Nihilism—Nothing Works

There are still cynics and naysayers, even in our professions, who question the validity of any claims, scientific or otherwise, that psychiatric and psychological disorders really exist, or that aberrant behavior can (or should) be modified or manipulated by psychiatric or psychological means. Their pernicious view is that any behavior that is deemed to be aberrant or problematic is solely based on volitional self-indulgence, arrogance, or insensitivity. They are, in general, impatient with those who cannot conform to society's standards of demeanor and propriety. They tend to view with suspicion any psychotherapeutic endeavor; changes in society or directive interventions are more to their liking. Widely disparate theoretical stances in this genre represent perspectives such as these: There is no such thing as mental illness (Szasz, 1974); madness merely reflects an appropriate and normative, even healthy, adaptation to a sick society (Laing, 1991); psychotherapeutic intervention is tyrannical (Masson, 1988).

Prevention Programs Are a Waste of Time, Money, Effort, and Resources

Contrary to the fatalistic pronouncements of some cynical mental health professionals, we do have excellent evidence that comprehensively and properly done, sufficiently funded, and longitudinally pursued prevention and early-intervention programs do, in fact, have remarkably successful short- and long-term effects, influences, and outcomes. Some prevention and early intervention programs have been shown to optimize the environment for children and adolescents and to greatly diminish the appearance of self-destructive or antisocial behaviors (Zeigler, Taussig, and Black, 1992; Henggeler et al., 1996; Karoly, 1999; Schorr, 2000).

Not only are these programs effective for targeted symptoms, syndromes, or behaviors (e.g., violence, scholastic achievement, sexual acting out, vandalism, teen pregnancies, substance abuse), but generic improvement is the rule rather than the exception. Enthusiastic, energetic programs that, in addition to providing classes and lessons directed at the miscreant or offensive behaviors, are also designed to involve and support the family, implement strong educational enhancement, provide necessary medical and psychological care, and use intensive case management, usually show a significant reduction in other (nontargeted) behaviors that have been awry.

The documented efficacy of prevention should serve as a wake-up call to our policymakers and leaders. A significant investment of resources at the front end of life will indubitably pay off immense generic long-term dividends for society as a whole in later years. The crucial question is whether we have the motivation to implement these programs. From a merely monetary perspective, prevention programs are initially very expensive to institute, implement, and pursue, but they will save us enormous amounts of money in the long run. The oft-seen stories of success tend to culminate in adults who are law-abiding, gainfully employed, tax-paying, generative, and productive citizens. To put this another way, they (as adults) tend not to be unemployed, on welfare, institutionalized, incarcerated, on drugs, or dangerous. It is well-nigh time in America to institute these programs.

Mental Health Professionals Have No Useful Role to Play in the Human Condition, that is, in Existential (Philosophical) or Religious (Spiritual) and Ethical (Moral) Issues

Except by a relative few of our colleagues, the aforementioned issues are not considered within our purview or expertise. None of these issues

335

is mentioned in the realm or domain of *DSM-IV*, except as a potential symptom or pathological entity (e.g., religiosity, cults). Many feel that these concepts smack of deism and theology and certainly have no place in scientific (data-based) discourse, research, or interventions.

Yet, there is overwhelming evidence that most human beings hunger for comfort, solace, and fulfillment in these domains. If millions of normal people are searching for beliefs that are of profound meaning to them, should not this be an area of our concern and study? Is it not remarkable to the reader that there are many more Americans in various forms of alternative and spiritual healing experiences than in all traditional psychotherapies combined? If life is, in part, a quest, shouldn't we, of all people, be playing a major role in that search for meaning?

We are avowed experts in the areas of behavior, feelings, symptoms, syndromes, adaptations, deviance, dysfunction, and pathology, yet have we so little to say about matters of crucial importance to humanity such as existential issues, evil versus good in humanity, love and hate, and morality? Can and should we only involve ourselves in difficult existential dilemmas solely on the basis of implied or apparent psychopathology? Surely we should not shy away from the word soul in working with our patients or in contributing to complex deliberations about behavior, motivation, and ethical conundrums.

To the extent that human beings have an overriding belief system (beyond subsistence, materialism, and so on), and a loftier raison d'être bringing some enobling meaning to their lives, and to which they feel that they are integral members of a group with similar values, their quality of living is perceived by them as significantly enhanced (Frankel, 1984; Friend and Editors of *Life*, 1991; Levine, 2000).

MYTHS OF MANAGED CARE

Hierarchical Status and Worth of Mental Health Professionals

If one were to rate perceived competence and effectiveness of mental health professionals solely on the basis of their relative incomes, then clearly psychiatrists are deemed to be the best, and psychologists are next on the totem pole, followed by licensed clinical social workers, marriage and family therapists, and counselors. Paradoxically, in the contemporary world of managed care, the for-profit health maintenance organizations (HMOs) have chosen to make decisions that fly in the face of this fallacious logic. They systemically choose as their preferred providers of psychotherapeutic and counseling services those disciplines and professions at the (fiscal) lower end of this conventional-wisdom hierarchy. Only a cynic would say that these fonts of wisdom and seers of medical and psychological expertise (the HMOs) would select providers solely on the basis of who costs less. They must believe, then, that in terms of relative efficacy and outcomes, the data are at best equivocal. Using standard outcome measures, there is scarcely any discernible difference in quality and effects of psychotherapy on patients and clients between the different levels of therapist disciplines or training (Stein and Lambert, 1984; Smith and Sechrest, 1991; Dawes, 1994; Berman and Norton, 1995). Perhaps it has more to do with our limited abilities to assess and measure the process and results of psychotherapies, but there are no studies in the domain of psychotherapy that unequivocally demonstrate that this cost-based hierarchy has any real-world validity.

Patient/Client Satisfaction and the Myth of Clinical Success

"If my patients are satisfied, my work must be good." The mantra of patient satisfaction in HMO-oriented health care is an unavoidable consequence of unfettered competition for market share and profit margins. Of course, we all want our patients to be satisfied with the quality of care they receive (in terms of improved comfort, amelioration of symptoms, and successful outcomes), the manner in which they are treated (respectfully, with adequate time and attention, with personal interest), and the logistics of their care (immediacy of phone response, appointments scheduled in the near future, lack of inordinate sojourns in the waiting room).

But elevating the criteria of patient satisfaction to the level of apotheosis of care can be extremely misleading and even destructive (Levine, 1985; Young, Nicholson, and David, 1995; Stallard, 1996; LaSala, 1997; Staniszewska and Ahmed, 1999; Garland, Saltzman, and Aarons, 2000). There are many consumers of treatment who express respect, loyalty, and even adulation for their doctors/therapists/healers, in spite of the public knowledge that the particular object of their admiration is incompetent, negligent, or dangerous. There have even been public demonstrations in support of various practitioners who have been charged and indicted for various types of malpractice. Mere personal attestation by a large number of recipients of a healing or therapeutic service should not inevitably lead to the conclusion that the provider and his or her quality of work are meritorious.

Managed Care Ensures Quality of Psychotherapy

Anyone who believes this is clearly in need of not-for-profit, nonmanaged-care psychotherapy. Unfortunately, there are even such gullible or disingenuous individuals in our own professions, too often in the employ of for-profit HMOs. If there is any validity to Harry Stack Sullivan's important concept of engendering a therapeutic alliance between a therapist (or provider—an egregious term; see section on HMOs and medical terminology) and a patient (i.e., "covered life")—and there are now considerable empirical data in support of this (Sullivan, 1953; Frank, 1993; Bickman, 1996)—then it is important to note that managed care has systematically gone out of its way to destroy this extraordinarily vital aspect of psychotherapy. By curtailing and constricting the extent, meaningfulness, and continuity of involvement with our patients and clients, *time* (one of the very lifebloods of the therapeutic alliance) is egregiously exsanguinated.

Managed care was developed as an antidote to physicians' lack of fiscal accountability, profligate use of medications, expensive investigations, and doctrinaire and costly interventions having no basis in data of efficacy or successful outcomes. One might cynically say that there was a transfer of greed from some in the medical and related professions to rapacious for-profit insurance companies. Although there may have been a decided improvement in physicians' and therapists' awareness of the bottom line (and fiscal accountability as a result), there has also been a palpable and sad deterioration in patient care and in physicians' and other professionals' autonomy, and in this crucial element of our professions: the available time spent together by patients and therapists.

Managed Care and Medical Terminology

The for-profit managed care organizations have turned medical terminology on its head, using business terms to supplant medical ones:

338

1. Patients are now referred to as "covered lives."
2. Psychiatrists and psychologists are euphemistically called "providers."
3. Specific systems of care are replaced in discourse by "product lines."
4. "Market share" and "profitability" vie with clinical outcomes (and often win) as goals and criteria for success.

We in the health care professions, and our patients, are in the midst of a critical and potentially tragic time. It is inconceivable and unconscionable that this, the most affluent country in the world, in an era of unprecedented success and power, has a generic second-rate national health care delivery system. As good as the medical schools and physicians are, the blind fiscal management of health care, and the perception of service delivery as no better than an industrial product may prove disastrous for contemporary American medicine (and for society as a whole, because this dehumanizing of our basic relationships and functions permeates the entire fabric of our culture).

CONCLUSION

There are obviously other possible examples of our professions acting as if beliefs in our practice reflect absolute truths (e.g., validity of the Rorschach, or the so-called false memory syndrome). Nobody is accusing proponents of these questionable practices of malfeasance. Deception implies malevolence and manipulation; that is decidedly not the intention of this chapter. Rather, what I have attempted to demonstrate are examples of the best of intentions of some of our colleagues, gone awry.

It is clearly within our capabilities, our mandate, and our responsibility to ensure that dogma and doctrinaire thinking do not constrain and supersede our open communications, vigorous exchange of ideas, and (especially) empirically validated research. We must eschew zealous promulgation of magical avenues to complex cognitive, affective, behavioral, and existential questions. Our avowed talents for discourse, dialogue, and dialectic are never more important than in our professional attitudes, pronouncements, and behavior. Even if it might make us uncomfortable, we must in our words and work continually put ourselves to the test of always seeking the closest approximation to reality. (Isn't this one of our hallowed mantras for patients?)

REFERENCES

American Psychiatric Association (1994), *Diagnostic and Statistical Manual of Mental Disorders,* 4th ed. (*DSM-IV*). Washington, DC: American Psychiatric Association.

Berman, J. S. & Norton, N. C. (1995), Does professional training make a therapist more effective? *Psych. Bull.,* 98:401–407.

Bickman, L. (1996), A continuum of care: More is not always better. *Amer. Psychol.,* 51:689–701.

——— Nurcombe, B., Townsend, C., Belle, M., Schut, J. L. & Karver, M. (1998), *Consumer Measurement Systems for Mental Health.* Brisbane, Australia & Nashville, TN: University of Queensland and Vanderbilt University.

Bird, H. R. (Submitted), The prevalence and cross-cultural validity of attention deficit hyperactivity disorder.

Breda, C. S. (1996), Methodological issues in evaluating mental health outcomes in managed care. *J. Ment. Health Admin.,* 15:1–18.

Brown, C. (1965), *Manchild in the Promised Land.* New York: Macmillan.

California Mental Health Planning Council (1997), *Performance Outcome Study: Wave 1 to Wave 2.* Sacramento, CA: California Mental Health Planning Council.

Dawes, R. M. (1994), *House of Cards: Psychology and Psychotherapy Built on Myth.* New York: Free Press.

De Oliveira, I. R. (1998), The treatment of unipolar major depression: Pharmacotherapy, cognitive behaviour therapy or both? *J. Clin. Pharmacy & Therapeutics,* 23(6):467–475.

Faust, D. & Ziskin, J. (1988), The expert witness in psychology and psychiatry. *Science,* 241:31–35.

Fava, G. A., Rafanelli, C., Grandi, S., Conti, S. & Bellaurdo, P. (1998), Prevention of recurrent depression with cognitive behavioral therapy: Preliminary findings. *Arch. Gen. Psychiat.,* 55:816–820.

Festinger, L. & Carlsmith, J. M. (1959), Cognitive dissonance. *J. Abnor. Soc. Psychol.,* 58:203–210.

Frank, J. D. (1993), *Persuasion and Healing,* 2nd ed. Baltimore: Johns Hopkins University Press.

Frankel, V. (1984), *Man's Search for Meaning.* New York: Simon & Schuster.

Freud, A. (1966), *The Ego and Mechanisms of Defense.* New York: International Universities Press.

Friend, D. & Editors of *Life* (1991), *The Meaning of Life.* Boston: Little, Brown.

Garland, A., Kruse, M. & Aarons, G. (In press), Clinicians and outcome measures: What's the use? *J. Behav. Health Serv. Res.*

—————— Saltzman, M. D. & Aarons, G. A. (2000), Adolescent satisfaction with mental health services: Development of a multidimensional scale. *Eval. Prog. Plan.,* 23:165–175.

Garmezy, N. (1991), Resilience and vulnerability to adverse developmental outcomes associated with poverty. *Amer. Behav. Scient.,* 34:416–430.

Henggeler, S. W., Pickrel, S. G., Brondino, M. J. & Crouch, J. L. (1996), Eliminating (almost) treatment dropout of substance abusing or dependent delinquents through home-based multi-systemic therapy. *Amer. J. Psychiat.,* 153:427–428.

Karoly, L. (1999), *Early Childhood Programs: Promoting Optimal Development.* Los Angeles: Rand Corporation.

Kazdin, A. E. & Wassell, G. (2000),. Predictors of barriers to treatment and therapeutic change in outpatient therapy for anti-social children and their families. *Mental Health Serv. Res.,* 2:28–40.

Kessler, R. C. & Mroczek, D. K. (2000), Measuring the effects of medical interventions. *Med. Care,* 33:109–119.

Laing, R. D. (1991), *The Divided Self.* London: Penguin.

LaSala, M. C. (1997), Client satisfaction: Consideration of correlates and response bias. *Families in Society,* 78:54–64.

Levine, S. (1983), The role of the mental health expert witness in family law disputes. *Can. J. Psychiat.,* 28:255–258.

—————— (1985), Who should do psychotherapy? *Amer. J. Soc. Psych.,* 5:60–65.

—————— (1997), The development of wickedness—from whence does evil stem? *Psychiat. Annals,* 27:617–623.

—————— (1999), Wraparound programs: A review of clinical roles, responsibilities, constraints, and possibilities, a report for the County of San Diego Health and Human Services Agency. Unpublished manuscript.

—————— (2000), The Tao and Talmud of adolescent trajectories: Being, belonging, believing, benevolence. *Adolescent Psychiatry.* 25:45–58. Hillsdale, NJ: The Analytic Press.

—————— & Ion, H. W. (2001), *Against Terrible Odds: Lessons in Resilience from Our Children.* Palo Alto, CA: Bull.

Mann, E. M., Ikeda, Y., Mueller, C. W., Takahashi, A., Tao, K. T., Humris, E., Li, B. L. & Chin, D. (1992), Cross-cultural differences in rating hyperactive-disruptive behaviors in children. *Amer. J. Psychiat.,* 149:1539–1542.

Masson, J. M. (1988), *Against Therapy: Emotional Tyranny and the Myth of Psychological Healing.* New York: Atheneum.

Mele, A. R. (1997), Real self-deception. *Behav. Brain Sci.,* 20(1):91–102.

Offer, D. & Sabshin, M. (1984), *Normality and the Life Cycle.* New York: Basic Books.

Peterson, C. B. & Mitchell, J. E. (1999), Psychosocial and pharmacological treatment of eating disorders: A review of research findings. *J. Clin. Psychol.,* 55:685–697.

Richters, J. & Martinez, P. E. (1993), Violent communities, family choices, and children's chances: An algorithm for improving the odds. *Dev. & Psychopath.,* 5:609–627.

Robins, L. N. & Regier, D. A. ed. (1996), *Psychiatric Disorders in America.* New York: Free Press.

Rutter, M. (1990), Psychosocial resilience and protective mechanisms. In: *Risk and Protective Factors in the Development of Psychopathology,* ed. J. E., Rolf, A. S. Master, D. Cicchetti, K. H. Nuechterlein, & S. Weintraub. New York: Cambridge University Press, pp. 181–214.

Schorr, L. (1988), *Within Our Reach: Breaking the Cycle of Disadvantage.* New York: Anchor Press.

Skeels, H. M. (1966), Adult status of children with contrasting early life experiences. *Monographs Soc. Res. Child Dev.,* 31:1–65.

Smith, B. & Sechrest, L. (1991), The treatment of aptitude X treatment interactions. *J. Cons. Clin. Psychol.,* 59:223–244.

Stallard, P. (1996), The role and use of consumer satisfaction surveys in mental health services. *J. Mental Health,* 5:333–348.

Staniszewska, S. & Ahmed, L. (1999), The concepts of expectation and satisfaction: Do they capture the way patients evaluate their care? *J. Adv. Nurs.,* 29:364–372.

Stein, D. M. & Lambert, M. J. (1984), On the relationship between therapist experience and psychotherapy outcome. *Clin. Psychol. Rev.,* 4:127–142.

Strupp, H. H. (1989), Psychotherapy: Can the practitioner learn from the researcher? *Amer. Psychol.,* 44:717–724.

Sullivan, H. S. (1953), *The Interpersonal Theory of Psychiatry.* New York: Norton.

Szasz, T. (1974), *The Myth of Mental Illness: Foundations of a Theory of Personal Conduct.* New York: Harper & Row.

Taylor, E., Sanberg, S., Thorley, G. & Giles, S. (1991), *The epidemiology of childhood hyperactivity.* Maudsley Monographs, #33. London: Oxford University Press.

Thase, M. E., Greenhouse, J. B., Frank, E., Reynolds, C. F. III, Pilkonis, P. A., Hurley, K., Grochocinski, V. & Kupfer, D. J. (1997), Treatment of major depression with psychotherapy or psychotherapy-pharmacotherapy combinations. *Arch. Gen. Psychiat.,* 54:1009–1015.

Trivers, R. (2000), The elements of a scientific theory of self-deception. *Ann. N.Y. Acad. Sci.,* 907:114–131.

Van Balkom, A. J., Bakker, A., Spinhoven, P., Blaauw, B. M., Smeenk, S. & Ruesink, B. (1997), A meta-analysis of the treatment of panic disorder with or without agoraphobia: A comparison of psychopharmacological, cognitive-behavioral, and combination treatments. *J. Nerv. Ment. Dis.,* 185:510–516.

Walsh, B. T., Wilson, G. T., Loeb, K. L., Devlin, M. J., Pike, K. M., Roose, S. P., Fleiss, J. & Waternaux, C. (1997), Medication and psychotherapy in the treatment of bulimia nervosa. *Amer. J. Psychiat.,* 154:523–531.

Werner, E. E. & Smith, R. S. (1992), *Overcoming the Odds: High-Risk Children from Birth to Adulthood.* Ithaca, NY: Cornell University Press.

Young, S. C., Nicholson, J. & David, M. (1995), An overview of issues in research on consumer satisfaction with child and adolescent mental health. *J. Child Fam. Stud.,* 4:219–238.

Zeigler, E., Taussig, C. & Black, K. (1992), Early childhood intervention: A promising preventative for juvenile delinquency. *Amer. Psychol.,* 47(8):997–1006.

14   ADOLESCENTS IN PSYCHOTHERAPY

THE IMPORTANCE OF THE BELIEF SYSTEM
OF THE FAMILY

JAMES H. GILFOIL

Psychotherapy has been studied extensively, and factors relevant to successful outcome such as (among others) motivation, a good therapeutic alliance, a skilled therapist, and "mutuality of expectation" (Heine and Trosman, 1960, pp. 275–278) between patient and therapist have been identified. Psychotherapy with adolescents, however, presents special problems. Not only do parents have to support treatment by encouraging it, but they also have to pay for it. At the same time, they are unlikely to see an immediate benefit, and in fact, bringing their son or daughter for therapy involves potential loss and narcissistic injury. Will they allow the adolescent to attach to someone else, that is, will they encourage the process of separation? Parents whose children are having problems tend to feel guilty and ashamed about what they unconsciously perceive to be their failure, and, consequently, they behave defensively in various ways. They may dump the kid on us, or conversely, try to control us as they have tried to control the child. In fact, there will always be some element of parental resistance, for the parents recognize at some level that a successful treatment will confirm the notion that they have failed to some extent in their parental roles.

It is rare indeed for an adolescent to ask to see a psychiatrist; he or she is usually forced to do so by parents, the school, or other authorities. Given this, along with the age-appropriate rebellion (or, at least, resistance to authority) of adolescents, it is no wonder that they approach treatment without much enthusiasm. The adolescent's attitude is hardly the one of "expectant faith" that Frank and Frank (1991, p. 109) have identified as integral to the healing process, noting, "At least part of

345

the efficacy of psychotherapeutic methods lies in the shared belief of the participants that these methods work" (p. 3).

Those who work with adolescents appreciate that optimal preconditions such as these seldom exist. Teens usually approach us with an admixture of fear and loathing and a belief that we have nothing worthwhile to offer. Though Freud (1917) believed that "nothing can be done against prejudices" (p. 462), he also noted that "the contrary state of mind, in which expectation is coloured by hope and faith, is an effective force with which we have to reckon . . . in all our attempts at treatment and cure" (1905, p. 289).

It is my contention that the belief that psychotherapy can effect change is intricately related, as are motivation and responsibility, to the culture and belief system of the family. Despite an adolescent's developmentally appropriate antagonism to the familial worldview, he or she still retains the common framework of that worldview, just as the communist and the fascist are flip sides of the same authoritarian coin. I will examine my personal experience with psychiatry in adolescence and compare and contrast that with a series of case vignettes from my practice focusing on this issue and how it influences treatment. I will conclude with some thoughts as to how we therapists may be able to influence the adolescent's belief system.

PERSONAL EXPERIENCE

I grew up in a small, Delta town in rural, northeast Louisiana. Like most people, I had virtually no contact with psychiatry and thought psychiatrists were, in the words of an infamous governor of Louisiana "crazier'n the man they're examinin' " (Long, 1961). It happened that one of my relatives was a psychiatrist; when I was a child, he was referred to as Dr. _____, and no one ever mentioned his specialty.

In my early teens, my mother became depressed, although I don't remember noticing any change. My father took me aside and spoke to me of how she was depressed as "many women get at that age," and he encouraged me to be understanding. He also told me that she was seeing a psychiatrist. Shortly before this time, I was angry with my parents and had begun to argue with them about various issues. This was a change for me, and these were, in retrospect, my first stirrings toward independence.

Over the course of the next year or so, my mother started to change. I noticed that when I would take issue with her or criticize some hypocrisy I had noticed, she would agree with me. After I had gotten over my initial shock, it dawned on me that she was changing and that it had to do with her experience with psychiatry. She and I began to talk about it. She told me how she felt better and more relaxed and how she saw through some of the same adult hypocrisies I saw through. She stopped putting pressure on my siblings and me to attend church and left this and many other decisions to us.

I had always been tightly wound and a real worrier. My grades were excellent, but I had to make As because of the pressure I put on myself. I was a good athlete, but I worried that I would lose my starting position in football. I worried about masturbation and drinking affecting me. I worried about being successful with girls. Finally, in one of the discussions with my mother, I told her I wanted to see the psychiatrist. She said, "Fine," and then arranged an appointment.

When I walked into the psychiatrist's office, I noticed the couch, but I sat down in a chair. I started to tell him what was on my mind and what had been bothering me. As I did so, my trunk began to twitch almost convulsively. The twitching shocked me somewhat. After it continued for a few minutes, I told the doctor that I had to lie down on the couch to try to relax, and that helped.

The psychiatrist took an active role and informed me that masturbation wasn't harmful, smoking was a noxious habit he wished he didn't have, but drinking in moderation could enhance one's enjoyment of life. He added that being able to drink and commiserate with his buddies had made the Army tolerable. His candor and openness were refreshing, but, above all, his empathic understanding helped me feel better by reassuring me that I wasn't crazy. He was also able to help me modify some of my superego injunctions so that I could tolerate better the impulses and feelings with which I was struggling.

When I walked out of his office, I felt as though an anvil had been lifted from my shoulders. This process seemed magical, and it was powerful. I wanted to do this to help others, and, unconsciously, I wanted to experience it more so I could be more relaxed. On the ride home, I turned to my mother and said, "Mama, I want to be a psychiatrist." I have never wavered from that decision.

I chose a medical school largely on the basis of electives and being able to study more psychiatry. In medical school, I also encountered the enormous prejudice against psychiatry in other branches of medicine. My classmates, like most students in medical school, initially weren't well disposed toward it either, though many later changed their attitudes because of an unusually dynamic teacher.

It happened that the psychiatry department was a bit moribund, but a skilled, energetic clinician became chairman in my sophomore year. The third-year psychiatry clerkship was amazing. The psychiatrist in charge was vigorous, challenging, and interesting. He was given the Golden Shovel award for teaching excellence—the first time the award had been given to a psychiatrist. Members of the other departments were chagrined and skeptical, but we students had seen what psychiatry could do. We had felt some of the magic, especially when this teacher demonstrated hypnosis to us. His impact and that of the chairman's impact were so great that 20% of my class chose psychiatry, and 25% did so the following year.

CASE EXAMPLES

Like Father, Like Daughter

Because psychiatry had been so influential in my life, it seemed only natural for me to be interested in helping other teens and young adults with the important issues of that age. With my personal experience as a background, I had the naive impression that psychotherapy would be easy. The first adolescent I treated in practice appeared to confirm this notion. The patient's father was a physician. This young woman looked up to him, and, furthermore, he had had a very positive experience with psychiatry. She came into therapy primed to have it be helpful.

At the time I had a half-time job at a hospital where I would often have lunch with other doctors on the staff. I became friendly with another physician who eventually asked me if I worked with teenagers. I told him I had a special interest in them, though I didn't tell him this was because of my experience with psychiatry as a teenager. He then asked if I would see his daughter Peggy. He explained that he and his wife were concerned about her. They had suggested that she see someone, and she had agreed.

Peggy was a very sharp, likable girl who was a bit overgrown and hefty with an awkward, ill-at-ease style. Her appearance was not

348

enhanced by the oversized plaid flannel shirts, baggy blue jeans, and work boots she wore to deemphasize her femininity. This young woman was depressed, cynical, and confused about what she wanted to do, but primarily about who she was and whether she was okay.

Initially, Peggy was quite shy and reticent with me and reluctant to talk about herself and her feelings. She didn't fight her parents about the visits, however, and it was obvious to me that she got something out of them. I persisted with gentle encouragement, and she began to trust me. During this phase, I helped her understand how she could use the process of psychotherapy and share her big secret—that she had had a lesbian experience with her closest friend. When she first mentioned this, she tossed it off rather lightheartedly as though it were no big deal. I confronted this stance, because it was characteristic of her and her parents. Over the ensuing weeks, she talked about it more honestly and began to share her shame, especially her fear of what the experience meant about her own sexual identity.

I met with her parents two or three times during the course of Peggy's treatment to assuage any anxiety they had about her, as well as to get to know them in order to understand their daughter better. Though I didn't mention it, the parents knew about Peggy's sexual experience with her friend. They tried to be lighthearted about it also, but they were panicked. The father also blamed himself for his daughter's depression. He told me his secret—he had been depressed and had gotten treatment for it.

I was able to reassure the parents and help alleviate their guilt. In time, Peggy settled down and began to appreciate this sexual experience and the relationship with her friend as part of a developmental stage. We also looked at some of her difficulties with her mother, who had an alcohol problem and had been unavailable for her daughter in many ways. Peggy's appearance became more feminine; she acquired a boyfriend and finally terminated a successful treatment.

For this young woman, I had served in the transference as an avuncular figure providing fatherly counsel, superego modification, and a holding environment in which to work out her conflicting feelings about her identity and her sexuality. She identified me with her father, and, because her feelings for him were so positive, she was open to me and what I had to say. He had paved the way by having a positive experience with his own treatment.

Like Father, Unlike Son

The following case illustrates that things are not always what they seem. This young man had two competing models of psychiatry—one very positive, the other not so good. The challenge was to help him get past some resentment of psychiatry so that he could use it for himself.

This youngster was referred to me by a colleague who was seeing his mother. In fact, both parents were in treatment and presented themselves as believers in psychiatry, their trust based on positive experiences with it. I met with the boy and his mother at the first interview, in which the mother told me she was concerned about how Jack was handling the divorce she and her husband were going through. Despite this concern, she surprisingly painted a picture of an almost model son. When Jack and I spoke privately, he confirmed that his conduct was sterling, but he said that he was troubled by his anger toward and manipulation of his father. He said that he thought he needed to see a psychiatrist about it. This, needless to say, is not the typical behavior of a teen referred to a shrink. It struck me as an attitude similar to that of psychiatrists or residents who come into treatment and act as though they have already worked everything out. These individuals are tough to reach.

Despite his rather sophisticated assessment of his issues, as Jack and I worked together, he was guarded, with a fair amount of denial. During exams, he became upset with his mother for trying to schedule sessions when he thought they would interfere with his studying. This attitude, coupled with his obsessive accounts of rather mundane events, made it clear that I needed to find a way to engage him in the therapeutic process. In grappling with this impasse, I discovered that Jack had had a previous experience with psychiatry, and that, as he put it, "It didn't change anything." I acknowledged the limitations of psychiatry and also confronted his multidetermined passivity, raising the possibility that psychiatry might be able to help him with his anxiety about doing well. Jack responded to the idea that it would be good to feel less pressured and began a therapeutic dialogue with me. As a result, he began to appreciate that I understood the "pressure cooker" he was in, and I let him know that I knew a few things about taking exams and dealing with performance anxiety.

During this impasse phase I discovered how Jack blamed psychiatry, to a degree, for his father's infidelity to his mother. The way Jack saw it, the psychiatric treatment ought to have stopped that behavior and helped his parents stay together. The mother's experience with psychiatry had been much more positive, in that it had helped her deal with her husband and stand up for herself. Jack had a very ambivalent relationship with his dad. He admired his father's intelligence and success but hated him for having cheated on his mother and, in Jack's eyes, having destroyed the family. Despite appearing so positive about psychiatry, Jack had been quite wary, but he had denied that anxiety. I had to empathize with him and confront and interpret his passivity and obsessiveness before he could trust me and allow me to function in a helping role—at various times in the transference as a big brother and at other times as a benign fatherly figure. With these issues worked out, Jack was able to relax and have a very positive therapeutic experience.

Father Knows Best

During my residency, I, like many of my peers, was influenced by the writings and interviews of Harold Searles. A teacher during my inpatient work also stimulated an interest in intensive psychotherapeutic work with severely disturbed teenagers and young adults. After being in practice for a few years, I began to concentrate more of my energies in that area and moved my office to the Institute of Pennsylvania Hospital, at that time one of the best-known tertiary-care centers in the nation. A case I struggled with there highlights some of the issues I'm addressing, albeit with a more negative outcome. The case illustrates how difficult therapy is when a power struggle exists between parents and therapist, especially when the therapeutic process arouses anxiety in both the patient and the parents.

A psychotic adolescent girl was referred to the institute from a Christian psychiatric hospital in a rural area of the state. The girl's parents were from another state, but they were understandably concerned about their daughter's well-being and, therefore, willing to drive a long distance every two weeks for family meetings. A brother of the patient also participated, because he attended a Christian college in the Philadelphia area. The parents were fundamentalist Protestants and devoutly religious, though they never asked me about my religious beliefs. In fact, religion surfaced surprisingly infrequently as a topic, given their espoused conviction.

The patient, whom I shall call Sue, was an attractive young girl, though she didn't use makeup and appeared rather plain—akin in appearance to women in some of the ascetic sects such as the Amish, but without the distinctive clothing common to those groups. She seemed fairly intelligent, but she was distant and a bit cool with me.

As therapy progressed, many interesting details emerged about the family and the parents' marriage. There was tremendous discord between the parents with intense verbal battles, although no physical fighting. Sue's brother described these scenes and, indeed, family life itself as a "smoldering volcano," likening the periodic outbursts to explosions that "could destroy almost everything." Not surprisingly, Sue had symptoms related to anger—severe headaches and constipation.

Sue's parents were preoccupied with the influence of food and vitamins on their daughter's health. It seemed pointless and self-defeating to go head-to-head with them in confronting their bias. My style in such a situation is to agree (after all, food and vitamins are integral to health). It was my hope that, by joining with the family in such a situation, they would not see me as so threatening. They might then be able to hear what I had to say about other factors, such as their (particularly the father's) need to control almost everything about their daughter's life.

At one point, the patient began to refuse food and became mute. During this period I would attempt to be with her experientially and free-associate about what she might be feeling. In addition, I would bring to our sessions some peanut-butter crackers that I knew she liked. Sometimes I would eat a few, commenting about how good they were and offering her some. When she refused, I would marvel at her impulse control and wonder aloud how she had the willpower to do this. At the end of the session, I would leave the crackers behind "just in case you get hungry."

Though the patient resolved this issue fairly quickly, the parents panicked over their daughter's refusal to eat. At our next family meeting, they demanded that I let the patient be taken for evaluation to a nearby orthomolecular center, or they would transfer her to another hospital. Reluctantly I agreed to this request, feeling as though I were being blackmailed, and subsequently followed the center's recommendations for vitamin treatment.

Later in the course of her therapy, Sue shared with me letters her mother wrote to her in which the mother spoke in hyperbolic, mystical terms of the glories of Jesus, heaven, and whatever other religious themes came to mind. As I read these letters, I was aware of how trance-inducing they were. In some of our sessions, I read them to the girl and commented about the altered state of consciousness they produced. These seemed to be part of the process of brainwashing whereby the parents tried to continue controlling their daughter. It reminded me of what I had read about how the Chinese tried to control their citizenry during the Cultural Revolution with hymns of praise to Chairman Mao (Chang, 1991). The letters clearly seemed a renewed mobilization of the family's defenses.

As time went on, the patient started to address sexual issues, albeit in a quite circumspect way. The increasing level of trust evidenced by her ability to talk about sexuality was not without conflict, however, a conflict she resolved by insuring that her parents, never fully supportive of her treatment, would end it abruptly. She told her parents about some of our sessions in such a way that they, especially her father, became further disenchanted with my treatment. Contending that I was too focused on their daughter as being sick, they decided to fire me and took their daughter to a Christian psychiatrist.

My understanding of what happened was that, as treatment progressed, the patient had experienced increased anxiety on several levels. Her emerging sexuality terrified her, as did developing a more trusting and intimate relationship with me. She must have been frightened that I would ignore her strivings for independence—and on a more primitive level, that I would overpower and devour her, as her parents had symbolically done. In the transference, I represented an extremely threatening amalgam of mother and father. She was more manipulative than she appeared and played on her parents' anxiety. These parents were very rigid and controlling; indeed, I experienced them as impossible. They were too threatened by psychiatry to let go of their daughter.

Mother Knows Best

In recent years, I have moved from working with the type of patient described in the previous section to working with a seemingly healthier population, mainly outpatients. The following case illustrates some of the same dynamics and issues as the last one, but with more flexible and less neurotic people. Here again was a power struggle between therapist and parents, but the parents' anxiety was not as extreme as in that case. The therapist, therefore, had more options available.

Bill was a 13-year-old youngster in eighth grade. His parents had been concerned because of his temper, the quality of his peer group, and the fact that he had begun to seem "out of it" both at home and at school. Bill had a history of encopresis for which he had been treated by a psychiatrist at the age of four or five. After several years of treatment at a respected child center in the area, the parents had become disillusioned and had taken Bill to see a local gastroenterologist who supposedly worked wonders with medicines only. In fact, the symptoms had lessened, but Bill had continued to have bowel problems.

As one would expect, Bill was markedly constrained and didn't readily open up. His mother brought him to the sessions, and after my initial evaluation, she soon started a pattern of wanting to speak to me privately at the end of each. Bill okayed these talks, but he didn't want to sit in. He had begun to relax and open up a bit, but soon after these visits with his mother became routine, he clammed up again. I thought this was related to his feelings about his mother's visits, so I insisted that we hold the meetings with Bill in the room. The very next week, she requested that I give her some sort of medical excuse so she could stay home and keep an eye on Bill because she was concerned about him. This crystallized her need for control over Bill, me, and his treatment. I informed her with Bill present that I couldn't do that because there seemed to be no real medical reason to do so.

Although Bill's mother was angry about this, Bill began to trust me after I refused his mother's request. He started to talk about his anger and his headaches. He brought in some of his CDs so we could listen to some of the heavy metal music he liked. I explained the dynamics of anger, guilt, and punishment to him. He told me that he had been smoking pot frequently during the past year but was doing so rarely now.

By no means did Bill's mother back out of the picture. She characterized her husband as troubled and abusive, though the boy denied this. She proposed sending Bill to a private school without considering the boy's input. Both parents changed their minds when I suggested to them that a unilateral move such as this, without Bill's cooperation, was doomed to failure. Another gambit was to get Bill tested for attention-deficit hyperactivity disorder. When I reviewed this request and pointed out that he didn't have and, indeed, had never had some of the key symptoms, she disagreed with me, though she did agree to hold off temporarily. Then she scheduled the testing anyway.

Bill's mother wrote me many letters, primarily about how best to handle Bill's teachers. Several months after beginning the letters, she started to share some personal anguish with me and requested an individual session. As a result of that meeting, I referred her to a colleague, whom she began seeing. At the end of a subsequent session with Bill, he asked if I would bring his mother in so he could tell her how he felt that living at home was like living in a communist state. Surprisingly, she listened without being defensive and actually seemed to hear him. So, major strides had been made.

In Bill's case, as in that of Jack, I had to empathize with the patient before he could trust me and form a therapeutic alliance. With Bill, empathic action was warranted: I had to demonstrate—by confronting and setting limits with his mother—that I understood his predicament. Then he could enter treatment and allow a transferential relationship to develop. Despite their anger, the parents seemed to respect my stance and began to allow me to be in charge.

DISCUSSION

What can we learn from these cases that will help us clinically? My own case shows the impact on other family members of successful treatment. There is a ripple effect, if you will, that may lead other family members to consider psychiatry in times of distress. When they turn to it, there will be a belief that the process can succeed and that they can get well. This certainly seemed to be the case with the doctor's daughter. The family truly believed in medicine and psychiatry, because they had had a very positive experience with it, so the treatment went fairly smoothly.

Jack's case had some of the same dynamics as that of the doctor's daughter, but it was trickier. Jack had had conflicting models of psychiatry's effectiveness. Though his mother had a successful experience, his father hadn't appeared to benefit, and, indeed, Jack blamed psychiatry to a degree for his father's escapades that led to the breakup of the family. Jack's previous treatment hadn't worked wonders. There was an element of his wanting to defeat psychiatry. I had to win Jack over to the idea that psychiatry could be helpful to him so that he could relinquish his neurotic desire to beat it.

In Sue's case, the operative belief system in the family was that the parents, especially the father, knew best. The parents would let me have some control, but, if I got out of line, they would step in. In retrospect, it is apparent that their belief system precluded successful psychotherapy. For success to occur, the doctor needs to be in charge. I believe that I only delayed the inevitable by okaying their taking their daughter to the orthomolecular center. If I had it to do over, I would agree with their plan and transfer her care to the center in as diplomatic a fashion as possible. Given that they would have either transferred her or sought another doctor, I would still have provided the daughter with a model of how to deal with impossible parents. As I understood the case, she didn't know how to separate or be deprogrammed, and, with her level of rage and ambivalence, psychosis was the result.

Bill's case presents many of the same issues in a situation that could have led to severe decompensation. Like Sue's parents, Bill's mother thought she knew best, but she was not as controlling as Sue's parents. In providing a model to the boy of how to handle this tyrannical mother, I showed him a path of escape. He came to believe that psychiatry could help, in contrast to his expectation of no benefit that was based on his earlier experience with it as a child, when it failed to help his bowel problems. His mother was troubled by her unhappiness and willing to take some responsibility for it, so she was somewhat open to the idea that psychiatry could be helpful.

CONCLUSION

Although work with families is demanding, it is, in my view, necessary in working with adolescents. For healthier families, it may consist only of meeting with the parents occasionally to assuage their anxieties or to better appreciate the context in which the teen has developed. The more dysfunctional families are more challenging. Their structure is more rigid, and they have more trouble letting go of their children, but they must if therapy is to succeed. I meet more often with these families, for I know that my work with the adolescent hinges on whether or not I can win the parents' support.

Jim Cox provided important influence and guidance in some of my dark hours of working with some very difficult patients at the Institute of Pennsylvania Hospital. He helped me have the courage to trust my instincts and to be much bolder with these patients and their families. Whenever I was struggling with a patient, which was quite often, I would consult Jim. The patient and I would meet with him, and I almost always left that meeting feeling freed and less burdened by the struggle. He helped me appreciate the process of treatment—a process in which all patients, but especially adolescents and their families, are constantly testing us and neurotically hoping to defeat us. Addressing that dynamic is paramount in treatment.

Just as we need to be sensitive to a patient's values, we need to be sensitive to and aware of his or her cultural and familial biases, especially when these are antitherapeutic. Though they may not initially be apparent, we must address them, because they are part of the patient's and the family's resistance to change.

Adolescents are wary, mistrustful, and testing. They want to see if we really care about them, and they have an exquisite radar for hypocrisy. We face the challenge of helping the adolescent make the transition from pretreatment (J. E. Taylor, 1990, personal communication) to actual treatment itself, that is, to the point at which the patient believes he or she can benefit from treatment. Various techniques such as an anticipatory socialization interview (Orne and Wender, 1968) or a role-induction interview (Hoehn-Saric et al., 1964) have been devised to help with this transition. We must go further than this, however, because, as Frank and Frank (1991) noted, "The success . . . of psychotherapy depends on the patients' conviction that the therapist cares about them and is competent to help" (p. 154). It's all in the convincing.

REFERENCES

Chang, J. (1991), *Wild Swans: Three Daughters of China.* New York: Simon & Schuster.

Frank, J. D. & Frank, J. B. (1991), *Persuasion and Healing: A Comparative Study of Psychotherapy,* 3rd ed. Baltimore: Johns Hopkins University Press.

Freud, S. (1905), Psychical Treatment. *Standard Edition,* 7:289. London: Hogarth Press, 1966.

——— (1917), Introductory Lectures on Psychoanalysis. *Standard Edition,* 16:462. London: Hogarth Press, 1966.

Heine, R. W. & Trosman, H. (1960), Initial expectations of the doctor-patient interaction as a factor in continuance in psychotherapy. *Psychiatry,* 23:275–278.

Hoehn-Saric, R., Frank, J. D., Imber, S. D., Nash, E. H. Jr., Stone, A. R. & Battle, C. C. (1964), Systematic preparation of patients for psychotherapy: I. Effects on therapy behavior and outcome. *J. Psychiat. Res.,* 2:267–281.

Long, E. K. (1961), *The Voice of Earl Long,* ed. & narrated B. Read & B. Hebert. Baton Rouge, LA: News Records, Inc.

Orne, M. T. & Wender, P. H. (1968), Anticipatory socialization for psychotherapy: Method and rationale. *Amer. J. Psychiat.,* 124:1202–1211.

PART V

POSITION PAPER OF THE
AMERICAN SOCIETY FOR
ADOLESCENT PSYCHIATRY

15 YOUTH VIOLENCE: ITS MEANINGS TO SOCIETY IN THE 21ST CENTURY

POSITION STATEMENT OF THE AMERICAN SOCIETY FOR ADOLESCENT PSYCHIATRY PASSED BY THE HOUSE OF DELEGATES, MARCH 22, 2001

CHARLES W. HUFFINE

Youth violence is on our minds. We are worried, despite evidence that the incidence of youth violence has actually been decreasing steadily since the mid-1990s. Recent highly publicized school shootings; reports of gang violence; young people obsessed with violent video games, movies, and song lyrics; and media prone to publicize all incidents of violence no matter how tragic or trivial have left us with a sense of crisis and eminent danger. Individual incidents of violence involving youth are compelling, because they bring forth all our fears for our children. They mobilize our instincts to do whatever is necessary to protect them from a seemingly hostile world. Media attention to violence by youth has created a grossly distorted but socially important focus on this problem. As tragic as the school shootings are, the numbers of deaths is small to the point of statistical insignificance. But the social significance is great. Seeing the halls of learning turned into shooting galleries has understandably galvanized the American public's attention. The meanings go beyond the issues of school safety. These incidents have provoked a great deal of soul searching and anguishing about the health of our society. Such a public reaction can, and should, prompt a more sober look at certain social phenomena that surround such incidents as school shootings. They should raise questions about how such unhappy children can be unrecognized by their families, schools, and communities until tragedy happens.

Uninformed reactions, born of frustration and a lack of understanding of adolescence, may have the effect of leading to policies that become part of the problem. In this atmosphere of fear, the U.S. Congress and many state legislatures have passed laws designed to protect our communities from youth who are out of control. A policy of zero tolerance has been a key feature of many of these laws. Legislative action in the area of juvenile justice has emphasized more harsh punishments. Some new laws aim to strip younger adolescents of their historical rights to protection in juvenile courts by allowing prosecutors to remand them to adult courts without hearings and providing them with adult punishments. Such reactive laws satisfy some in our society who wish to throw all troubled youth into a punitive system that will contain them forever. These new laws are vulnerable to being selectively practiced with youth of color, with the poor and the unattractive. In contrast to the barrage of harsh punitive measures, few resources have been allocated to understanding the phenomena of youth violence or to understanding etiology or changes in prevalence, the meanings of violence to the youth involved, or the appropriate societal response when tragic incidents occur.

The American Society for Adolescent Psychiatry (ASAP) is an organization devoted to the study of adolescents and their difficulties. ASAP advocates for conditions that allow healthy adolescent development and promulgates best practices in the treatment of mental disorders in adolescents. ASAP has long been a leader in understanding the interplay between individual psychological issues and their manifestation in a social context. This has led ASAP to study and define appropriate policies in areas related to youth violence since its founding in 1967. In concert with many other groups concerned with the welfare of children and youth, ASAP offers the following observations on the current phenomenon of youth violence and our societal response to it. We offer our thoughts in the hope that they will contribute to a wise and effective response to serving our youth and our communities.

YOUTH VIOLENCE: HISTORICAL CONTEXT AND PREVALENCE AT THE MILLENNIUM

It has been said that the American society has always been a violent one. Historians trace a tradition of civil strife born of a strong value on independence, suspicion of the state and the value of personal honor. These traits in our forefathers led to the founding of our country through violent revolution. These traditions were nurtured by white males in the social order of the old South. They were exported to the West with the march of settlers in the 19th century and exploded in the American Civil War (Butterfield, 1995). The institution of slavery, endemic to American society from the beginning, has been called as brutal and violent an institution as has existed in the history of man. Traditions of proud, independent men claiming and defending their territory, or fighting the social order to redress grievances, are part of our 20th and 21st century life. Labor organizers warred with company agents, Southern men lynched blacks for presumed breaches of honor and the Black Panthers horrified us all by waving guns and threatening retribution. America is the great hope for the dispossessed around the world. Many immigrate to our country and contribute much to American society. But they also bring the residua of their trauma from civil strife in their home countries. Some bring with them the effects of severe psychological trauma and an urge for retribution. Sometimes their continuing conflicts with their countrymen explode on our streets and become the content of a newspaper story on violence. Gangs of home grown socially disadvantaged youth roam the streets of poor neighborhoods and engage in fratricidal warfare; the poor killing the poor. But in the process, such youth menace us all with their posturing. They play out a social drama whose meanings transcend the sad issues of who "disses" who in the "hood." Most of us can insulate ourselves from this frightening drama. We don't want to know the history or have to acknowledge that it is there now, in front of our faces. When forced to deal with the ugliness of violence and its social context, we see it as aberrant and monstrous. We seek to isolate such terrifying drama because it scares us.

There was a striking rise in youth violence from the mid-1980s to 1993, when the rates reached a peak. It began to decrease in 1994. Prothrow-Stith and Weissman (1991) make a convincing case that social violence is endemic to American society. They define the rise in violence in the 1980s as an epidemic on top of endemic violence and warn that the ingredients are there for another rise in violence. They believe that the subsiding of violence in the late 1990s is only a lull in the epidemic.

Since 1994, there has been a steady decline in reported incidents of violence by youth. Such acts (as measured in crime statistics) include murder, assault, rape, and burglary with associated threats or violent acts. Although rates have declined significantly in the last seven years, they are still substantially higher than the period between the mid-1970s and mid-1980s. The only factor that seems clearly associated with the rise and fall of violence in society is the state of the economy. Economic difficulties are associated with a rise in violence in society, whereas economic booms correlate with its decline. This is true for both adults and youth, although the amplitude of the fluctuations is greater for youth (Zimring, 1999). Only one subfactor has not declined with the overall improvement in youth violence statistics: murder by gunshot wound. The rate of death by gunshot has remained at essentially the same high rate despite a decline in incidents of assault. This is because an increasing number of assaults are associated with guns and thus more likely to be lethal, yielding a stable rate of assault-related deaths (Zimring, 1999). This suggests that the ready availability of guns to our youth creates a dangerous climate and leads to more deaths. Easy availability of guns to adults assures easy availability to youth.

What is not on the public's agenda is striking, given the horror over shootings in schools. Social affiliation patterns seem to be changing in our society. Families are ever more fragmented and overwhelmed as social institutions offer them less and less support. Youth spend less time with friends, and when they do, this time is less structured or focused. Little attention is given to evidence of alienation in our society, although sociological evidence abounds regarding our lessening degrees of social affiliation (Putnam, 2000). Little attention is drawn to the social impact of welfare reform despite growing data on the impact of psychological stress on a new cadre of working poor. Many in this group have inadequate child care, less mobility, and fewer resources for solving family problems (Loprest, 2001). Domestic violence and its most disturbing subset, the sexual and physical abuse of children, barely stay on our societal radar screen. Suicide remains one of the highest causes of death in the younger age groups. Violence toward oneself is much more often lethal when guns are readily available. These acts of violence are met with a societal denial reaction. It is the acts of violence by young men, often of a different race, perpetrated randomly on unsuspecting innocents that strike fear into our hearts and get us to take notice. We focus our fear on the boogie man, a dark force that embodies unknown evils. The failure to consider more common issues is an important social aspect of the phenomenon of violence in our society. The modern-day boogie man is a social construct that is a derivative of both common psychological defenses and sociological forces. Adolescent psychiatrists, as part of their clinical work, must integrate an understanding of psychological and social dynamics. We are, therefore, in a good position to comment on these phenomena as they relate to youth violence.

WHY YOUTH COMMIT VIOLENT CRIMES

The vast majority of youth engage in the social developmental process of adolescence without endangering themselves or others (Offer and Offer, 1976). But most adolescents do suffer stress as they meet their many challenges. Many keep their worries to themselves; others tell them to their parents or close friends. Many express their complex feelings about the society they are entering through their hairstyles, dress, or tastes in music. For some, a fascination with violence in movies and song lyrics is a functional way of coping with their own concerns about aggression. By and large, they are successful in school, have friends, are mostly respectful to their families, and emerge as productive young adults. Even most youth suffering the indignities of poverty, racism, or the adjustments demanded of recent immigrants seem to pass through the travails of adolescence without committing serious offenses. Many other children suffer from terrible family difficulties. They witness violence in their homes and are the victims of physical and sexual abuse. We know that such children are at much higher risk for expressing their frustrations in violence when they become adolescents (Carter, 1999). It is remarkable how many individuals who suffer such horrendous hardships do not pass on the violence by victimizing others. An amazing percentage of our teens seems to be resilient, somehow finding the ingredients for successful adolescent development.

Social conditions alone cannot explain why youth succumb to rage and alienation. It is more likely that acts of violence are the product of a complex interplay between constitutional factors and social forces. The stress/diathesis hypothesis embraces this idea: Constitutional vulnerabilities, or a diathesis, interact with social forces that impinge negatively on an individual, creating stress. Violent action is only occasionally the final outcome of this interplay. There is a risk of violence, however, when an individual is stressed and blinded by complex emotions for which the end result is confused anger. Such an individual feels like a bad person. Society teaches him or her what it is to act bad. Violent acts are shaped in accordance to what is perceived by a troubled individual to be most troubling for our society. Violent responses in a vulnerable individual often reflect, quite unconsciously, an accurate reading of what in our communities is most feared and what most fascinates. Collective fear and fascination with violence are very effectively communicated in our media nightly on the evening news, by our entertainment media, and in casual talk in our communities. For a teenager exposed to these influences, it is not hard to know how to act like the boogie man. It is even easier if one is from a minority culture. One learns what is expected of someone like oneself and proceeds, unconsciously, to act the part when the stress/diathesis complex is activated.

Psychiatrists have contributed a great deal to our knowledge about certain forms of diatheses and to the analysis of their complex interactions with stress. These contributions are reflected in the system of psychiatric diagnoses that are elaborately defined in the American Psychiatric Association's (1994) *Diagnostic and Statistical Manual of Mental Disorders*, fourth edition (*DSM-IV*). There is no single diagnosis that explains youth violence, just as no set of social factors explains it. Many individuals with severe psychiatric illness are never prone to acts of violence. However, if unrecognized and untreated, there are some indications that psychiatric illness can be a serious risk factor for acting violently. If a teen is in the throes of a psychiatric illness, the behavioral expression of the symptoms of the condition may very well be aggressive and offensive to society. Adolescent development is primarily a social developmental phenomena; thus, behavior is the social means through which an adolescent communicates stress and symptoms (Rakoff, 1989; Huffine, 1999).

ASAP has contributed suggestions for understanding common diagnostic syndromes in view of social developmental factors. We believe that more work is necessary on the diagnostic system for children and adolescents (Huffine, 1999). Often, the formal diagnostic criteria for our most common diagnoses do not account for teenagers' expressing their symptoms in their behavior. For instance, depression and suicidal ideation in a teenager may be expressed in terms of recklessness and the abandonment of regard for self or anyone else. A depressed and hurting teenage boy may recklessly direct rage at a peer. If guns are available, his undisciplined rage and agitation may result in a homicide.

Guns are a potent symbol in our culture. They convey a sense of power and control. Their misuse is often noted in the media with horror. For an angry, depressed teenager, enveloped in feelings of powerlessness and self-loathing, the negative social meanings of misusing a gun may be very congruent with his depressed feelings. Anxiety and fear may be socially humiliating. If social slights and disrespect have been cues for anxiety, a teen may react violently toward a perceived tormentor in a desperate struggle to compensate for feeling humiliated and anxious. In adolescent mania, impulsivity and poor judgment mixed with social developmental stress may be exceptionally troublesome. If a teenager has been badly treated as a child and carries the scars in the form of posttraumatic stress, the memories of trauma may be expressed behaviorally in the form of perpetrating violent acts on others similar to what the violent individual has suffered. Each of these psychiatric conditions can be addressed with effective treatment. Teenagers affected by these conditions can be helped, with a careful reading of their behavioral messages, to avoid continuing expression of illness through dangerous behavioral symptoms.

A small number of young people have a personality constellation, formed early in their lives, that appears to predict a poor prognosis for ever becoming socialized. Encountering an adolescent with sociopathic features is a chilling experience for most mental health professionals. These teenagers are different from others we see who may commit acts as heinous, or manipulate as narcissistically, but are not sociopathic. It is a reasonable hypothesis that the few true monsters in our society had to be young once and that on occasion they will appear as adolescents in our system of care. Although we may offer a poor prognosis for such individuals, the rule of law applies to them as well. Few mental health professionals believe we know enough to predict that they will be unredeemable and justify holding them forever in jails. Most are at large in our communities between detentions. Although we may have a chilling feeling about these rare individuals, we look for cracks in their hardness, for some cultural explanations, or for some form of leverage in order to attempt rehabilitation. A very few will remain menacing and deeply troubling to us all.

Unfortunately, the rare sociopathic teenager stands as an icon for many in society. Like Dracula, the nonsocialized predatory teen has been mythologized by our culture. All who have been bitten and bear resemblance to the iconic monster will be seen as warranting separation from the human race. This is our social boogie man.

Most teens who commit acts of violence do not have unredeemable personality profiles. They include many adolescents with treatable mental illness. But their behavior, chosen unwittingly to create the most exquisite and horrifying social drama, invariably makes them superficially indistinguishable from sociopaths. Their behavior creates a powerful effect because of its great social meaning. By committing an act of violence, the confused and distraught teenager—perhaps overwhelmed by life stress, perhaps vulnerable due to a mental disorder—has created a nightmare for himself and society. He lives out the social meaning in the act of doing violence, often feeling quite justified with twisted moral logic (Garbarino, 1999). Later, as the consequences of their violent acts accrue, violent teens may become aware of the meanings of their acts and suffer great remorse. Everyone struggles to understand. Why would a teenager commit the act most feared, most expected of rampaging youth, and which draws the most horrified fascination? It is as if that child has been bitten by Dracula, in the mind of most. They have become the boogie man and have committed the very act guaranteed to push them out of the social order.

MEASURED PUNISHMENT VERSUS SOCIAL RETRIBUTION

What, then, is the appropriate societal reaction to such sad youth? Adolescents who, while suffering from mental disorders, commit terrible acts must be regarded in two ways at once. We must understand that a teen needs to complete the expected social drama through an appropriate and constructive punishment. We must always be attentive to community safety in the process. No one who values the social order will dispute this basic tenet. Certain youth are dangerous and must be separated from society. Other youth do disturbing or obnoxious things and must suffer the consequences. We must also remain aware, however, that these young offenders are still in the throes of a developmental process. We must be diligent in ensuring that they are given effective treatment for their underlying difficulties. There is no essential conflict between protecting the social order from the misbehavior of youth and providing appropriate treatment of those whose mental illnesses manifest in disordered behavior.

Differences may occur over strategies and timing. Should we opt for a consistent application of the law, ensuring a fair application of justice? Or should we apply individualized approaches to all youth in trouble, recognizing their unique situations and needs? Faced with an individual adolescent in trouble, psychiatrists and other mental health professionals tend to focus on aspects of care that will lead to rehabilitation. But addressing offensive behavior with appropriate consequences is also part of the rehabilitative process. Failure to provide measured and appropriate responses to such behavior is a form of child neglect. The opportunities for intervention with a troubled child after an offense, even a violent and dangerous one, cannot be missed or squandered. Adolescent psychiatrists, with good evidence and considerable passion, favor individualized interventions in the behavioral difficulties of youth. Skillfully applied treatment interventions will do more to prevent future offenses, thereby better attending to the public's safety, than will blind retributive punishment.

CREATING AND ASSURING ACCESS
TO ADEQUATE CARE AND TREATMENT

Our juvenile detention facilities are filled with young people with clearly diagnosable conditions such as those noted previously (Trupin et al., 1988; Atkins, Pumariega, and Rogers, 1999). Sometimes the relationship between the diagnosis and the socially offensive behavior is missed. Most often the diagnosis is missed altogether. Diagnoses such as conduct disorder or oppositional defiant disorder are widely used to categorize behaviorally disruptive youth. These are seen by many adolescent psychiatrists as of doubtful utility in understanding an adolescent's psychological functioning and may hinder accurate diagnosing of treatable conditions (Huffine, 1999). As adolescent psychiatrists, we know it is crucial that the population of youth who have committed acts of violence be evaluated by individuals with the training to know how psychiatric illness manifests in teenagers. It is tragic if a clearly indicated treatment is withheld from an individual when a good outcome hangs on the psychiatric illness being addressed. True access to treatment demands that those delivering the treatment have the time and setting to properly make an evaluation. It is even more important that there is sufficient opportunity for developing a relationship with the juvenile offender to forge a treatment alliance. Forming a treatment alliance with an angry, hurting, jailed teenager clearly requires special talent and training for the therapist. Allowing therapists to do effective work will take some thoughtful programming on the part of planners and administrators. There are some models in practice. Multisystemic therapy (MST) offers a method of gaining access to youth and their families to enable a viable treatment process (Henggeler, Borduin, and Schoenwald, 1998). Psychiatrists can have meaningful involvement in the evaluation and management of young offenders by working on teams, as modeled in MST, with youth workers trained in a mental health discipline. Psychiatrists and the teams with which they affiliate will succeed if they are supported in establishing close ties to the families of these young people. Cultural barriers to adequate care abound in a youth-offender population (Pumariega et al., 1999). Access to appropriate cultural consultants and members of the youth's community is emerging as a key ingredient in the creation of meaningful access to treatment (Isaacs and Benjamin, 1991).

Vulnerable youth who may become violent can be identified on the basis of good information we now have on risk factors (Carter, 1999). Populations of at-risk youth must have access to screening and, when indicated, appropriate psychiatric care. Rarely do such youth and their families seek mental health services on their own. Fears of the stigma of mental illness are most exquisitely felt by members of society who are already marginalized due to racism, poverty, or other adverse social conditions. Violence-prevention programs must include creative ways of accessing such vulnerable youth for psychiatric evaluation and treatment. Such vulnerable youth must be engaged in the communities where they live, play, and go to school. The keys involve allying with family advocates, seeking cultural consultation, and forming teams with youth workers and younger outreach workers who can most easily relate to the young people at risk.

Psychiatrists cannot create such conditions alone. We desperately need more creative programs that allow teams of clinicians and youth workers to provide meaningful care for vulnerable youth. Psychiatrists should be a part of such policy teams, along with family advocates and other community leaders. Adolescent psychiatrists with practical clinical experience have a perspective that is critical in planning effective programs. Ensuring that psychiatrists are optimally used in programs for violent teens demands the presence of program medical directors empowered to create programs that support good clinical work.

The availability of guns to youth is intolerable in our society. One cannot review the literature on youth violence without coming to this conclusion. Gun availability to teens leads directly to adolescent death. As physicians with a passion for the welfare of our adolescents, ASAP stands with many other medical groups and social advocates in calling for much tighter controls on the availability of guns in our society. We also seek reevaluation of a social value that places more importance on the freedom to have guns available than on the needs of youth for protection. Might our beliefs in gun ownership and using guns for protection be a factor that will prove Prothrow-Stith and Weissman (1991) correct regarding a pending new wave of the youth violence epidemic?

ADDRESSING THE PUBLIC'S FEARS

Psychiatric interventions are only a part of the strategies for reducing the risks for offending or reoffending. Psychiatrists who work with teenagers appreciate the complex nature of an adolescent's relationship to family and the larger society. Effective programs strive to intervene with youth by addressing the complex social and economic issues impacting their lives and those of their families. Psychiatrists can be helpful far beyond their clinical role. They should participate in comprehensive intervention programs by being included in cross-system planning and coordination. They can work with administrators interested in policy change. They can be deployed in meetings with family advocates and community leaders. They can influence public policy by educating the public, especially lawmakers.

Part of the solution to the complex problem of youth violence is toning down the public dialogue on the subject of youth violence. There is a great need for a public dialogue that thoughtfully considers the complexity of the phenomenon of violence and fosters discussion in a way that promotes clear thinking. Psychiatrists are ideally suited for this role. Those trained in understanding family systems are more likely to be able to understand larger social systems, including the ways in which legislative efforts can aggravate problems they are designed to solve. Psychiatrists can be effective public educators and excellent spokespersons to the media for youth intervention programs. Clearly, all of us in the human services professions must join in the task of ensuring that public horror concerning acts of violence by youth is channeled into constructive directions. We must help our society avoid the trap of stigmatizing all troubled youth as boogie men who spread their malignancy like Dracula. Collectively, we must ensure that our society has the motivation and skills for effectively addressing the problem. Adolescent psychiatrists and all others serving youth are in their professions due to a love for youth. We need to help restore a sense of optimism and belief in our young people in the rest of our society. It remains all of our responsibility to nurture and care for even the most troublesome and least attractive children in our communities, including those who must be separated from society or monitored closely due to their potential for violence.

REFERENCES

American Psychiatric Association (1994), *Diagnostic and Statistical Manual of Mental Disorders,* 4th ed. (*DSM-IV*). Washington, DC: American Psychiatric Association.

American Society for Adolescent Psychiatry (1999), *Official Action: Proposal to Abolish the Diagnosis of Conduct Disorder.* Dallas, TX: American Society for Adolescent Psychiatry.

Atkins, D. L., Pumariega, A. J. & Rogers, K. (1999), Mental health and incarcerated youth, I: prevalence and nature of psychopathology. *J. Child Fam. Stud.,* 8:193–204.

Butterfield, F. (1995), *All God's Children.* New York: Knopf.

Carter, J. (1999), *Domestic Violence, Child Abuse, and Youth Violence: Strategies for Prevention and Early Intervention.* Position paper. San Francisco, CA: Family Violence Prevention Fund.

Garbarino J. (1999), *Lost Boys: Why Our Sons Turn Violent and How We Can Save Them.* New York: Free Press.

Henggeler, S. W., Borduin, C. M. & Schoenwald, S. K. (1998), *Multisystemic Treatment of Antisocial Behavior in Children and Adolescents.* New York: Guilford Press.

Huffine, C. W. (1999), Social developmental issues in adolescence. Presented at the Institute on Psychiatric Services, New Orleans, LA.

——— (2002), Conduct disorder should be eliminated from the *Diagnostic and Statistical Manual of Mental Disorders. Adolescent Psychiatry,* 26:215–236. Hillsdale, NJ: The Analytic Press.

Isaacs, M. R. & Benjamin, M. P. (1991), *Toward a culturally competent system of care: Programs which utilize culturally competent princi-*

ples. Washington, DC: National Technical Assistance Center for Children and Youth, Georgetown University Child Developmental Center.

Loprest, P. (1999), *Families Who Left Welfare: Who Are They and How Are They Doing?* Washington, DC: The Urban Institute, discussion paper No. 99-02. Available at http://newfederalism.urban.org, accessed September 15, 2002.

Offer, D. & Offer, J. (1976), Three developmental routes though normal adolescence. *Adolescent Psychiatry*, 4:121–141. Chicago, IL: University of Chicago Press.

Prothrow-Stith, D. & Weissman, M. (1991), *Deadly Consequences: How Violence Is Destroying Our Teenage Population and a Plan to Begin Solving the Problem.* New York: HarperCollins.

Pumariega, A. J., Atkins, D. L., Rogers, K. M., Montgomery, L., Nybro, C., Caesar, R. & Millus, D. (1999), Mental health and incarcerated youth: II. Service utilization. *J. Child. Fam. Stud.,* 8:205–215.

Putnam, R. D. (2000), *Bowling Alone: The Collapse and Revival of American Community.* New York: Simon & Schuster.

Rakoff, V. A. (1989), Adolescent behavior in historical perspective. Presented at annual meeting of the American Society of Adolescent Psychiatry, San Francisco, CA.

Trupin, E., Low, B., Forsythe-Stephens, A., Tarico, V. & Cox, G. (1988), *Washington State Children's Mental Health System Analysis, Final Report.* Seattle, WA: Division of Community Psychiatry, Department of Psychiatry and Behavioral Sciences, University of Washington.

Zimring, F. E. (1998), *American Youth Violence.* New York: Oxford University Press.

Daniel F. Becker, M.D., is Associate Clinical Professor of Psychiatry at the University of California, San Francisco, and Medical Director of Behavioral Health Services, Burlingame, California.

Melita L. Daley, M.D., was a GAP fellow during her child and adolescent psychiatry fellowship at the University of California at Los Angeles, and is now Medical Director of Youth Services, Merced County Department of Mental Health in California.

Lois T. Flaherty, M.D., Editor of *Adolescent Psychiatry*, is Adjunct Associate Professor in the Department of Psychiatry, University of Maryland School of Medicine, Baltimore, MD, and lecturer on Psychiatry, Harvard Medical School.

Warren J. Gadpaille, M.D., is Clinical Professor Emeritus at the University of Colorado Health Sciences University.

James H. Gilfoil, M.D., is a Clinical Associate in the Department of Psychiatry at Thomas Jefferson University, Philadelphia and is in Private Practice in Bryn Mawr, PA.

Monica R. Green, M.D., is Instructor of Medicine in the Department of Internal Medicine, Johns Hopkins University, Baltimore, MD and Instructor, Department of Psychiatry and Behavioral Sciences, Johns Hopkins University, Baltimore, MD.

Robert L. Hendren, D.O., is Professor of Psychiatry and Executive Director, Medical Investigation of Neurodevelopmental Disorders Institute, and Chief, Child and Adolescent Psychiatry, University of California, Davis.

Charles E. Holzer, III, Ph.D., is Professor in the Department of Psychiatry and Behavioral Sciences at the University of Texas Medical Branch at Galveston.

375

Charles W. Huffine, M.D., is Assistant Medical Director for Child and Adolescent Programs, King County Mental Health, Chemical Abuse and Dependency Services Division, Seattle, Washington, and Immediate Past President, American Association of Community Psychiatry.

Philip G. Janicak, M.D., is Professor in Psychiatry and Pharmacology, Medical Director of Psychiatric Clinical Research Center, University of Illinois at Chicago.

Michael G. Kalogerakis, M.D., is Clinical Professor of Psychiatry, New York University School of Medicine, and Past-President, International Society for Adolescent Psychiatry.

Robert King, M.D., is Editor of The Psychoanalytic Study of the Child and Professor of Child Psychiatry at Yale University and the Yale Child Study Center, New Haven, CT.

Patricia Lester, M.D., is a researcher at the Center for Community Health, Department of Psychiatry, University of California, Los Angeles, and consultant to the UCLA–Duke National Center on Child Traumatic Stress.

Saul Levine, M.D., is the Chairman, Department of Psychiatry, Children's Hospital and Health Center; and Professor and Director, Division of Child and Adolescent Psychiatry, University of California, San Diego.

Michael W. Naylor, M.D., is Professor in Child Psychiatry, Interim Service Chief of Division of Child Psychiatry, University of Illinois at Chicago.

Silvio J. Onesti, M.D., is Emeritus Director of Child and Adolescent Psychiatry at McLean Hospital in Belmont, Massachusetts, and Assistant Professor of Psychiatry at Harvard Medical School.

Mani N. Pavuluri, M.D., FRANZCP, MD (Otago), is Assistant Professor in Child Psychiatry, and Director of Pediatric Mood Disorders Clinic, University of Illinois at Chicago.

Theodore A. Petti, M.D., M.P.H., was the Arthur B. Richter Professor of Child Psychiatry, Indiana University School of Medicine and Medical

Director of Youth Service, Larue Carter Hospital. He is Director of Child and Adolescent Psychiatry, Robert Wood Johnson School of Medicine, Piscataway, New Jersey.

Mary Schwab-Stone, M.D., is Associate Professor of Child Psychiatry and Psychology, Yale Child Study Center, New Haven, CT.

Linda Sims, M.S.N., R.N., is Associate Director of Nursing, Larue Carter Hospital, Indianapolis, Indiana.

John Somers, Ed.D., is Associate Professor of Education in the School of Education at the University of Indianapolis.

Max Sugar, M.D., is Emeritus Professor of Clinical Psychiatry at Louisiana State University Medical Center and Clinical Professor of Psychiatry at Tulane University Medical Center, New Orleans, LA.

John A. Sweeney, Ph.D., is Professor in Psychology, Psychiatry and Neurology, Director of Center for Cognitive Medicine, University of Illinois at Chicago.

Christopher R. Thomas, M.D., is Professor in the Department of Psychiatry and Behavioral Sciences at the University of Texas Medical Branch.

Julie A. Wall, Ph.D., is an evaluation consultant for *The Open Book Initiative*, the "pilot implementation" of a state-wide school-based reading reform model, sponsored by the J. A. Kathryn Albertson Foundation, Boise, Idaho.

Susan W. Wong, M.D., is Assistant Clinical Professor of Psychiatry, Columbia University College of Physicians and Surgeons.

Author Index

Friedman, M. J., 217, *221*, 227, 242, *255*, 296, 297, *302*
Friend, A., 168–169, *194*
Friend, D., 336, *341*
Frost, A. K., 145, 146, *159*
Fuller, K., 63, *81*

G
Gadpaille, W. J., 187, 216, 289
Gair, D. G., 84, *110*
Galatzer-Levy, R. M., 50, *57*
Galea, S., 291, *304*
Gallo, C., 181, *197*
Galvin, M. R., 179, *195*, 204, *222*
Ganzel, B. L., 177, *194*
Garbarino, J., 154, *159*, 368, *372*
Garcia, I. G., 173, 183, *199*, 202, 205, 209, 212, 218, *223*
Garcia, J., 118, 123, 125, *130*
Gardner-Haycox, J., 97, *111*
Garland, A., 334, 337, *341*
Garmezy, N., 272, *279*, 327, *341*
Garrison, C. Z., 146, *159*, 185, 186, 189, *195*
Garrison, W. T., 84, *110*
Geller, B., 118, 123–125, 128, 129, *132*
George, L. K., 167, *194*
Gerring, J. P., 206, *221*
Gerson, S. C., 267, *277*
Ghurabi, M., 146, 147, *159*, 180, *195*
Giaconia, R. M., 145, 146, *159*
Giedd, J. N., 118, *132*, 259, *276*
Gilbertson, M. W., 265, *278*
Giles, S., 328, *343*
Giller, E., 266, 268, *282*
Giller, E. L., 295–296, *303*, *304*, 313, *321*
Giller, H., 76, *80*
Gilles, E., 268, *278*
Gillis, H. M., 285, 288, 291, *302*
Glass, A. J., 308, 312, 313, *319–320*
Glazer, J. P., 182, *200*
Glazer, W. M., 298, *305*
Gleser, G. C., 147, *159*, 167, 168, *195*, *196*
Glod, C. A., 168, *195*
Glynn, S., 147, *158*, 186, *193*

Gochman, P., 125, 130, *131*
Goenjian, A. K., 146, 147, *159*, 179, 180, 185, *195*, 204, *222*, 261, 268, *277*, *280*, 288, 291, *302*
Goff, B., 150, 151, *162*
Goisman, R. M., 182, *198*
Goldenberg, B., 156, *161*, 183, *197*
Golding, J. M., 242, *257*
Golier, J., 270, *278*
Golomb, A., 149, *160*
Goodwin, D. C., 124, 128, *134*
Goodwin, F. K., 124, 128, *132*
Gordon, C. T., 118, 120–122, *130*, *132*
Gordon, D., 229, 230, *255*
Gordon, M., 61, *79*
Goren, S., 102, *110*
Gorman, J. M., 264, 273, *279*
Goupil, G., 182, *196*
Grace, M., 272, *278*
Grace, M. C., 147, 148, *159*, *160*, 167, 191, *195*, *197*, 207, *222*, 313, *320*
Gracious, B. L., 129, *131*
Grad, G. J., 7, *26*
Grados, M., 206, *221*
Grady, D. S., 310, 313, *320*
Grady, T. A., 275, *279*
Grandi, S., 331, *340*
Granholm, E., 118, 120, *130*
Green, B. L., 147, *159*, 167, 168, 191, *195–197*, 244, *255*, 272, *278*
Green, M. R., 217
Green, W. H., 119–120, 129, *132*
Greenberg, D., 296, 297, *301*, *304*
Greenberg, M., 308, *321*
Greenberger, E., 202, *223*
Greenfield, H., 312, *320*
Greenhouse, J. B., 331, *343*
Greening, L., 181, *199*
Grega, D. M., 119–120, 129, *132*
Griffin, M. G., 261, *278*
Grillon, C., 261, 264, *278*, *280*
Grilo, C. M., 181, *195*
Grimley, P., 299, *303*
Grinker, R. R., 310, 311, *320*
Grochocinski, V., 331, *343*
Grossmann, K., 269, *281*
Gruenbaum, E., 230, 231, 234, 240, *255*

Subject Index*

A

adolescence. *See also specific topics*
  sturm und drang as inevitable in, 326–327
adolescent-onset bipolar disorder (AO-BD), 123–125, 129
adulthood, young. *See* postadolescence
American Society for Adolescent Psychiatry (ASAP), 362
amitriptyline, 295–296
amygdala, 263, 264
anterior cingulate, 263–264
anticonvulsants, 299
antidepressants, 274, 295–296
antipsychotic medication, 122, 170, 297–298
antisocial behavior following trauma, 183
anxiety following trauma, 180
anxiety management, 287
attachment, neurobiology of, 269
attention-deficit/hyperactivity disorder (ADHD), 173, 183
attribution of responsibility for traumatic events, 174, 234–235, 237, 241
authority, respect for, 9
avoidance of thought, 174

B

behavior, pathological *vs.* "bad," 329–330
behavior disorders, disruptive

following trauma, 183
  "He's Not Bad, He's Mad," 329–330
behavioral therapies, 285–287
benzodiazepines, 297
beta-blockers, 298–299
bipolar disorder. *See* pediatric bipolar disorder
Black Liberation Army, 36
Bosnian refugees, 150–151
Boston Gun Project, 17
Broca's area, 264
Buddhism, 227

C

Cambodians, 233–235, 244
carbamazepine, 299
cerebellar vermis, 265
child-adult sexual activity
  cultures that accept, 232
  differing views of, 236–237
  greater or lesser trauma from, 240–241
child maltreatment, 154–157, 169–171, 190, 232. *See also* female circumcision; sexual abuse
circumcision, female. *See* female circumcision
clonidine, 296–297
cognitive-behavioral therapies, 285–287
combat, returning from, 310–311
combat exposure of officers and OR, 309–310
combat PTSD, 307–308, 318. *See also* war trauma

*The contents of Volumes 1–26, indexed by author, may be found on the ASAP website, www.adolpsych.org.

W

war trauma, 149–152, 203–204, 238.
  See also combat PTSD
  identification with victims in warfare,
    235
Weather Underground, 45, 48, 55
witchcraft, cultures that believe in, 228
witchcraft beliefs, acceptance of,
    235–236
world order
  destruction of existing, 31–32
  envisioning new, 32

wraparound services for youth and fami-
    lies, 332–333

Y

young adulthood. *See* postadolescence
youth movements, 51–52

Z

Zionism, 39, 41